The Fallacy of Mother's Wisdom

A Critical Perspective on Health Psychology

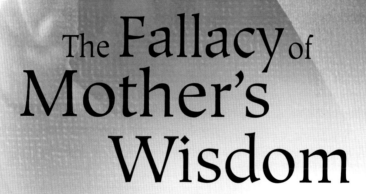

The Fallacy of Mother's Wisdom

A Critical Perspective on Health Psychology

Michael S Myslobodsky

Howard University, USA

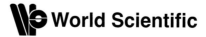
World Scientific

NEW JERSEY · LONDON · SINGAPORE · BEIJING · SHANGHAI · HONG KONG · TAIPEI · CHENNAI

Published by

World Scientific Publishing Co. Pte. Ltd.

5 Toh Tuck Link, Singapore 596224

USA office: 27 Warren Street, Suite 401-402, Hackensack, NJ 07601

UK office: 57 Shelton Street, Covent Garden, London WC2H 9HE

British Library Cataloguing-in-Publication Data
A catalogue record for this book is available from the British Library.

THE FALLACY OF MOTHER'S WISDOM
A Critical Perspective on Health Psychology

ISBN 981-238-457-X
ISBN 981-238-458-8 (pbk)

Typeset by Stallion Press
Email: Sales@stallionpress.com

Printed in Singapore by World Scientific Printers (S) Pte Ltd

Contents

Preface

By many accounts, the quality of medical care available today in the US is the best in the world and is at an all-time high. The US is leading in innovative research, technology, and training, and the number of drugs available to physicians for providing safe, rapid, and effective treatment is greater than ever before. And yet, even as the medical profession strives to redefine itself and reform the delivery of health services and professional education, there is a growing belief that all is not as healthy as it seems in the health care area.

The 'territory' of medicine is getting bigger by the day, as it spreads beyond its traditional borders of hospitals and university research facilities to reach out to the legion of patients who are *not* there. The needs of these patients will not go away simply because the medical profession has become increasingly sophisticated, busy, or turned to new ideologies of doctoring and various empirical healthcare alternatives. In one charming cartoon by Peter Steiner for the *New Yorker*, a somber doctor stares at the patient who shares a neat hospital bed with a dog: "Under our holistic approach, Mr. Wyndot," he explains, "we not only treat your symptoms, we also treat your dog." It is impossible not to feel sorry for the patient, a sadness acutely perceived by many in psychology. Indeed, the dissatisfaction with individual-oriented practices of contemporary medicine is a trigger for the relatively recent efforts of health psychology to edge into the arena.

In 1969, William Schofield pioneered the view that psychologists have a unique opportunity to go beyond their traditional alliances with psychiatry and think of adopting somatic disability as their working arena; to offer assistance in such a hitherto ignored area as somatic disorders. Many would consider such an initiative as a waste of effort, time, and money. But Schofield's plea yielded, at least among some psychologists, to a strong desire to do something that could be immediately seen as helpful to the patient. In less than a decade, that vision has given birth to what is known as *health psychology*. As one of the fast-growing sub-specialties, it has now outstripped other divisions of psychology in terms of excitement in the public eye.

The Mission Statement of the APA Division 38 (Health Psychology) explains that the new professionals will not differ much from 'classical' psychologists, save for the fact that they will "*strive to understand how biological, behavioral, and social factors influence health and illness*" and will support "*the educational, scientific, and professional contributions of psychology to: understanding the etiology and promotion and maintenance of health; the prevention, diagnosis, treatment and rehabilitation of physical and mental illness; the study of psychological, social, emotional, and behavioral factors in physical and mental illness; the improvement of the health care system; and formulation of health policy*" (*www.health-psych.org*).

This statement conveys an image of a chimera, not quite a scientific direction, not quite a professional agency. It sounds like a cheerful postmortem to medicine with a promise for health psychology to be everywhere. However, anyone involved in research or thinking about health psychology is certainly aware by now that something serious is happening to the goals with which health psychology is concerned: the rebirth of germ theory has shattered the conviction that behavioral changes themselves are sufficient to eradicate somatic diseases; the notion of psychosomatic diseases has been so overtaken by events that it seems completely dated; the role of microbial and viral pathogens in somatic and neurological disorders is now being reconsidered; genome researchers are making progress in finding faulty genes, while in the past they could only guess the mode of transmission of the diseases that genes cause; there is a renewed interest in allergy; psychopharmacology has had a second wind with the novel paradigms of drug design; there are efforts to explain 'medically unexplained symptoms'; and the march of technology continues to upset doctor–patients relationships.

The impact of these events has not been fully appreciated within the health psychology curriculum, despite the declaration of the goals put forward in the Mission Statement. Consequently, there has never been a consensus as to what should be studied first, what to include and what should be omitted from the health psychology syllabus. Some students were fast to notice that health psychology was built on somewhat unrealistic, idealized assumptions, a critique of which is almost entirely missing. Health psychology's recommendations were reminiscent of the wisdom of our caring and health-conscious mothers and all their "dos" and "don'ts" and premonitions of "what," "when," and "why" something can go wrong.

Teaching health psychology in the ever-expanding world of medicine was becoming a demanding task. By letting students weigh available evidence and put forward sensible solutions, I came to realize that the messianic marketability of many *ex-cathedra* health pronouncements does not carry much weight. The mass media 'hype' over every novel drug or new therapeutic strategy urged students to ask no-nonsense questions as to what specifically can be done by a practitioner within the discipline's arbitrary boundaries beyond the valued, but tired cliché, the importance of compassion, sensitivity and a positive outlook on life. These questions did not challenge the authority of our mothers. Rather, they correctly implied that their wisdom was insufficient to qualify for a final grade in a course or for MD/nursing continuing education credit since, to paraphrase Ludwig Wittgenstein, almost everything the discipline states or recommends 'could also be otherwise.' Therefore, there were not many ready prescriptions up my sleeve for the various hypothetical health care scenarios. Those offered often have fallen short due to the core curriculum restrictions, or the 'dose' of information the students were ready to put up with given time limitations. This academic discomfort has often brought to mind my late mother, a passionate and dedicated teacher who used to remind me of the inevitability of justice: *"One day you'll have your own students ... and I hope they turn out just like you!"* That admonition, though tongue-in-cheek, proved prophetic. That day has arrived: this book is a reflection of efforts to standardize the boundaries for discussions in my own class.

Given the 'boundary problem,' the array of subjects in this book is organized into three tiers of discussion. The opening chapters (Chaps. 1 and 2) set the stage by explaining why the new discipline cannot stand still in the midst of a flood of findings that often conflict with the original vision of its founders. The second tier (Chaps. 3–5) attempts to answer the 'territorial' question, namely, who are the patients? The reader will be exposed to the theme of medically unexplained symptoms displayed by individuals with chronic or recurrent complaints for which no organic cause or positive laboratory findings is said to be available. The patients suffering from these symptoms do not constitute a uniform group. They have been a subject of controversy almost from the beginning of the systematic research on these conditions. General practitioners spend a great deal of their time examining individuals who are labeled 'frustrating,' 'difficult,' or 'frequent consulters.' As if to make up for decades of neglect, this group's conditions — labeled in the book as Q syndromes (with 'Q' for *question*) — is now favored above many disorders because they dominate in terms of health care costs, lost wages, disability and misery. Some topics include mass anxiety and the issues brought up by complementary medicine. Others are covered under the worn-out heading of 'epidemics' — a complex metaphor that is commonly used in writings on medical matters (e.g. dementia, obesity and suicidal death, and so on).

The third tier of the book (Chaps. 6–8) explores the question of whether health psychology has a systematic and pragmatic structure so as to qualify as a profession. The chapters give an appraisal of the current and potential impact of complementary medicine and holistic approaches to health psychology, with an examination of how well they accommodate its therapeutic and research goals. Given that the increasing role played by molecular biology in treating the sick effectively distances medicine from health psychology and threatens to reduce the latter to a minor player in community health, Chaps. 6 and 8 also examine how the practice of health psychologists dovetails with that of other health professionals. They discuss the strain in health psychology that is created by the need to bond with other health professionals who seek to achieve overlapping goals.

One would hesitate to add more to what already appears to be an alarmingly wide spread of subjects. A truly all-inclusive book would promise to swell to immoderate size and should be created by several contributors. Hence, the present volume does not aim to provide the most up-to-date information, nor is it capable of keeping up with the mounting number of relevant papers in professional journals that in themselves wastefully proliferate. Rather, it is targeted at a graduate level student of behavioral medicine or health psychology with the intention to discuss some troubling developments that are diverting professional (health) psychology away from scientific research in neurosciences and medicine. Some of the book's content should present no difficulty to undergraduates and even the general reader, who nowadays is well accustomed to reading all sorts of articles about medical innovations in their morning newspapers without pause to look up medical terms. For psychologists, medical terms are desirable acquisitions for communicating with other practitioners, and for establishing working relations with physicians. It is assumed that they took a course in abnormal psychology, and thus have a good deal of familiarity with the psychopathology and somatic disorders associated with psychological aberrations. The rest can be profitably supplemented by any medical dictionary. For medical students, the glossary is a small problem since most of the 'disease topics' are part of their curriculum.

Acknowledgments

This part recognizes the most important players in the book's production — regardless of the fact that the credits are likely to be wasted on many since this section is seldom read.

In the process of shaping the manuscript, I have been fortunate to have had critical reactions to its early drafts from so many people that it is difficult to acknowledge all of them fairly. The idea for the book might be traced to the time when Professor Leslie Hicks and I submitted a paper to *American Psychologist* featuring a critique of health psychology. It took a year for the editorial office to return the manuscript with a tepid compliment of a somewhat interesting contribution that could not be published. That work was never resubmitted, but it made me think about a format different from that of a clubby journal. Next, I must mention Professor Israel Nachson, who read a major chunk of the first draft. More than just appraising it, he drew my attention to the fact that the manuscript was unnecessarily detailed and technical, and gave me fair warning in instances where I chose to disagree with him. In the spirit of Antoine de Saint-Exupéry, he insisted that "In anything at all, perfection is finally attained not when there is no longer anything to add, but when there is no longer anything to take away." Consequently, I have done a lot of unforgiving chiseling on the draft until it was barely viable. I am grateful to a staunch friend and indomitable ally, Professor Irving Maltzman, who encouraged me not to discard this project when I could so easily have done. Irving is known to be utterly resistant to scientific indoctrination and his approval was priceless.

I am greatly indebted to many for the critical reading of sections of the manuscript. These are: Professors R. Dar, H. Frenk, A. Merari, N. Milgram, M. Mintz (Tel-Aviv University), J. Glicksohn (Bar-Ilan University), S. Glick (Albany Medical College), L. Hicks (Howard University), J.-A. Skolbekken

(Norwegian University of Science and Technology), A. Martin, D. Weinberger (National Institutes of Health), E. Fuller Torrey (Uniformed Services University of Health Sciences), E. Vallenstein (The University of Michigan), Dr. Lapidot and Dr. B. Konnikow (both in private practice). Furthermore, Dr. E. Fuller Torrey generously shared with me his extensive personal file of reprints and correspondence on the issues of prescription privileges for psychologists.

The foregoing recognition is not to delegate the responsibility for all my omissions and errors. I have known from the start that some of the scientific territory I have elected to cover would be controversial and it would be naïve to expect that all recommendations will be accepted. Criticism is a great aid, particularly when covering hotly contested issues, but it is also a precarious pole to lean on. On more than one occasion have I had to recall Denis Diderot, a creator of the modern craft of art criticism, who mused that the artist who wishes to incorporate all tastes and opinions might end up exhibiting the framed canvas.

My special thanks go to Dan Weinberger and Richard Coppola, who have been friends and hosts for almost two decades. I was privileged to have been given a second roof in the National Institute of Mental Health.

Dr. Francois Lalonde helped to prepare in a suitable form a number of figures reproduced in the book. With his permission, I quote material from our studies that is either under review or has yet to be completed.

Figure credits go to Drs. Philippa Uwins (The University of Queensland, Australia); John-Arne Skolbekken (Norwegian University of Science and Technology); Javier Nieto (University of Wisconsin Medical School); Thorkild (I. A.) Sørensen (The Institute of Preventive Medicine, Copenhagen University Hospital); Alber J. Stunkard (University of Pennsylvania School of Medicine); Wei-Xing Shi (Yale University School of Medicine). Nederlands Drogisterij Museum sent me a wonderful picture of the Gapers (*www.museum.com/jb/museum?sub=drogisterij*); I am also grateful to Dr. Maria Alessandra Umilta (Università di Parma) for figures granted, but not used due to limitations on the use of color, and to Professor Joram Feldon (Swiss Federal Institute of Technology) for locating for me *Monomanie de l'envie* by Théodore Gericault, a figure that was taken out with a chunk of text. Figures given by Tom Cox, M. Mahil, Erik Johnson (*http://edj.net/vgallery*), and Ido Mintz were also sacrificed in order to trim the size of the book.

My editor at *World Scientific Publishing*, Ian Seldrup, worked tirelessly on the volume. He helped in 'humanizing' the text, alerting me to many moot points, suggesting better wording as well as in editing and arranging the figures — a task whose magnitude can only be fully appreciated by someone who has experienced it. Ms. Yin Yin Pui, who briefly preceded Ian, took care of some early issues, including the design and layout of the text. My acquisition editor, Elaine Tham, stayed on throughout the project and was always there to help with a few administrative hurdles.

I am also indebted to the countless collectors of the unending witticisms attributed to our mothers. A few were appropriated without attribution to the source. I take solace in Jim Holt's assurance in his essay on the history of jokes (*The New Yorker*, April 19 & 26, 2004) that "jokes don't get invented; they evolve." The lineage of some reaches back several centuries.

Finally, Alexandra Parmet-Myslobodsky has been my major life support. She came up with an idea implemented in the cover of the book.

1

The Point of Departure: The Pillars of the Health Psychology Edifice

On one thing all authorities agree, the 20th century was an incredible century for science. It was also dubbed a 'century of psychology.' Health psychology was practically swaddled in expectation from its origin. It had seemingly accumulated scientific capital and was now anointed a challenger. And yet, notwithstanding its impressive lineage, its legitimacy was not readily recognized. Rather, it gained acceptance because in the middle of the 20th century medicine appeared to be dragging its feet. That does not mean that medicine at that time was helpless. Paradoxically though, public health measures, such as vaccination and perfection of the quality of water by filtration, coagulation and chlorination so significantly reduced the incidence of infections that they exposed cancer and heart diseases as the principal causes of morbidity and mortality. Medicine did not give the impression of being any nearer the expected goal of reducing the rates of cardiovascular disease, obesity, diabetes, neurodegenerative diseases, and cancer. It was better informed, more scientific and systematic, more dependent upon technology, but in a very important sense its glory days seemed already over. Physicians marched on by developing many elegant, often daring medical and surgical procedures. They were increasingly busy, but they did not abandon their conventions and mores, and their efforts were not matched by a commensurate decline of morbidity. The crucial issue was not only how to achieve recuperation at the individual level, but how to improve adaptation of individuals and advance the health of society at large.

In the neighborly yard of psychiatry, which psychologists were competent to size up, medicine was historically at its worst. In the early years of the century, psychiatry was a peculiar area of medicine where many brilliant clinicians had to use quite irrational drugs and essentially punitive nonpharmacological tools, ranging from castration to nasal mucosal cauterization, 'faradic brush,' and more recently, lobotomy. The idea of 'brain disease' behind the façade of 'mental disorder' advocated by such neuropsychiatry greats as Theodor Meynert and Carl Wernicke was too radical to be trusted and a century before their peers were ready to accept its rationale. The best that psychiatrists hoped for a century ago, was the formation of some realistic preventive measures as well as moralistic or social changes to alter the public mood. These goals were reminiscent of those put forward by Luigi Cornaro of Venice (1484–1566) in his book, properly titled, *Discourse on a Sober and Temperate Life*, first published in 1558 and intended for a general audience. It was one of most popular among health guides at a time when doing something was much better than doing nothing. Since the publication of his book, many professionals have been saying much the same.

In 1909, the National Committee for Mental Hygiene was founded, which implicitly shared the goals of Johann Christian Heinroth (1773–1843) as reflected in his famous textbook of 1823 entitled *Mental Hygiene*. Although celebrated principally for being the first professor of so-called psychological therapy in Europe, he capitalized on the promise of Moses (Exodus 15:26)[a] and the Sanitary Movement driven by the proliferation of poverty and pollution in the early years of the industrial era. Heinroth recommended self-control, healthy nutrition, adequate sleep, fresh air, exercise, a clean habitat, psychological well-being, abstention from passions, and personal hygiene as key protections against disease. These recommendations were mixed with a heavy dose (albeit for our place and time) of spirituality and moralizing. However, his claim to fame rests with the recognition of 'psychosomatic' connections maintaining that moral health begins with overall community health, sanitary management of food and water, as well as human and animal waste. Heinroth's doctrine implied that morbidity is a

---

[a]Health care examined though pious eyeglasses shows its seeds in the promise of Moses: "If thou wilt diligently hearken to the voice of the LORD thy God, and wilt do that which is right in his sight, and wilt give ear to his commandments, and keep all his statutes, I will put none of these diseases upon thee, which I have brought upon the Egyptians: for I am the LORD that healeth thee." (Exodus 15:26)

function of poverty, thus making the achievement of health endpoints contingent upon economic and political changes. These ideas were anchored solidly in those of the Swiss-French philosopher Jean-Jacques Rousseau (1712–1778) that human beings are "essentially good and equal in the state of nature" and their ills and inequalities are brought about by the rise of civilization. They shaped much of 19th century Romanticism in Germany and influenced such figures as Kant and Goethe. They were certainly persuasive. Ironically, though, in Heinroth's Europe, diseases were mostly acute and so dangerous that there was no need for a health professional other than a compassionate physician to assist the sick or a priest to minister to the dying. A high probability of death due to morbid infections reduced the probability of sickness among survivors, thus limiting the need for instructors on changes of lifestyle. Even survivors did not live long enough to prove the efficacy of Heinroth's doctrine.

In the mid-twenties of the century, psychiatry was still quite an insecure profession, concerned mostly with the charting of its nosological territory. The best of its forces were in psychotherapy, and psychoanalysis. The dominance of psychotherapy, and psychoanalysis in particular, was irrevocably upset by the revolution in psychopharmacology. In 1949, John Cade described the efficacy of lithium salts in the treatment of mania and in 1952, Henri Laborit (1914–1995) and his colleagues paved the way to using chlorpromazine as a pioneer antipsychotic drug. The antitubercular drugs isoniazid and iproniazid were discovered to have antidepressant properties. New drugs were an eye-opener in revealing the path to biological psychiatry and neurosciences; they changed the practice of handling the mentally ill, but they did not cure the psychotics, as hoped. On the tide of psychopharmacology, neurology was back in the psychiatry courtyard. But neurology too fared no better. As one prominent neurologist[1] sullenly observed, "… although new correctives are being extolled almost daily with much pride and publicity, a stalemate is the outcome" (p. 85).

Psychologists were less familiar with the field of 'true' internal medicine. But they could surmise its dwindling authority from what physicians were unable to handle: quite a legion of the sick that had numerous symptoms, gastrointestinal, cardiovascular and autonomic, but with no detectable organic causes based on available methodologies. The art of medicine reminds one of playing chess. If a patient does not recover in response to the therapeutic plan, there is a need to go beyond a standard set of 'moves' looking for a more individualized algorithm based on general knowledge and experience. That is a time-consuming process. With an explosive growth of new technologies and information overload, physicians were no longer able to provide the major remedy available to previous generations — unlimited time for talking — necessary in order to promote a sense of sympathy, partnership and bonds. Ultimately, organically trained physicians were helpless in alleviating these symptoms and consequently felt deep antipathy towards these patients. The patients reciprocated by noncompliance, thereby defying the authority of medicine. In his excellent treatise on a history of psychosomatic illness, Edward Shorter[2] saw the mistrust of physicians as a relatively new theme in doctor-patient relations, dating back to the 1960s. Almost exclusively, patients with a 'psychosomatic' type of pathology were the ones who exhibited this mistrust. These patients were often handled by clinical psychologists.

Clinical psychology has evolved as a discipline which attempts to help individuals with psychological, educational, and behavioral aberrations, and thus it had natural bonds with neuropsychiatry in having the objectives of assessing and treating patients with mental and neurological disorders. In the aftermath of World War II, the profession underwent important changes, such as its departure from the emphasis on using the manuals of personality testing and tests of intellectual functioning. It expanded its curriculum: enhanced research efforts along with the requirement of a Ph.D. for practicing clinical psychologists; and gradually, it achieved a more prominent role outside of private practice, such as state and university hospitals, and Veterans Administration services. In light of these social and professional pressures, it is easily appreciated why in the early 60s, Schofield[3] pioneered the view that psychologists have a unique opportunity to go beyond their traditional alliances with psychiatry and think of adopting somatic disability as their working model, to offer assistance in such a hitherto ignored area as somatic disorders. Insofar as physicians alone cannot effectively help the sick, or so it appeared, deservedly or not, the breakdown of the classical system of healthcare seemed logically preordained unless all agreed that a change of behavior and lifestyle would make a difference in terms of prevention and management of disease. The era of lifestyle modifications had arrived. Health psychology was sure to be waiting in the wings.

In the early 70s, there was a growing belief that such a new discipline dealing with lifestyle modifications may evolve to a point where it will serve society, science and medicine far more effectively than medicine alone ever could. A profound and popular joke of science is that one can measure its progress by the problems that it cannot solve. It could be said that there are four fundamental thoughts implicit in the view that the successful progression of medicine is over, and that it has reached an asymptote in its ability to control morbidity:

- The medical profession, however successful in curbing infectious disease and acute disorders, is less effective in confronting chronic noncommunicable diseases (e.g. cardiovascular, gastrointestinal, and malignant);
- Drugs, the major device of physicians, appear to have limited powers; their failings are disappointing and do not balance their benefits at a time when manipulation of psychological factors is recognized for its ability to alter physical health, reduce stress, and improve the quality of life (the 'pharmaconihilism pillar');
- Patient-doctor relations are fragile. An illustration of poor patient satisfaction is the distrust in the allopathic approach to health matters and the increasing popularity of more benign 'natural' (herbal), diet-based treatments and unconventional (complementary) practices;
- The notion of treating 'isolated' disorders seemed an antiquated principle. Health was conceived of as affected by numerous factors in the immediate and remote environment, and thus can only be effectively handled *holistically*.

In the swiftly changing economical, scientific and moral climate, the notion of health psychology has been formed. In 1978, the American Psychological Association, driven by the perception that there is a need to fill the vacuum caused by the shrinking role of medicine, launched its Division of Health Psychology (38th division). It moved in the direction of solving these formidable challenges. Yet the foregoing four assumptions are not theoretical positions. What follows questions how unassailable the data are on which these founding principles rest.

Out of Sight/Out of Mind: The Comeback of Vanished Pathogens

The notion of invisible pathogens in human illness had been on the agenda of medicine ever since the time of 'modern societies' (in the sense of *Cambridge Modern History*). In his book "*De contagione et contagiosis*" (*On Contagion and Contagious Diseases*), Girolamo Fracastorius (1478–1553) speculated that each disorder is caused by a different type of minute body. It is amazing that, in those days, he was able to suggest three modes of disease transmission: by direct contact; by carriers such as soiled clothing and linen; and through the air. This germ theory of disease was proposed 50 years before the invention of the microscope and more than 300 years before its empirical formulation by Robert Koch and Louis Pasteur. Yet the ideas of Girolamo Fracastorius were largely overlooked. There were other more intuitively appealing models of maladies phrased in terms of offensive stench, dysfunctional organs and tissues and there was no available paradigm to prove him right. Caesar's 'epileptic attack' is attributed by Shakespeare to his being choked by the 'stinking breath' of his audience, which alludes to the belief that epilepsy, too, was a contagious malady. The theme of contagion briefly reappeared in 1658 when the Jesuit priest and scholar, Athanasius Kircher (1601–1680) of Rome was able to detect a semblance of organisms through a primitive microscope. Giovanni Batista Morgagni (1682–1771), professor of anatomy in Padua was such a firm believer in contagion of phthisis that he cautiously kept a long distance from the corpse when performing post-mortem examination. Physicians of that time were reluctant to sample the bad odor of their patients in fear of falling ill, and this lasted long through the end of the 17th century. The dominant miasmal theory implicated stench, mist, haze, and damp places in all diseases and evils. That was the first proto-ecological theory that focused on the need for maintaining health by controlling the systems of nature by modifying living conditions, providing breathable air, purifying water, eating healthy foods, restricting the sale of putrid meat, and ensuring the disposal of waste. Most of Europe followed the wisdom of the 'sanitation doctrine.' Only in the second part of the 19th century the sanitation doctrine was replaced, or rather compounded by the germ theory. With the discovery of some microscopic forms of life that cause disease, man was gradually able to confront the major factors that regulate the size of the population and its morbidity.

Bacteria comprise a very large percentage of the biomass on earth and they perform many important tasks in maintaining the balance of nature. They constitute an intricate ecosystem, or rather a sort of weird organ we carry that outnumbers the cells of our body, and that are essential for immune functions. Some bacteria are *'commensal'* — they populate the skin, mouth, and the upper respiratory, intestinal and female genital tracts. Most of "our" bodies, wrote Margulis and Sagan,[4] are "actually joint property of the descendants of diverse ancestors." Bacteria are one of the most likely claimants to be considered our ancestors, since they contribute a great deal to our dry weight. Only in specific conditions do such pathogens exhibit high virulence. That happens when the bodily defenses are weakened, and its peaceful coexistence with bacteria is punctuated by the declaration of bacterial wars. Commensal bacteria are then 'upgraded' to the status of *opportunist pathogens*. Although *Escherichia coli* is a representative of the common commensal of the bowel of human and domestic animals, it can cause a variety of gastrointestinal diseases. A separate group of bacteria belongs to the class of *true pathogens* that are adapted to invade the host by overcoming the normal defense mechanisms. Their discovery was the harbinger of the 'golden age' of microbiology. No longer was an extensive list of factors or mythological causes mandatory to explain disease. Germs provided physicians with an uncomplicated, mechanistic, and practical '*single pathogen → single disease*' model that was confirmed by a convincing victory over the majority of formidable infections. Immunization against major infectious diseases has saved more lives than any other public health intervention, apart from the introduction of rules of hygiene in home and hospitals, and the decontamination of water for urban consumption. Louis Pasteur (1822–1885) was convinced that "it is within the power of man to eradicate all parasitic diseases from the earth." The field took a number of scientific progressions to reach, by the end of the 19th century, today's situation whereupon the concept of microbes was firmly established in the field of medicine. It also hailed an interruption of the era of the unrelenting onslaught of the major members of the 'morbid' epidemics, such as cholera, bubonic plague, malaria, influenza, smallpox, tuberculosis, typhoid fever, and typhus.[5]

The faith in the victory over contagious pathogens was reinforced when Robert Koch (1843–1910), the German general practitioner and microbiologist of the University of Breslau was able to link the coal-black (and thus 'anthrax') cutaneous sores to a specific pathogen, *Bacillus anthracis*. He also tracked tuberculosis to an airborne bacterium, *Mycobacterium tuberculosis*. Koch revolutionized medical epidemiology by suggesting four simple requirements for bacterial causality:

(a) Finding the contributing organism in individuals with characteristic clinical manifestations;

(b) Its separation and growth in culture;
(c) Its ability to cause disease by inoculating experimental animals;
(d) Isolating the same pathogen from the diseased animal.

These were excellent prerequisites, which became the yardstick for many years to come, by which a given pathogen was tightly linked to a specific disease. By working back from the disease, generations of physicians were able to guess the pathogen and organized preventive and medication strategy before the disease was identified. This victory did not come overnight. The doyen of German pathologists and the author of the cell theory of illness, Rudolf L.K. Virchow (1821–1902), viewed the notion of infectious pathogens with considerable contempt. He fumed that the multiplication of microbe discoveries was a manipulative ploy for creating a new research institute for every *verfluchte Mircrobe*. In spite of the disbelief of this illustrious pathologist, the miraculous feat of bacteriology changed the practice of medicine. It won out over misconceptions and biases. Almost all industrial countries have seen an impressive decline in some notorious, previously common infections. Oddly enough, with its acknowledged victory by the early 1970s, the pace of development of microbiology began to decline. All chronic maladies and disabilities in Western countries were now understood as non-contagious. The unprecedented increase in life expectancy worldwide and the redistribution of mortality rate, with the rising death toll from cardiovascular pathology and cancer, amounted to a firm evidence for the great biomedical success of the century over the pathogens. The discovery of a presumed effective and inexpensive way of curtailing lung cancer by abstaining from tobacco smoking brought about a campaign for changing lifestyle variables and socioeconomic conditions, which essentially restated the principles advocated by Heinroth. Reports by the Surgeon General's Office reflected the mood of that time in asserting: "the leading causes of mortality in the U.S. have substantial behavioral components." These reports recommended that behavioral risk factors (e.g. drug and alcohol use, high risk sexual behavior, smoking, poor diet, a sedentary lifestyle, stress) be the focus of efforts in health promotion and disease prevention. Many practitioners felt that physicians were left to deal with such maladies as drug addiction, cardiac pathology, hypertension, as well as sexually transmitted diseases, particularly HIV. The pursuit of healing by non-medical means gradually became a dominant feature of modern reasoning.

Social theorists have cherished the idea that society alone can determine the rate of death from disease by imposing its own standards of life and behavior. In the 70s, many psychologists drew their inspiration from this conviction. The movement to help the chronically ill was born. The goals of health psychology were expressed urgently and enthusiastically, grand promises attracting interest and money. Money created career demands and positions, stimulated personal and group ambitions, and generated research programs aimed at investigating the impact of behavior on health as well as the weight of disease states on psychological factors. Finally, the changing views on the etiology of human disorders made a world of difference to the stigma attached to those disorders and the social reactions to stigmatized persons. Whereas a patient with viral or metabolic disorders is considered a victim and elicits compassion and help, the attribution of a disease to unhealthy practices reduces these feelings and attenuates the apparent legitimacy of the ailing person's need for assistance. The public reacts less sympathetically to a disease for which the individual is held responsible. Such a disease becomes 'abnormal' in Freidson's[6] parlance as opposed to 'normal' disease (e.g. non-sexually transmitted infections).

Sadly, nobody could have guessed that medical achievements would contribute to a chronification of sickness (Fig. 1.2) and the decrement in mortality would cause an increase in morbidity.[5] It is not difficult to predict the future; the trick is to predict it correctly. Running ahead of the story I am tempted to add that Lundberg,[7] a former editor of *JAMA*, maintained that a disproportionate effort to treat acute, rather than chronic, illness is largely responsible for the "severed trust" between doctors and patients. Alas, combating pathogens and acute diseases always felt like real doctoring. Emerging data from epidemiological studies show that as patients survive longer, they face a range of complications from the disease itself or consequent to its treatment. In addition, there were also some sobering signs that infections did not vanish. The border between 'infections' as opposed to non-infectious disease was chartered on the basis of Koch's postulate. Thousands of researchers have published small tweaks of the postulate. However, its borders were porous. If these postulates were so revolutionary, what was wrong with them? Plenty.

For some time, the blind faith in Koch's authority prevented anyone from seeing that his principle was an overstatement. It made no specific predictions about the size of the infected population, the latent period of illness, chain of transmission, size of the pathogens, or the state of the host. It permitted the establishment of a causal relationship between a pathogen and a given syndrome only for a very few specific conditions. It worked best when "the most conspicuous transmission chains occur when disease manifestations are extremely apparent in a high proportion of infected individuals, when they occur soon after the onset of infection, and when contact between infected and susceptible individuals is easy to observe"[8] (p. 409). Many diseases eluded, however, the label of infections because in the past physicians simply had no proper methodology to deal with them adequately. Likewise, it was not appreciated that infections are capable of setting in motion a series of changes that produce manifestations of disease several years or decades after the invasion of a pathogen; for example, an invasion which occurs prenatally might cause very selective damage that will be noticed only in adulthood. Some pathogens may actually need a "helper" to trigger disease. For example, delta hepatitis requires infection with both hepatitis D and B. Given the limitations of Koch's principle, it was pointless to exercise diagnosis by medication (diagnosis *ex-juvantibus*) because of its theoretical incongruity with etiological expectations. But the major thing was that these principles were constructed with the bold finality of laws with no protective shield of exclusions or disclaimers. Koch himself recognized the limitations of his postulates so that with each newly discovered pathogen, the rules were modified and broadened, thus weakening the validity of his criteria. There were other problems with the postulates that are summarized in Table 1.1 in the modified version.

With such a hiatus of ignorance about infectiousness, it was easier *not* to fulfil Koch's requirements for infectious causation than to prove them when infection was present. That was not a simple omission. It caused the juggernaut

Table 1.1   Limitations of Koch's Postulates of Causation (modified after Evans[9]).

- Not applicable to all pathogenic bacteria
- May not be applicable to viruses, fungi, parasites
- Do not include the following concepts
  - a asymptomatic carrier state
  - biological spectrum of disease
  - epidemiological elements of causation
  - immunologic elements of causation
  - prevention of disease by elimination of putative cause as elements of causation
  - multiple causation
  - a given syndrome has different causes in different settings
  - reactivation of latent agents can cause disease

of the germ paradigm to ultimately run into the sand. In the philosophical climate of the Popperian philosophy of the early 60s, the limitations of Koch's postulate were paramount in the failure of the causality hypothesis since, according to Karl Popper (1902–1994), a hypothesis cannot be proven. Rather, only by disproving a hypothesis, can science be effectively advanced. There was consequently a natural temptation to attribute any disease, not proven to be infectious, to any other cause: genetic liability, neurodevelopmental problems, vitamin deficiencies, faulty diet, malnutrition, xenobiotics, environmental insults, and socioeconomic inequalities, natural wear and tear, stress or various combinations of these factors. No longer were the ill exposed to public scrutiny or kept secluded for treatment. The feverish and chronically ill became significant parts of the work force with no specific sickness label and soon the catalogue of pathogens began to grow. During the last two decades, at least 30 new candidates were entered into that catalogue. As an example, although Lyme disease was first detected in the US in 1975, its presence in the afflicted remained difficult to diagnose. It may be camouflaged for years with a cluster of medically unexplained symptoms, ultimately leading to chronic disability (Chap. 3).

A few infectious diseases were associated with population movements due to wars, political change or the tendency for economic circumstances to improve. Infections reemerge due to changing behavior, and recreational or sexual practices. There are new diseases caused by pathogens that we have not known about before (e.g. the sinister Ebola and Marburg viruses or a previously unrecognized virus from the coronavirus family, presumably associated with the deadly global outbreak of "super-pneumonia" or "severe acute respiratory syndrome" of 2003). There are a myriad of dangerous subviral agents such as prions (proteinatious infectious particles) whose nature has yet to be understood. They may well change the style of managing neurodegenerative diseases. Previously unknown encephalitis viruses (e.g. Nipah and Hendra viruses), or an extension of the range of well-known infections, such as West Nile virus outbreaks in such countries as Israel or as remote as the US suggests the high probability of future epidemics in different regions of the world.

Microorganisms can be spread by tourism, migratory birds, air travel, or illegal importation of exotic infected animals. The reemergence of tuberculosis in developing countries is an example. After 1984, the rate of new cases of tuberculosis in the US, which had decreased to 9.4 per 100,000, began to rise. Noncompliance with drug therapy, homelessness, and immigration from developing countries with endemic tuberculosis are major reasons for that rise. In addition, focal episodes of multidrug-resistant tuberculosis have been reported engrafted onto the pandemic of HIV infection. It seems as though we may soon be as helpless as we were in the pre-streptomycin era, investing in German-type sanatoria, and relying on lung-collapse surgery, hydrotherapy, and cod-liver oil.[10]

In short, the emergence of benign or dangerous pathogens is an ongoing process. Their conversion process is prone to frequent errors that lead to mutations. Consequently, a successful vaccine developed against a parent virus may not help in fighting a disorder caused by a mutant. The visibility of these infections is such that the current wave of public anxiety has been described as a "viral panic." It made us all realize that the threat of pathogens, chiefly in the form of viral infection has been miserably overlooked.[11]

A Paradigm for an Epidemic

In 1998, Philippa Uwins and her colleagues[12] from the University of Queensland (Australia) discovered novel nano-sized organisms which live in colonies on Triassic and Jurassic sandstone. Quite appropriately, they called them *nanobs*. Their cellular structure is similar to actinomycetes and fungi (spores, filaments, and fruiting bodies) (Fig. 1.1). They seem to be an exotic form of life developed in rarely-studied thermophilic habitats. The role of *nanobs* for the health practitioner is still enigmatic. Given that we know only a fraction of the medically-relevant parasites, they represent a useful reference to calibrate our ignorance of biological diversity. Their existence cautions that we know very little about the microscopic world around us, and that there may be more surprises to come.

Uwins and her colleagues were active bacteria hunters. More often, though, the pathogens are looking for a host. Such finds are noticed mostly when they cause epidemic morbidity and mortality. This scenario occurred during the recent outbreak of a flu-reminiscent disease when an elderly Chinese doctor coughing and sneezing while waiting for an elevator on the ninth floor of the 'Metropole' Hotel in Hong Kong apparently felt he "just had a cold." The flu is commonly viewed as a 1–2-week annoyance, even though each year as many as 40,000 Americans die due to influenza virus infection and its complications, particularly among people with symptomatic or subclinical lung, heart, and kidney disease, and diseases that result in

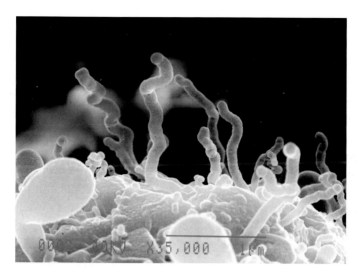

Fig. 1.1 Novel nano-organisms ('nanobs') described by Philippa Uwins.[12] Such nanostructures have dimensions of the order of a billionth (10^{-9}) of a meter. Yet, they are capable of maintaining themselves. These surprising organisms cause conceptual vertigo in microbiologists and evolutionary biologists. Their uniqueness poses a question as to whether they are not a discrete phylum in their own right. Despite their small size they seem to have genetic material that is considered essential for independent life. With this bare minimum of machinery to function, they may have been around as long as the hills.

immunosuppression. The influenza viruses that caused the Hong Kong pandemic in 1997 may have originated in poultry and ultimately jumped to humans. However, the doctor in Hong Kong was identified as the person who was among the first who ignited the outbreak of a life-threatening new sickness dubbed *severe acute respiratory syndrome* (SARS). It began, indeed, with flu-like symptoms, fever, cough, and difficulty breathing, and quickly progressed to lethal pneumonia. This syndrome is shared with so many disorders that guessing an impending epidemic from a clinical presentation may be unsafe. Parenthetically, one might observe that older adults, when suffering from pneumonia, are often thought to exhibit nonspecific symptoms instead of more suggestive pulmonary symptoms. When cultures in laboratories grew something resembling a paramyxovirus or the coronavirus, a known cause of a variety of pathological conditions, the plot began to unfold.

A virus is a small particle consisting of a nucleic acid molecule surrounded by a protective protein coat, the 'capside.' But unlike a nonobe, it does not have a metabolism of its own, and being devoid of the capacity of self-maintenance it becomes an obligatory pathogen: it has to colonize a living cell (bacteria or cells of an animal) to survive and multiply. While in the cell, the viral chromosome makes the cell's metabolism produce ('replicate') new viruses, thereby actually killing the host cell and moving on to populate new cells, fueling the infection in the process. As an example, the herpes simplex virus (HSV) can remain with its host for life in a latent state. Only occasionally does it induce skin lesions. Herpes simplex virus type 1 has been identified as a cause of skin or ocular infection among athletes involved in contact sports; in this context it is known as *herpes gladiatorum*. An outbreak of *herpes gladiatorum* was recorded among 34% of wrestlers in July 1989.[13] The herpes simplex virus has become a paradigm of pathology when a disease is an end-point of a process which may begin prenatally, and début clinically with advancing years, ultimately contributing to encephalitis or dementia.

Returning to the mortal coronavirus, it must be added that it belongs to a family whose members cause one third of common colds. Despite that, its emergence was pronounced 'an ugly surprise.' In fact, the surprise was in the speed with which the virus was detected and identified (note, it took three years to identify the agent of AIDS). Were it not for being sensitized to the anthrax threat, the world would have probably only learned of the current SARS epidemic after it had acquired a pandemic character. The understanding of the etiology of this "super-pneumonia" has become a societal and epidemiological priority on more than one count. SARS demonstrated that the début of mortal sickness may be easily misperceived as a benign health problem.

Bioterrorism

There are a number of pathogens to fear: *Variola major, Bacillus anthracis, Yersinia pestis, Francisella tularensis* to name a few. B.W.J. Mahy opened a special issue of *Antiviral Research* (v. 57, 2003; *www.elsevier.com/locate/antiviral*) on the smallpox (*Variola major*) virus with the question, 'Why smallpox?' He gave several good reasons. Among others, it is highly transmissible and deadly (30% mortality). This assessment is given based on the image of smallpox epidemics in the past. Today, those who are immunocompromised (say, as a result of treatment with immunosuppressive drugs or due to HIV infection) would be the prime candidates of mortality. Almost everyone should be considered potentially susceptible since nobody was immunized after 1980 when the World Health Organization (WHO) declared that "smallpox is dead."

These reasons alone must be viewed as sufficient to treat smallpox as a low probability/high impact event, i.e. one that is sure to create a devastating epidemic unless all potentially infected persons are located and vaccinated. Initially, that would include emergency services personnel and hospital-selected health care providers, and later include all of their contacts, and contacts of their contacts and so on. It is like demanding to manufacture all houses in the areas of endemic tornado occurrence to survive a twister's direct hit.

Such a demand has already generated apprehension among health practitioners. Vaccination alone could cause a spectrum of minor complications, such as rashes, fever or malaise (about 1,000 in every 1 million people inoculated). In about 14–52 of every 1 million people inoculated, smallpox vaccination can cause serious complications, such as ocular and neurological problems, as well as death.[14] Although these might happen in a vanishingly small percentage of people, the vaccine is described as the most unsafe inoculation available today. It would surprise nobody if the general public were less than enthusiastic about such protection. Mack[14] estimated that preventing all potential deaths from smallpox would require universal compliance with vaccination, with as many as 800 deaths from complications. That may delay inoculations of health professionals for several months not only because of their anxieties, but largely because of the unresolved question about potential liability lawsuits of individuals with untoward effects as well as provisions for treating those who suffer such reactions. Clearly, the current doctrine that conceives of bacteriological warfare as a low probability/high impact event implies the need for excessive resources. Even sporadic terrorism will require deploying and maintaining a gigantic defense infrastructure, binding the resources and workforce of the state.

The ballast water discharged from vessels in our ports is capable of distributing microorganisms worldwide thereby affecting plants, animals, and humans. Contaminated waste from ships is among the suspects that contributed to the epidemic of the foot and mouth disease in the UK of 2001. The lesson to be learned according to the WHO is that it is neither possible nor perhaps even necessary to prepare specifically for attack by *all* possible agents. The WHO report, *Public Health response to biological and chemical weapons: WHO guidance*, second edition (Prepublication draft *www.who.int/emc/book_2nd_edition.htm*) maintains that the humanitarian community may need to learn new skills to confront the organizational, ethical and medical challenges posed by weapons of mass destruction.

Consider *Salmonella*. It is a pathogen to be reckoned with for it can be produced using relatively inexpensive technology and used subtly as a "poor man's bio-weapon." An even better bet for a terrorist would be to churn out a flu virus. Robert M. Krug's analysis on why the influenza virus could be of potential use as an agent for bioterrorism was relegated to the last section of an *Antiviral Research* issue. He explains that the virus is highly contagious. Its antigenic mutability ('antigenic drift') necessitates annual vaccination, particularly of vulnerable groups. The reservoir of susceptible individuals allows common source epidemics to evolve rapidly. Therefore, having a strain of flu virus, a terrorist might also cause an epizootic with a high mortality (say, in chickens) that can be transmitted to mammals, and eventually to humans, on the model of an outbreak of the "bird flu" pandemic originating in Hong Kong. Scientists already have the tools to assemble viruses that are tailored for virulence in a desired host. Such a newly emerging virus would be highly virulent for humans, causing pandemics of fatal disease.[15] All a terrorist needs to start a new pandemic is an acceptable strain and a menial job at a poultry farm, or perhaps, to wait to sneeze in a crowded elevator.

It is difficult to say what the authorities can do. One might argue that all the resources and energy needed to build the foundation for a response to the 'unthinkable' is likely to be wasted. In the case of a massive attack or sustained biologic warfare, a 'limited' response would likely be to default into old-fashioned quarantine hospitals and decontamination camps whose already trained and vaccinated personnel need to be engaged in a spectrum of medical decisions. The authorities are certainly aware that there is no country that is fully prepared to face a bioterrorist attack effectively. There is an urgent need for a nuanced biomedical doctrine of defence, but even more so for the formulation of conceptual tools providing ideas in ethical, social, and psychological response to such a threat. Thus far, a sure doctrine of individual defenses is limited to the bare bones: "Your mother was right," informs Bruce Clements of the Center for the Study of Bioterrorism and Emerging Infections at Saint Louis University, "when she told you how important it is to wash your hands. Good hygiene and good health are your best weapons."

A Pillar of Pharmaconihilism

"The only goal of the physician," lectured the famous neuropsychiatrist, Kurt Goldstein (1878–1965), is "to provide the patient with the possibility of existing in spite of his defect." New antipsychotic drugs do precisely that. They do not cure psychoses, but they change the fate of the mentally ill and their families by controlling many socially damaging and personally disturbing symptoms. The achievements of psychopharmacology as a discipline can be fairly assessed by the same yardstick one measures the success of anti-cancer drugs, such as Gleevec, discussed in Fig. 1.2. That does not obscure the fact that the old and recent history of psychopharmacology remains that of a trial and error effort where gains have been small, triumphs temporary, disenchantment and losses painful, costly, and common.

Harmacology?

It is not a typo for Pharmacology. Lay opponents of drug treatment still have good reason to mock doctors and pharmacists, repeating the acrimonious line of Voltaire that doctors pour drugs of which they know little, to cure diseases of which they know less, into human beings about whom they know nothing. The wrong-headed dogmas of the etiology and pathophysiology of diseases and grotesque treatment practices of the times of Voltaire took this tease further to a powerful weapon that still stays venomous centuries after those lines were written. There is a renewed tide of publications exposing the real and often exaggerated menace of drugs, which have fueled public anger, triggered liability suits and drug withdrawals, and undermined the trust of patients. In addition to alleged bodily harm, the damage is done to the consumers' wallet since the cost of prescription drugs is rising. As always, when pharmacotherapy does not deliver on its promises the attitude of ambivalent condemnation takes over. The conviction that psychiatry did not really benefit from drugs prompts a kind of negative normativity — a type of pharmaconihilism — that can function to set psychiatry at odds with the great fund of neurosciences. We will come to the core of this ambivalence in due course. For now, it will suffice to concede that a good number of psychologists, as well as physicians, are worried when reading of the numerous cases of failed treatment. That rate, indeed, is still unacceptably high. However, telling the sick that pharmacotherapy is poorly justified or precarious is surely a way of *scaring* rather than *caring*. In keeping with *The Doctor's Dilemma* of George Bernard Shaw, if people are persuaded that night air is unhealthy and that fresh air makes them catch a cold, it will not be possible for a doctor to make a living by prescribing ventilation. One wonders, to what authority patients should entrust their health — writers of inflammatory papers and semi-popular books, talk show hosts, radio DJs, testimonials, lawyers, the Food and Drug Administration, or none of the above?

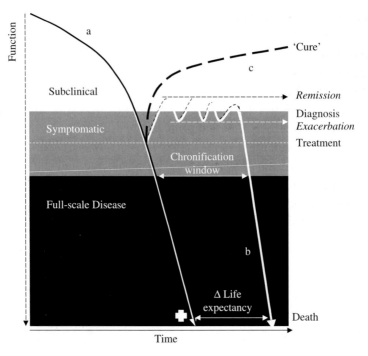

Fig. 1.2 Cumulative changes of function ('healthy state' or subclinical disorder) related to time of clinical symptoms (full-scale disease, diagnosis, treatment, and odds of survival). When no treatment is given to a very sick person, the outcome is likely to be unfavorable. The treatment curve shows that when functions recover to a subclinical state, a person may return to work and family responsibilities. Occasional intrusions of the curve into the symptomatic area communicate a situation when disease is in its chronic state. The idealized outcome of a complete 'cure' is shown as the dashed line. The gain of longevity is determined by the width of the 'chonification window.'[5] *The Washington Post* of January 29, 2003 ran an article about a patient eloquently illustrating the effect. That patient forgets at times that she actually *has* cancer. She is neither cured, nor impeded by her disease. "I feel great," she admits, "I don't even remember I'm sick." That spectacular difference was not made by her stoic buoyancy, but a few capsules of *Gleevec*, an inhibitor of platelet-derived growth factor, which suppresses the migration of smooth muscle cells, and which she swallows every morning. The new drug has kept her leukemia in check for more than three years and let her enjoy her work and family. For her, living with cancer has become as 'normal' as for many now surviving with any other condition, such as asthma or diabetes, when medication cannot cure, yet allows living a life of a fairly good quality. Treatment with Gleevec, should one add, was shown in preclinical studies to greatly retard the development of atherosclerosis. Collectively, such effects show the tragic destiny of medicine in the decades following the defeat of perilous infections, i.e. the fear that physicians would bring about a protracted process of dying or produce at best a chronically sick individual.

Admittedly, despite all the rigors that go into drug design and manufacture, no drug is ever perfect, nor will it be in the foreseeable future. Drugs are never 100% helpful for 100% of people, every time they are given. Nor are they often a pleasure to ingest, such that some people might surely fail to be compliant. An oft cited appeal to humility is that of heroin, which was synthesized at the Bayer laboratories in Germany and put on the market in 1898 with the conviction that it represents a non-habit forming alternative to morphine. The story of thalidomide, however tragic, is another common reminder of the tortuous path of pharmacological discovery. Thalidomide was designed in 'Chemie Grunenthal,' a company in Germany that manufactured the drug under the name of Contergan in 1956. It was promoted as a *safe sedative* and as a remedy for morning sickness in pregnant women despite the fact that it was not tested for embryotoxicity. Unwary women ingested thalidomide during pregnancy, at the most sensitive period of about the first trimester of gestation. It contributed to malformations of extremities in newborn babies named phocomelia (for the resemblance of limbs foreshortening to seal's flippers). Should this result have been anticipated? It is fair to say that such testing was not mandatory at the time. Yet, even if the drug had been tested as required today, it is not certain that teratogenicity would have been discovered. The rat embryo (the major laboratory 'litmus test') is apparently insensitive to the drug. By 1962, thalidomide was removed from the market in response to the public outcry mostly in Europe and Australia, and the shock of the medical community that realized how inadequate safety control over the drugs had been. With traumatic memories of the birth defects it caused, the drug is now controlled as tightly as are narcotic agents.

That was certainly an overreaction. With the benefit of hindsight we can say that the indictment of pharmacology based on this tragic incident was wrong and the hasty decision to ban thalidomide was erroneous. In 1965, an Israeli dermatologist, David J. Sheskin administered thalidomide to a manic patient with lepromatous leprosy (Hansen's disease) who happened to be in a manic state. There is nothing wrong when doctors choose to prescribe a drug for "off-label" reasons if they think it might be of assistance. But in doing so he actually disregarded a different potential side effect of thalidomide: neuropathy (a rather significant oversight, one might add, since the bacillus, *Mycobacterium leprae*, affects not only the skin but also nerves). With regard to side effects the irony of phobias is that we do not require what we eat and what we drink to comply with requirements as tough as those imposed on drugs. Much to the doctor's surprise, leprosy was markedly improved by virtually the next morning. To shorten the story, suffice it to say that thalidomide is gradually coming back and is currently very popular in treatment for leprosy. Leprosy still remains a public health problem. For example, Brazil has a large leper community (of over 95,000) that is second only to India. Recently, the Food and Drug Administration approved thalidomide for the treatment of Erythema Nodosum Leprosum, an inflammatory complication of leprosy. In spite of its being exceptionally harmful when ingested in pregnancy, thalidomide proved to have a unique spectrum of beneficial properties,[16] which was not overlooked. It has some promise in controlling HIV infection, as well as in increasing transplant tolerance, treating urogenital ulceration, rheumatoid arthritis, and a list of other conditions. Thalidomide has jumped from the status of a promising experimental cancer drug to that of the "first line" treatment for multiple myeloma, a blood cancer that is diagnosed in 14 million Americans a year. In addition, the drug works at doses lower than expected, thus reducing the heavy sedative side effects, which 50 years ago were its primary indication. If proven effective against solid tumors, such as brain tumors, prostate and colorectal cancers, its market may be as big as that for aspirin. There are numerous fresh "me-too" compounds created by tweaking the thalidomide molecule and laboratory testing the efficacy of each new version that is likely to reduce the risk of teratogenicity. In fact, that hazard is easily avoidable by simply not prescribing the drug to women of child bearing age.

Taxonomic Problems and Psychopharmacology

Wilhelm Griesenger (1817–1868), an outstanding figure in the history of psychiatry, unwittingly laid the foundations of the current crisis. Before the word 'psychopharmacology' was coined, he insisted that psychiatry must be an integral part of medicine. Such integration, he hoped, would only be possible if the discipline were to acquire a credible nosology, modeled on the architecture of diseases in medicine. In such a new world, psychological diseases were expected to acquire the status equivalent to any other medical problem in neurology or internal medicine. Although German psychiatrists pioneered the task of erecting fences between the major psychiatric aberrations, this was not a secure undertaking. Unlike neurologists who are capable of diagnosing 'silent strokes,' or cardiologists who can identify (subjectively) 'silent infarctions,' psychiatrists' notion of larval or 'subthreshold' psychopathology is based on the imperfect constellation of symptoms that satisfy criteria for specified deviations that are deemed unacceptable to society. Consequently, psychopharmacology has the added complication of taxonomic uncertainty. Psychiatrists and psychologists commonly deal with a spectrum of aberrant behaviors of people whose responses do not fit the pattern of contemporary classification systems. The word 'aberrant' was deliberately used since, according to Merriam-Webster, it means straying from the right or normal way or deviating from the usual or natural type. By suggesting the presence of aberrations, one may not necessarily be compelled to place them into the current taxonomic boxes or make dubious attributions to mental as opposed to biological since all of them *are* biological. Aberrations of sensory experience (e.g. body image aberration), antisocial behavior (e.g. aberrant drug-taking attitudes and driving behaviors) or cognitive aberrations could be real diseases regardless of the fact that they are often more descriptive than prescriptive. In psychiatry, the arbitrary borders between psychopathology and the garden variety irrationality may be easily crossed. Troubling psychological episodes often evolve into mental disorders that require psychiatric attention.[17]

Science is a constant rivalry between those who tend to see any phenomenon as a kaleidoscope and those who use a wide brush to construe the picture of nature, and pack the world together in order to reduce it to more easily classifiable lumps of black and white. One of the most illustrious 'splitters' in neuropsychiatry was Carl Wernicke (1848–1905), who attempted to tie each psychiatric syndrome to an anatomical 'region of interest.' His imagination and authority notwithstanding, such taxonomy was much too complicated and cryptic to survive. Wernicke's system was so unappetizing that it was discarded before it was properly examined. Those who promise simplicity can always count on their peers' approval. One of a few convincing 'lumpers' in psychiatry was Emil Kraepelin (1856–1926). He provided us with a dichotomous classification of severe mental disorders, i.e. *dementia praecox* (with a variety of sub-syndromes) and affective psychoses. There were additional diseases, to be sure, but this great oversimplification was a major achievement. Predictably, Wernicke did not think that Kraepelin's doctrine would last long, but his stake in complexity was a hopelessly lost cause. Until very recently, or rather after schizophrenia (the schizophrenias) acquired a unique group-disorder status, the splitters were a fading minority in psychiatry. Affective disorders seemed less sanctified, and more and more subcategories of anxiety, ache, anguish and disablement have been recognized. The 10th revision of the *International Classification of Diseases* (ICD-10) listed 48 categories of depressive disorders. The common algorithm for managing depression recommends a succession of trial and error efforts (designated as drug changes, adjustments and augmentations). These are lasting, and are fruitless in a good number of cases. Van Praag has championed the departure from the shackles of the nosological structure of psychiatric taxonomy, an effort reminiscent of that of Karl Kleist (1879–1960). His choice was to steer the diagnostic process, and consequently psychopharmacological strategies towards psychological dysfunctions. He saw the future in the denosologization of psychiatry and management of disorders based on goal-directed, "functional psychopharmacology."[18]

However tempting, psychology and psychopathology are not easy to classify. It is even more difficult to translate their polychrome into the language of neurochemistry. There is nothing in psychiatry close to Koch's postulate to link a given outcome to a specific alteration of molecular machinery. Besides, this knowledge is always in flux. In 1970s, van Praag was hoping to see three major advances in a few decades:

- More precise indication of psychotropic drugs;
- The development of psychotropic drugs with greater biochemical specificity and hence, presumably, greater therapeutic specificity;
- 'Goal-directed polypharmacy,' because with regard to the pathogenesis of mental disorders, it seems more reasonable to think in terms of disturbed functional equillibria than of circumscribed lesions.

Drug specificity was the greatest disappointment. The well-known diagnosis ex-juvantibus, mentioned earlier, was proposed based on the idea that medicine has a sort of Rosetta stone against which doctors could test their diagnoses. Then the discovery came that the specificity illusion cannot be sustained. Recalling his expectations almost 30 years later, van Praag admitted that they did not fare well.[18] Although much had been learned at that time, the necessity of some neurotransmitters was doubted, the presence of dozens of neuromodulators and numerous families of known receptors were not even suspected to exist; almost nothing was understood of the basic rules governing the way they might interact with each other in the body. "The greatest of all the accomplishments of twenty-century science," held Lewis Thomas famously, "has been the discovery of human ignorance." In reality, human ignorance is discovered *de novo* every decade after a period of cognitive vertigo of confidence caused by previous breakthroughs. The hopes of physicians today still continue to exceed their abilities to deliver a successful drug. The sheer variety of psychological phenomena weighs heavily against any simple unitary account.

Unlike depression, the 'schizophrenias,' although originally referred to in the plural remained a monolithic block. It was psychopharmacology that helped to expose the inadequacy of the diagnostic labels, and to focus on the need to use drugs in the context of specific syndromes rather than of the 'whole disease.' Anxiety symptoms in schizophrenia may be controlled by neuroleptics. Yet, neuroleptics are hardly effective in anxiety as what is called 'anxiety' may not be precisely the same entity from one case to another. It is thus useful to follow the path of psychiatric nosology with a good deal of caution, much as Van Praag admonished. Even if one were able to define the syndrome of interest more precisely, one may have to wait for the development of a new generation of specific drugs or new ways of their targeting. The same drug may be deceptively helpful in rather dissimilar clinical cases. Thus, bipolar disorders would not be considered a kin of epilepsy because they respond to some anticonvulsants, much as narcolepsy is hardly in the family of affective psychoses because it responds to fluoxetine. Likewise, the fact that calcium channel blockers may alleviate premenstrual syndrome, headaches, irritable bowel syndrome, schizophrenia, tardive dyskinesia, anxiety and Tourette's syndrome does not mean that these drugs can be categorized together. Although drug designs are guided by a precise idea of the biochemical system that is likely to be involved in a given disease, the definition of disease may still remain flawed. One must take a leap of faith to accept the pathophysiological foundation for drug effects in psychiatry. The truth is that drugs are only as good as the understanding of the maladies they are designed to treat and as the ability to tell them apart from one another.

Therefore, inevitably, pharmacology that has inherited the logical structure of organic chemistry had to loose its toughness in the context of psychopathology. Psychopharmacology can thus be easily subverted by public discontent or political pressure. Coverage by the mass media and consumer activism weighs heavily with both industry and regulators. Physicists often criticize neurobiologists for the lack of general laws and rigorous broad-spectrum descriptions of behaviors. But it is easy to see why the latter have not been forthcoming. What differentiates physics from biology is that many of the scientific theories that describe living things, while ultimately resulting from the fundamental laws of physics, cannot be rigorously derived from physical principles. When offered a glass of soda, one might notice that a straw in it appears bent on the boundary of water. This phenomenon familiar to every high school student as the law of refraction, or Snell's law, describes a ray of light across a boundary that separates two different, but optically transparent media. Neurosciences has reached the state where it might dare portray how perceptual experience is bent across human psychology with the crispness of Snell's law. The problem is we have yet to learn how to measure psychopathological 'distortions' with the same accuracy. Psychology and psychiatry are far less able to provide answers not hedged about with qualifications arising from the intrinsic individual variability which is confounded by time and circumstances. Few psychopathological theories of our illustrious predecessors are bound to be immutably true. A great deal of what is correct holds water only for a specific indication and then for a limited period. That is why Rene Descartes (1596–1650) maintained that disorders of spirit and mind are entirely matters for clergymen to deliberate on.

Box 1.1, modeled on the comparison between physics and ecology[19] shows the oversimplified differences between psychiatry and physics. One can clearly see the difference on all counts. The metaphor of spin or molecular

Box 1.1 Physics and Psychiatry compared.

Physics	Psychiatry
The more you look, the less complicated it gets	The more you look, the more complex it gets
Primacy of initial conditions	Primacy of contingencies; rife with risk factors, feedbacks, nonlinear synergies, and correlations
Search for laws	Reliance on unmanageable complexities
Predictive events (chaos and quantum mechanics notwithstanding)	Mostly descriptive, explanatory
Central role for 'ideal' systems (ideal gas, harmonic oscillator)	Disdain for closed systems and simplified ('caricature') models

collisions in gas phase are more meaningful than our understanding of 'logogens,' or just a pang of pain, because the former is built on a tightly knit theory of quantum mechanics where even metaphors are supported by mathematical computations. One might thus easily grant that psychopharmacology, too, cannot reach the predictive power of theoretical physics because its subject is chemical transformations affecting human perception, cognition, volition, memory, and affect. And yet, however imperfect, psychopharmacology has become a catalyst for insights into the nature of mind and its aberrations, and it does an excellent job in this regard. It has transferred the practice of psychiatry into a routine that is typical of any medical discipline and pulled it into the realm of science; it has become both its paradigm and its testing ground.

In sum, some pharmacohinilists[20] are on target when they maintain that our notion of psychopathology mechanisms has a very limited shelf life. However, this criticism is ultimate proof that pharmacology is a serious science. For now, pharmacology cannot pretend to have a grand unifying theory and its shortcomings are not at all surprising. Besides, a theory that tends to apply to all possible drug-disease situations may apply poorly in each. This situation would not be unexpected for any representative of Big League science where ironically, "most of what we do as scientists is wrong most of the time. This shouldn't worry us — after all, it is the ability to be incorrect that makes science a progressive venture."[21]

Doctor-Patient Relationship: Did We just Arrive There?

Doctors have always been concerned with their image in the eyes of their patients. Their expertise aside, tact, understanding, and civility were not only good manners, but were on occasion, an instrument of superior health outcomes. Folk tales used to portray doctors as eager to maintain professional demeanor and decorum, wisdom, compassion, warmth, forgiveness, altruism and competence. Early physicians promulgated this rendering. Hippocratic Decorum[22] assured the reader:

"Between wisdom and medicine there is no gulf fixed; in fact medicine possesses all the qualities that make for the wisdom. It has disinterestedness, shamefastness, modesty, reserve, sound opinion, judgment, quiet, pugnacity, purity, sententious speech, knowledge of the things good and necessary for life, selling of that which cleanses, freedom from superstition, pre-excellence divine."[22]

Lately, physicians have come under attack for being callous and excessively frugal in providing the full range of services necessary for the well-being of their patients; for no longer being autonomous in their decision making, and seldom ultimately responsible for their patients. Hippocratic moral dictum that physician should always do what is best for the patient is constantly confounded by the requirements and limitations of contemporary practice. It reduces trust in professionalism, violates compliance of patients, encourages excessive doctor shopping, and prompts patients' migration to alternative practices, ultimately working against the best interests of the public. But is it really a sign of the times, as is often held? Unlikely.

Centuries before the 'family physician' became a certified image of goodness, the best practitioners were repeatedly assaulted as blunt and arrogant bullies. Roy Porter[23] tells us that the philosopher David Hume (1711–1776) complained about the inveterate bickering of a gaggle of leading physicians. Doctors were commonly blamed for being patronizing and lofty, in the habit of distancing themselves from their patients and from other paramedical occupations which were considered inferior. The explosive appearance of self-medication and "quackery" in urban areas during the latter part of the 19th century was attributed to doctors' indifference and distance from their patients.[24] In fact, more "humane" professional care was provided by "botanical healers" and midwives, and supplemented by barber-surgeons, apothecaries, and all kinds of self-proclaimed practitioners. The claim by many that medicine is driven by selfless altruism is a plain nonsense. It was practiced mostly, if not exclusively, because it was fun, challenging, and rewarding — in a monetary sense too. These are all selfish motivations.

To be sure, the ambivalence of the public about the wisdom of doctors can be traced to antiquity. With a penchant for rigor, Galen subdivided motives for practicing medicine into four categories:

- for the love of humanity,
- for the love of honor,
- for the love of glory,
- for the love of money.

Galen was Roman and the 'love of money' must have been a veiled allusion to alien practices. The citizens of ancient Rome would not pay fees for having their sick cured. Treatment entailed propitiating the gods or frustrating malevolent forces or various wicked deities, and these acts were compensated for by promises and offerings rather than by money. Alien physicians, most commonly Greeks, institutionalized the fees for medical help. With tongue-in-cheek, Haggard[25] commented, "This fact impressed the Romans with the virtue of the treatment, on the principle of that which costs money must be worth having." Centuries later, the unmitigated greed of some fashionable practitioners was a common target of satire and kept the historians of medicine and the industry of the arts busy.[26] The founder of homeopathy, Hahnemann, is also known for being quite particular about demanding financial reimbursement from his patients, long before regular physicians propagated cash payments: "We are not allopaths who have high medical fees and can legally demand high sums for evil deeds," he is said to have advised one of his pupils in defiance of the legendary Hippocratic idealism, "We must take what we have earned on the spot, since we are not considered worthy of ordinary justice." In an earlier letter to the same addressee, Hahnemann wrote, "No one enters my house if he does not have with him the money to pay me, unless he is paying me monthly"[27] (p. 19).

So if greed was an acknowledged feature of some practitioners since time immemorial, what is new? To properly function in the contemporary environment at the accelerated pace of emerging knowledge, a young physician earns respect by also being an active researcher. This expectation, although dictated by professional interests, has shifted practitioners' minds from the individual in distress to a specific medical issue, itself in need of a solution, as well as to concerns of scientific publications that ultimately lead to recognition. This shift is an outcome of a long process affected by many factors, technological and social, but chiefly a transfer from the subjective to the objective in making sense of quantified bodily noises.

Patients and doctors have continued talking to each other for decades while ignoring something terribly important that was happening around them, until it became obvious that a conflict between the doctors' perspectives and patients' concerns is deep and probably beyond repair. That is why the "recent efforts to infuse the experience of medical students with recognition and appreciation of the psychological and social dimensions of health and illness have little currency in a system that favors technology and biology"[28] (p. 314). Once the advantage of technology was appreciated, it irrevocably changed physician-patient relations into that of a tripartite doctor-patient-technology conundrum.[29] As the most sophisticated procedures are concentrated in hospitals, physicians have gradually accumulated ever greater powers over hospital resources. This process was spurred by a trust in physicians' professional competence, which was not necessarily matched by a trust in their high moral integrity.[30]

The other aspect of the technological revolution is anchored in balancing ethics and cost. No instrumental diagnosis is ever fullproof, such that the doctor can be completely sure something crucial that might have accounted for the patient's symptoms has not been overlooked. This cannot reduce the authority of medicine, but it certainly increases its cost, since the need for an extra test may linger. Medicine is a "quasi-science — more science than, say, political science; less science than physics." We shall return to this issue again in Chap. 8 for it is at the core of many problems in health care. Here, suffice it to mention that patients do not realize that 'diagnostic certainty' may be an illusory objective even in presumably simple conditions. And thus, if faithfully pursued, it threatens to become the major component in increasing health costs. For a physician, the level of diagnostic certainty should only be increased when the risk of an unfavorable outcome is perilously high. But the catch is, as Wildawsky[31] quipped, that "uncertainty is resolved by doing more: the patient asks for more, the doctor orders more. The patient's simple rule for resolving uncertainty is to seek care up to the level of his insurance." The danger of throwing everything into such a health equation is a costly decision-making policy, since it assumes that society or the sick have unlimited resources and all the time necessary to make a comprehensive examination. In the current climate of managed care, such examinations are not always possible, since they are viewed as setting a precedent of ordering more tests than are mandated by the case or scheduling exploratory surgery and hospitalization just to avoid malpractice suits.

To overcome multifactorial uncertainties, medicine tends to limit postulated processes to the most relevant components. As a result, the pendulum may swing in a direction of the parsimonious. When health management organizations protect themselves, ultimately, such protection does deteriorate into a policy of economizing on patients.[32] (The opposite swing of the pendulum is in the direction of a complementary medicine and that 'swing' is discussed in Chap. 6.)

These problems were easy to tolerate for decades, if not centuries, since doctors traditionally viewed the sick as passive, miserable ("poor things"), and ignorant consumers of professional wisdom, and patients tolerated the role. Historically, they were unable to see a doctor other than in times of emergency, relying at all other times upon the power of prayer. They were expected to be grateful for medical help even when offered by narrow-minded doctors and certainly to be uncritical about its rationale.[6] Until very recently, patients have seldom been able, let alone requested, to voice a competent disagreement or disenchantment with their treatment. The less often cited part of Hippocrates' dictum ("Life is short, …") posits: "It is not enough for the physician to do what is necessary, but the patient and attendant must do their part as well, and circumstances must be favorable." Patient's compliance, if not complete trust and respect, was part of the bargain inasmuch as having the confidence to confront the doctor implies a reversal of responsibility. There were some illustrious exclusions, such as that of Samuel Johnson (1709–84), who used to propose a self-diagnosis to his physicians and expected them to confirm his diagnosis, or to challenge it, if they were courageous enough to do that.[23]

The contemporary sick are increasingly more knowledgeable and more demanding in matters that concern their health and often ask physicians to justify the drugs they prescribe. Searching for explanations of bodily sensations, the public is better prepared to guess about the relevant problems, discuss them with physicians, and hazard suggestions of possible treatment strategies. They are more aware and apprehensive of potential ecological hazards (e.g. environmental pollutants, contaminants, ionizing radiation, infections, and improper diet) and are better equipped to make connections between their bodily sensations and a host of possible harmful events. Contemporary patients often prepare themselves as good students do, before they visit their doctors. An overexposure to medical information and current medical studies have triggered what could be defined as an excessive 'body watch' of the public in the US and other industrial countries. An overstated omnipotence of medicine (often deliberately made to help researchers who compete for funds) prompted the sick to look for 'word of mouth' and ponder over health reports in the mass media in making personal decisions in matters of health. We cannot say that our generation complains more often, but when it does, it is certainly louder, more competent, and its indignation is more costly.

A Pillar of Psychoimmunology

As early as in the 17th century there was a conviction that consumption originates in passions of the mind. This is why there was plenty of good advice to improve patients' moods, such as that of John Locke (himself a doctor, and a famous philosopher), who recommended horseback riding as a cure of phthisis. A Japanese scientist, Ishigam, was reportedly the first who made immunological sense of these observations when he suggested in 1919 that psychological stressors might contribute to susceptibility to pulmonary tuberculosis. In a study of chronic tuberculosis patients he noticed a decrease in the phagocytic activity of leukocytes synchronized with the periods of greatest psychological stress. Sir Pendrill established in 1928 a psychiatric clinic to counsel despondent patients to increase their morale and sense of well-being. He was widely prized for individualizing care for consumptive patients, but as Dormandy[33] dryly commented in his elegant treatise on tuberculosis, his achievements were "somewhat disappointing in practice."

These pointers and many others sprinkled about interrelations of emotions and predisposition to sickness suggest that the phenomena were not unknown and that their incidence was probably not rare. However, their examination had to linger for the discovery of transplantation immunity and the development of immunology as a distinct discipline in the 1960s. The purpose of this brief section is to discuss critically the findings and convictions of the role of the emotional state of those afflicted with cancer.

Immune System in Stress and Cancer

Cancer is the second leading cause of death (after heart disease) in the United States. There is an ongoing debate within the scientific community and outside of it regarding the best way to reduce morbidity and mortality from malignancies. The disquiet of the public is reflected in the language of struggle that is often borrowed from the military glossary. In 1972, President Nixon declared a "war on cancer"; some findings in cancer research caused an "explosion" of interest and enthusiasm; numerous scientific problems were being "attacked" by the "army" of researchers lead by the National Cancer Institute. Health psychologists are participants in many of such activities that mostly revolve around behaviors that may alter cancer incidence and slow down its progression. They comprise of those who give advice to the sick; those who read about the latest studies and hope to understand for themselves what to make of the findings; neuroscientists who conduct applied research; clinical psychologists who implement recommendations by others in managing their clients, and so on. Most of them address the studies attempting to affect the immune mechanisms that are viewed as the major 'combatants' with malignancies.

The immune system is a relatively novel evolutionary acquisition that was needed to protect us from pathogens (infectious microbes, viruses, bacteria, fungi, protozoa, and multicellular parasites). Only vertebrates have evolved such an elaborate system for distinguishing 'self' from 'non-self' molecules and cells, and they further expanded the system's competence by adding 'memory' for all previous encounters with such antigens, and recognizing altered self components in order to neutralize or eliminate them from the body. These functions of policing the internal environment require a complex structure of an executive organ based on a crew of cells, mainly of hematopoetic origin, which have overlapping jobs and a hierarchy of complex interactions (see also Chap. 2). The brain, endocrine organs, and immune cells share common signal molecules and receptors, and a brain-immune system dialogue appears to be an ongoing process. A discovery of that 'dialogue' has led the renaissance of immunology research that contributed to the foundation of the new discipline, known now as *psychoneuroimmunology*. Ader[34] recalls that the neologism was first used in his presidential address to the American Psychosomatic Society in 1980. His brief account of studies on the brain-immune system interface modestly concedes that

However inconclusive, these initial studies inspired the sister discipline of *psychoimmunology* to posit more boldly that the immune system and behavior are interactive, and that by altering mental states, one can reverse the pathological condition. There were many exciting anecdotes of recovery that required rationalization. Nowhere has an effort to promote psychoimmunology been as enthusiastic as in those studies of aborted malignancies. They were adopted by health psychology and have become its guiding principle, the major bastion of the 'mind-body' doctrine. Some reports indicated that patients who showed high scores on self-report scales of dysphoric emotion and grief, which were administered one to three years prior to testing, had unfavorable disease outcomes.[35] Signs of immunosuppression, following an exposure to surgical stress[36] were also mentioned in support of the notion that there is some sort of unfavorable profile of emotions that accelerates the growth and metastasis of residual cancer cells. Regrettably, fear of

> *"No one study was or could have been responsible for psychoneuroimmunology. In fact, it is likely that no one study would have had quite the same impact had it not been for the converging evidence of brain-immune system interactions that were appearing in the literature at about the same time."*

cancer and distrust of conventional practices opened the door to enthusiastic questionable therapies as well as shrewd quackery. Many people did not require hard evidence regarding the feasibility of the idea of empowering the self as an anticancer remedy.

Dr Siegel,[37] known to his patients by his first name, Bernie, saw his therapeutic mission not only in providing cures as a "body doctor," but also in sharing himself emotionally and "getting involved" with the patients. His book helped to fashion the word "love" into a buzzword representing a shift in medicine's objectives. For the likes of Siegel, psychoimmunology offered the needed explanation of why maintaining positive expectations and controlling stress might heal; it also made available required ideology against the inroads of "pure" but callous molecular science. The promotion of common-sense maneuvers based on stress control, screening of specific personalities, and improving mood had become an engine of the new field before it was able to lay down hard data. While one cannot deny that some sick people may be more likeable than others and that all deserve compassion, loving a patient, and particularly showing it, might often be counterproductive. Maintaining that doctors also expect to receive their patients' love is nothing less than a brazen narcissistic portrayal of the medical profession. The idea of psychoimmunology went completely out of control when a radiation oncologist, Simonton and his wife, Matthews-Simonton who were Siegel's inspiration, wrote a popular book in which they instructed patients to visualize cancer cells being destroyed by their immune system. In addition, the patients were counseled to stay optimistic and relaxed. The results of their studies are presented in popular books and videocassettes instructing patients on their picture technique. Today, that technique has largely been discredited; yet, the idea was so irresistible that many researchers continued to work hard to find the role played by emotional trauma and tension in malignancy, to the disadvantage of other more gainful programmes. Demands for such studies is high in view of the expectations encouraged by the media that affecting immune mechanisms may cure cancers: "After all," asked Borberg and colleagues,[38] "haven't immune defenses against cancer been invoked by guru after guru on national television?"

Are psychological interventions, such as cognitive behavioral therapy, supportive-expressive therapy, relaxation and guided imagery, of benefit to patients? Do they increase survival or improve coping response and quality of life? The literature on the survival time of cancer patients is contradictory and plagued by numerous methodological confounding factors.[39] Among the studies, those that take a guarded pro-psychological interventions stance are based on smaller samples (63–94 patients). Those that fail to demonstrate their efficacy have greater statistical power (66–235 patients). A group of Danish researchers[40] examined, in a prospective study, the effect of personality, as measured by the Eysenck Personality Inventory, on the incidence of cancer among 1,031 persons. No evidence was found in support of the hypothesis that a high degree of extroversion and a low degree of neuroticism increase the risk of cancer. Likewise, supportive-expressive group therapy did not prolong survival (as opposed to earlier reports) in women with metastatic breast cancer. That is notwithstanding the fact that women assigned to supportive-expressive therapy in that multicenter trial (158 women) had a greater improvement in psychological symptoms and reported less pain than women in the control group (77 women), which received no such intervention.[41] This result is consistent with the fact that although optimism is usually conceptualized as a buffer against stressor-related changes in the immune system, it appears that optimists fare worse than pessimists immunologically when facing academic-social goal conflicts.[42]

Recently, a team of British scientists led by Mark Petticrew[43] revisited a popular faith that psychological factors can influence survival from cancer. They provided a comprehensive systematic review of published and unpublished prospective observational studies dealing with the role of psychological coping styles (e.g. 'fighting spirit,' helplessness/hopelessness, denial, and avoidance) on survival and recurrence in patients with cancer. There was little scientific basis for the view that psychological coping styles play an important part in survival from or recurrence of cancer. In general, the studies that investigated belligerence or helplessness/hopelessness found no significant associations with survival or recurrence, while the association of outcome with other coping styles was meager. Positive findings commonly rested on small or methodologically flawed studies. Although the popular lay and clinical beliefs prod patients to adopt coping styles to improve survival or reduce the risk of recurrence, such maneuvers are hardly rational. "People with cancer should not feel pressured," concluded the researchers, "into adopting particular coping styles to improve survival or reduce the risk of recurrence." The study was so compelling that the story even made it onto the front pages of *The Washington Post* with a cross reference to the web site *www.bmj.com/content/vol325/issue7372*. Hopefully, patients feared less that merely assuming the 'mood of vulnerability' — and that is their prevalent mood — would seal their fate.

The fundamental methodological flow of this area is in that it proposed a predictor variable (e.g. perceived stress, emotional profile, traits, and coping) to impact on health outcome (e.g. onset, course or severity of disease) without the painstaking analysis of some relevant dependent measures (related to the status of immune function) but attributing to the observed outcome. The notion that psychological factors and cancer are interrelated was fertilized by two major discoveries. One is the discovery of interferon (cytokine) labeled as α, β, or γ and the search for its medical applications. All three interferons inhibit the intracellular multiplication of DNA and RNA containing viruses. Another related discovery was that of a specific subset of lymphocytes, 'natural killer' T-cells in the early 1970s, as well as the fact that interferons enhance their cytotoxicity.[34,44] NK cells have been postulated as major bodily immune surveillance directed against tumors, and whose activity can be affected by stressors. With these dependent variables recognized, one only had to establish some theoretically relevant psychological predictors. Most influential among them were cancer-prone personality, depression, and repressive coping style.

The evidence *against* any oncogenic relationship was the strongest for such variables as depressed mood, stress, psychosis, and bereavement. If unhappiness were to contribute to distress-related immune dysregulation, malignancy might be found more often in chronically depressed individuals who contemplate suicide as compared with unperturbed community counterparts. Such an association was not unambiguous. Perhaps, the uncertainty about the presence, length, and severity of comorbid depression, particularly in the elderly has contributed to conflicting reports.[45,46] For such comparisons one might be better off by examining patients with Parkinson's disease, since in about 40% of the cases it is associated with depression,[47] disordered sleep,[48] painful dystonia and burning sensations, as well as marked somatic disabilities. Parkinson's disease is also a chronic and hopeless condition leaving a patient bedridden and requiring full assistance to lessen the presence of unrelenting psychological stress, and it is common among people over the age of 65 when immune functions are in decline. These factors notwithstanding, the rate of malignancy in Parkinson's disease appears to be surprisingly low. However, such projects are always tenuous. To be population based, they must either include all members of a specified group, or select a sample of that group chosen in a random and unbiased manner.

To circumvent the problem, one group,[49,50] turned to the computerized registers of death data of the National Center of Health Statistics. That permitted the extraction of all records with a diagnosis of Parkinson's disease in the US population for the years 1991–1996. Of the 12,430,473 deaths of persons aged 40 years or older, it was possible to extract 144,364 (1.2%) such cases. The study did indeed obtain *reduced* rates of cancer mortality in Parkinson's disease. There is, however, always a risk of misclassifying depression in Parkinson's disease. Depression is a fairly soft endpoint, but death by suicide is unequivocal. Since suicidal ideation is rare in the absence of affective illnesses and some psychologically significant stressors, individuals who committed suicide may be considered as more certifiably depressed or stressed. Lalonde and Myslobodsky[49,50] therefore compared suiciders with and without comorbid depression. Figure 1.3 shows that suicidal individuals

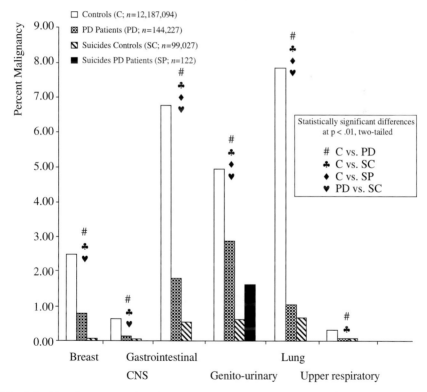

Fig. 1.3 Plots by group and malignancy in Parkinson's patients and referent population without (*C*) and with (*S*) comorbid depression and suicide. Note the low rates of malignancy in Parkinson's patients. Legends show group coding and statistically significant comparisons. After Lalonde & Myslobodsky.[50]

in the referent population with depression show significantly greater rates of malignancy. It clearly reveals an overall reduced rate of all types of cancer in patients with Parkinson's disease. However, the number of malignancies among suicidal PD patients is so small that any further comparisons within this subset are statistically meaningless.

This result is consonant with a study of comorbidity in patients afflicted by recurrent, early-onset unipolar major depressive disorder, the most heritable form of this disorder. As could be expected, this group showed a high rate of psychiatric comorbidity, as well as reduced longevity of patients and their family members. That was associated with a several-fold increase in the proportion of deaths by suicide, homicide, and liver disease, rather than malignancy. In fact, the rank order of the three most common causes of death, i.e. heart disease, cancer, and stroke, remained unchanged. The differences in the proportions of deaths from the other causes were small.[51]

The study by Bovbjerg and colleagues[38] mentioned above does not reject the possibility that immune responses to cancer cells can be demonstrated in individuals with malignancy. Yet, they argue that the results obtained thus far are not impressive enough to matter in considering their therapeutic utility. They have not been shown to be either theoretically valid or experimentally corroborated. The reasons for the reported miracles have yet to be understood. "Among the medical community," they adjudge, with considerable skepticism, "the huge scientific literature examining the interactions between cancer and immune system is replete with examples of exciting findings from initial studies that have failed to fulfill their early promise" (p. 479). One cannot deny that the negative results of casual relationship also indicate the low sensitivity of the paradigms that have been used up until now or an inclusion of variables that could be confounding. A confounding variable is associated with the influence under scrutiny and the outcome. Therefore, overlooking the need to control for the variable either analytically or through the study design, might result in a spurious estimate of the strength of association between the factors and even their direction.

In theory, one could propose an excellent design for such a study, but in practice, as Table 1.2 suggests, it would be impossible to fulfill. One question that comes logically to mind after perusing so much of contradictory data: are there guidelines which could be proposed to provide a reliable indication of a choice for the variety of requirements arising among non-selected patients in general practice? A significant difficulty with the studies examining

Table 1.2 A short list of factors confounding malignancy outcome that should be explored before progress to clinical trial is considered.

Characteristics of malignancy
  Type
  Stage of progression
  Anatomical location
  Symptoms intensity
  Long-term prognosis

Characteristics of the host
  Age, sex, genetic profile, concurrent morbidity, nutritional status
  Immune functions
  Hormonal profile (e.g. exposure to estrogen, testosterone, growth hormone)
  Medication variables, if any (type, duration, category of agents)
  Socio-economic status, education, lifestyle and risk behaviors (e.g. alcoholism, cigarette
    smoking)
  Family factors, social support
  Personality

History of stressors and environmental exposures
  Nature, avoidability
  Timing (prenatal or postnatal exposure)
  Duration and intensity (dose-response relationship)

Study design
  Prospective, Blind of adequate statistical power
  Time-window therapy studies to confirm efficacy
  Studies should be published in peer-reviewed professional journals

emotion-cancer associations is that they do not, and cannot easily take into account the complexity of malignancy (e.g. the stage of progression of tumors, its anatomical site and types, differences in the molecular mechanisms of immunity, and features of the host) without greatly diminishing their statistical power. Cancer is a complex malady. It is a collective name for a family of disorders arising from a variety of factors including genetic influences, environmental exposure, and trigger agents. Psychologically, cancer patients are not a homogeneous group, either. They differ in severity of anxiety, depression, and hostility, and personality-related lifestyles. They also vary in additional factors of disease such as fatigue and insomnia that are treated as manifestations of depression or sickness behavior. Yet they are symptoms of disease severity that correlate with immune markers.

Retrospective psychological studies based on reports of stressful life events or suicidal ideation periods that precede malignancy may also be questioned because awareness of the frightening illness might affect the patient's mood, thereby contributing to the endorsement of stress items in questionnaires, as well as for the selective retrieval of painful items from past events. People have dissimilar notions of the origin of their afflictions. Their attitude regarding cancer theories can be a significant confounder in psycho-oncological studies. Unavoidably, the majority of patients tend to rationalize their state, search for a plausible explanation as to why things came out as they did. Whereas some emphasize their diet or heredity, psychosocial factors and personal stress are more commonly singled out as cancer causes. Although depressed patients in such studies are likely to be carefully diagnosed, controls, however, may not be properly tested, other than to ascertain that they are not depressed. That does not tell us whether the samples are carefully matched with respect to evocative memory, temperamental factors such as frustration tolerance and mood reactivity. More reliable in this respect would be prospective studies, but they are hardly a realistic alternative, since a multicenter effort is needed to provide a study with adequate statistical power, assuming that all confounding variables are well thought out (Table 1.2).

This leads to the last relevant variable, that of the dose of 'cheerfulness' needed for recovery. Any manipulation expected to lead to biological effects should show evidence for a clear dose-response relationship. A study claiming psychosocial efficacy should be designed such that the intensity and duration of therapeutic programs are specified for each 'modality' of therapy, tumor location and the stage of tumorigenesis. That is a difficult requirement to implement for cancer patients, but it can be and should be explored in ecologically relevant paradigms in experimental animals.

Statements about immune processes modulated in a desired direction are, essentially, theoretical statements about relationships between task environments (cues and conditions) and specific cell responses. One idea is that those who experience anger in response to life events, and suppress it, are likely to aggravate malignancy. Concealed anger towards others, according to such a viewpoint will be then aimed against oneself, thereby contributing to cancer. The psychodynamic of this idea is actually very simple. Since depression is said to come from one's failure to express anger appropriately, the internalization of hostility is a somewhat tortuous way of saying that anger cures depression and therefore reduces the risk of malignancy. The anecdotes of the salubrious effects of letting one's fury go, inflated expectations of successful outcomes in those who blamed their cancer on self-control. Women were recommended to fight back not for their roles in society, insecurities, and their personal dignity or to amend difficult bonds with boyfriends or husbands, but for the sake of their breasts and ovaries. In the vacuum created by the hopelessness associated with relatively little success in the treatment of breast cancer, the myth of the therapeutic effects of militancy had to fill the void. The idea still lives on, fueled as it happens, by occasional positive findings, but more so by sheer conviction that self-restraint does something bad to the body. Recent attempts to replicate anger-containment theory were unsuccessful.[52] Medicine did not give up on these women, as is supported by the synthesis of Tamoxifen, a member of the selective estrogen receptor modulator family, approved for treatment of estrogen-sensitive breast cancer (produced by the British firm *AstraZeneca* PLC). By contrast, fighting back to control breast cancer could only promise to ruin one's family much sooner than it would affect malignant cells. It is certainly a scandalous recommendation to make.

Operationally, attempts to link psychological variables to immune response are a typical example of a search for event-related effects. Their results can be subverted by the chronological relationships between the mental state, stressors and the degree of immunological reaction. If the specifications of the experimental task are incorrect, the claims for positive or negative outcomes become irrelevant. Either they do not matter for malignancy, or they suggest that cancer cells are capable of eluding immune responses; or that the immune system was already compromised by treatment. In light of the difficulties involved in task specifications in the laboratory — where the psychologist can use all of his or her acumen to control experimental conditions, consider the difficulties involved in studying humans in real-life situations. To implicate physiological pathways in malignancy one has to focus on somatic mutation and genomic instability, e.g. demonstrate the presence of poorer repair of damaged DNA, and alterations of apoptosis in suffering or depression and converse processes in social support and tension reduction.[53] The time interval between the manipulation of the psychological state and a desirable outcome also adds to the uncertainties that make stress-psychological state correlations meaningless. Chronic stress induces a range of effects, depending on the capacity of the people to cope with tension, and on their social environment. By pooling the participants in such studies one may not come up with a noticeable, let alone significant, modification of NK cell activity. Perhaps the most common pitfall in a great deal of the laboratory work on the effect of emotions in human volunteers arises from confusion between what the experimenter assumes regarding the nature of the experimental task, and what individuals who enter these tasks actually experience in their efforts to comply with the demands placed on them.

In sum, there is no proof of a favorable prognosis among those who are happy and optimistic when confronted with cancer. The resultant 'overselling' of psychoimmunology makes it difficult to convey realistic information to the sick and their families.

Can We Depend on Those Pillars?

It is clear that health psychology has made a case for its role as an adjunct to healing on four founding pillars. It has been the contention of this chapter that these founding notions were overstated. They were formulated at a time when the public was not aware of the possible potential of medico-biological research. These assumptions have fared variously in last decades. Medical treatment for centuries has merely been a feat of blind hope or trial and error efforts when doctoring meant a *post hoc* choosing of a theory as to why disease-modifying effects were successful when they were. Despite that fact, life expectancy went up from under about 30 years in the ancient world to around the impressive 80 year mark in the majority of industrial countries. Yet the lesson learned is that many diseases are still incurable and will remain so for a considerable length of time; that treatment is not a 'zero-sum game' of a doctor against a disease when the outcome is either complete defeat (death) or complete triumph over sickness. The fact is that treatment is merely an effort that may heal to a certain degree, and is largely directed to improve quality of life and increase longevity (Fig. 1.2). These effects account for the frequent confusion of the notion of treatability increasing the 'chronification window' and curability[54] (p. 585). Of the four assumptions, the first seems most embarrassing given that many current disorders are suspected to be caused by microorganisms on a 'hit-and-run' model, a suggestion that was difficult to predict when major epidemic disorders began to retreat. Overlooking the fact that in the majority of cases the "occurrence of [disease] is not primarily determined by chosen activity of the victim (other than being alive) and is caused by unexpected invasion by a microorganism or exposure to a particular agent in the environment"[55] was a serious omission in health psychology.

This shortsightedness can be justified, though, by the solid predictions voiced by many. It suffices for our purposes to note that Sir F. MacFarlane Burnet also subscribed to the conviction that infections belong to the past. In Burnet's[56] words:

Small wonder that only a year later, US Surgeon General William H. Stewart enthusiastically echoed: "The time has come to close the book on infectious disease."

Burnet, of course, was neither ill-informed nor lacking imagination. Why such a failure of caution? What changed things in a decade? Slovic[57] explored a number of psychological elements of frustrated risk assessments. The first one is most obvious. It was

> *"Psychosomatic and neurotic disease is clearly outside the laboratory's responsibility. So are addiction to alcohol, cigarettes, phenacetin, heroin, LSD and other drugs; so is overeating and lack of exercise and, for that matter, dangerous driving and war. Having essentially got rid of infectious disease as a significant killer, virtually all the agents responsible on a large scale for untimely death are on those lists of what the laboratory is, from the nature of its approach, unable to handle"* (p. 248).

defined as 'out of sight/out of mind,' i.e. the failure to appreciate the limits of one's personal capacity to assess 'available' data. There are others: the common tendency to underestimate frequent causes of misfortune; audaciousness when predictors tend to have great self-reliance in their judgments or forget that their knowledge is based on assumptions that are often quite tenuous; overconfidence in the current status of scientific knowledge; slowness in detecting chronic, cumulative effects and many other attributions of certainty in conditions when uncertainty prevails. All of us share in an intimidating task of arriving at interpretations of what observations or findings mean for some fundamental policy decisions regarding the most prevalent disorders. Today, physicians realize that duodenal ulcer or cardiovascular problems may need to be handled almost as though they are similar to pneumonia. Tomorrow, when physicians spend a larger proportion of their time examining the genetic profiles of their patients, more will be learned about the 'susceptibility genes' that may underlie diseases that, in Ewald's[58] parlance, are caused by 'self-destructive defenses' against invading pathogens.

The degree of virulence of germs is determined by characteristics such as transmission vectors, attendants and water. This makes it extremely difficult to find strong connections between specific diseases and pathogens, particularly since, as pointed out by Ewald,[58] some weak pathogens may not impede or even contribute to normal functioning. The beauty of Ewald's idea is that the virulence of pathogens can respond to environmental changes. If proven true, his concept could be as revolutionary in terms of saving millions of lives as was the advent of vaccination. Public health and preventive medicine would have a viable theory to combat infections. It could also be a mission of health psychology provided that psychologists are taught evolutionary theory and microbiology. It may seem ironic that we shall eventually come full circle and scrutinize our environment through Ewald's eyeglasses which permit as to discern that our environment is not necessarily an external domain outside of our skin, as it might reside in our heart and gut as well. As microbiology and the genome project extend their maps toward each other, medicine will shift gears towards improving health of the low-mortality population, and curing not only living individuals, but also the next generation of the sick inasmuch as the remarkable achievements of medicine in increasing longevity are mostly a phenotypic effect, leaving thus far the genotype only marginally affected.[59] It will evolve into a theory-driven discipline where *ad hoc* 'choosing' determines the strategy of healing.

The other proposition of health psychology — the helplessness of psychopharmacology — was highly risky before, and remains so. All disappointments with psychopharmacology notwithstanding, its progress is impressive. It is an immense improvement over the therapeutics for the mentally ill of previous generations. Despite their many flaws, drugs are still viewed as a desirable answer to many conditions and will continue to be such in the foreseeable future, regardless of the fact that the curability of mental illness remains a dream. Psychopharmacology has accomplished too much to be cast aside as useless or because unrealistic expectations of the public were not fulfilled. It has made an impact on the scale of vaccines and antibiotics. By discarding psychopharmacology, medicine would have taken a bad turn into the torpid backwaters of archaic psychiatry. We thus have to move away from the sterile and hostile debates between the critics and advocates of psychopharmacology, and look forward to a simple verdict for any proposed treatment on the basis of its efficacy, risks, and cost-effectiveness regardless of its provenance and likely mechanisms. It is undeniable that, as with any fast-developing area, psychopharmacology occasionally finds itself in a mess.[20] But a mess has some redeeming quality for those who are capable of learning a lesson from it.

Burnet's[56] aforementioned admission that laboratory science has accomplished all it could in handling rising morbidity and mortality must have been interpreted as a plea for help rather than an error of judgment. The plea coming from the ranks of medicine, so advanced scientifically, and seemingly firm politically and economically must have encouraged a self-satisfied stance of an articulate elite of psychology who wished to participate in health care delivery, but was inhibited by its technological backwardness. The initial objective was a problem of science: to explore whether a coping style and personality factors have immunologic consequences. This psychoimmunological problem subsumed the practical question of whether a person's coping style might be utilized as a way of achieving a superior psychological status such as happiness, security, a sense of control, relaxation and other 'positive emotions' thereby contributing to immune enhancement.[60] One of the widely shared convictions in psychology is that the mammalian brain is capable of responding with lasting changes of neuronal connectivity and functions not only in the process of post-lesional recovery or following 'bottom-up' (e.g. sensory) stimulation (a classical case of plasticity), but also as a result of 'top-down' (mental) activity. The potential of top-down effects on certain aspects of somatic functions is undeniable. The question as to whether 'top-down interventions' can be popularized as a miraculous therapeutic wand to patients facing imminent death is not only an issue of 'data' readiness, but also or chiefly a problem of the scientific, ethical and social merits of such modalities.

The beliefs in the power of positive psychological experience to control malignancy were a significant booster to the field of health psychology. Progress is being made, although those beginnings, so thrilling in the past, are still a long way from translating predictions into verifiable fundamental terms. Psychoimmunology owes its success to the influential status of modern molecular biology, and to the techniques of psycho*neuro*immunology. With a much better understanding of molecular immunology, this tide has began to recede. The conviction that "behavioral interventions (such as psychotherapy, relaxation techniques, imagery, biofeedback, and hypnosis) should be able to enhance or optimize immune function"[60] (p. 5) was seldom documented. Ironically, however, positive-emotion therapies were like a hydra-headed creature that raises an extra anecdotal finding for each skeptical query. A likely explanation of why these facts were fitted into a preconceived theoretical framework is that commonly, "the intensity of the conviction that the hypothesis is true has no bearing on whether it is true or not."[61]

The efforts to provide documented evidence of conditions for immunosuppression and immunostimulation should certainly continue. Their credibility could only be rescued from humdrum 'therapeutic' advice of hope and love if they are based on falsifiable theories that are amenable to direct experimental testing, and thus would clearly identify the procedures for their own refutation. If these effects are weak or made in a specific set of circumstances it would be unwise to generalize their worth beyond the specific environment observed.[38]

It is the third proposition — that the declining quality of the doctor-patient bond constituted an intolerable threat — which leaves us with the only solid health psychology pillar. We have tried to show, however, that it is a chronic problem, though irrefutably it has worsened in recent decades. A patient no longer feels that a physician will "come in and take over," as he had in the past and will be "responsible for the outcome *whether he could affect it or not*"[62] (p. 20, italics added). When medical help is slow in coming, the public is unforgiving. Admittedly, with a failing doctor-patient bond, medicine could have lost something essential, because the principle of benevolent paternalism is not just an ethical principle but it is, in a way, a remedy in and of itself. And yet, merely screening medical students for empathy and motivation, or adding a mandatory course on bedside manners to the medical curriculum, may not remedy doctor-patient relations, nor would they help returning them to a desirable harmony. Besides, the presence of a poor doctor-patient bond is the lowest bar possible for justifying the need for a new occupation. In subsequent chapters, an attempt will be made to show why the old ties might help a particular disorder in a particular patient, but this would hardly transform the current rate of morbidity.

In sum, given that health psychology's goal is about working together with medicine, one might question the wisdom of an occupation that needs to wrestle for its legitimacy and a place in the mainstream not on its merits but because medicine has not delivered the goods, as expected by the public. Meehl,[63] a man to whom psychology accords considerable respect, voiced the strongest concerns:

For most consumers of medicine its authority may not seem much in doubt. But its legitimacy is very much in doubt among too large a percentage of those who shape public opinion and fill the shelves of the bookstores with psychological health advice. Thus, the dispute over the territory of health psychology is merely a proxy argument of the larger question of who determines the development of concepts of health care. That larger question makes the embers of the profession flicker. This opening chapter is insufficient for its analysis and it will be continued in Chap. 7.

"The amazing thing is that there are actually scholarly monographs written, lectures delivered, and press releases made by university professors in the social and medical sciences which rely upon an argument whose structure is identical with the following: Medicine has always tried to prevent disease and death; but still people get sick, and everybody finally dies. We can safely conclude that the medical sciences are a waste of time. Would anybody be impressed with this argument unless he had some sort of ideological axe to grind" (p. 68).

SO WHAT?

In 1978, the American Psychological Association, hoping to fill the vacuum caused by the shrinking role of medicine, launched its Division of Health Psychology (38th division). Implicit in this motion was the certainty that following the eradication of major epidemic diseases, medicine has reached an asymptote in its ability to control morbidity; that pharmacology, the major instrument of physicians, appears to have inadequate powers; its failings are disappointing and its errors do not balance its payback at a time when manipulation of psychological factors are increasingly recognized for their ability to alter physical health, reduce stress, and improve the quality of life. This conviction was further reinforced in the climate of deteriorating patient-doctor relations.

The foregoing assumptions are not theoretical positions. Unlike theoretical physics that can get by with a few elegant basic principles without knowing many facts, in psychology, doing dictates a *post-hoc* choice of a theoretical stance more often than choosing a principle is translated into doing. Attempting to settle the matter, health psychology put forward its case by scrutinizing a small segment of an alarmingly large mountain of conflicting information. This introduction questions how unassailable the data are on which these founding principles rest.

2

---•---

'Bad Boys' and Prenatal Programming

> The childhood shows the man
> As morning shows the day.
>
> *John Milton (1608–1674)*

The 'bad boy' label is informally applied in the spirit of Durfee[1] for a collection of signs and symptoms of different origin hinting at some imperfections noticed in infancy or early childhood, which may or may not serve as markers for subsequent health problems in adulthood. These children, commonly boys, cause grief to their mothers, occasionally bully their peers or are bullied by them, and are likely to be unpopular. This combination has a tendency to unfold into a distressing disorder depending on the nature of a child's environment. The problem of 'bad boys' may begin with poor progress in school, a slow acquisition of interpersonal skills, a short attention span, an inability to understand social rules, impulsiveness, defiant and aggressive behavior, self-punitive incidents, and deficient responsiveness to caregiver's instructions. This group portrait overlaps with that of more antiquated terms, such as "classroom pathology," disruptive behavior, or newer terms, such as outward-directed irritability, attention deficit disorder, motor hyperactivity, or neurologically slanted "minimal brain damage." In isolation, none of the symptoms listed above are sufficient to suspect that the boy is not well, unless he is also somatically, neurologically or anatomically 'imperfect.' In this climate of atheoretical taxonomy, Durfee's[1] colloquialism seems preferable.

The signs of somatic imperfection may be delegated to adulthood whereas 'neurological imperfections' are often too trivial and scattered across systems and functions to be useful. They comprise any defect of proprioception, ataxia, awkwardness in finger opposition and other fine movements, vestibular hypoactivity, poor midline bimanual skills, laterality confusion, faulty scanning of space, eye-contact impersistence and motor impersistence, erratic ocular motility, excessive rates of blinking, clumsiness, poor grasp, deficient gait and posture, restlessness, and numerous other signs that may be detected in the course of specialized investigation. In short, a child with oddities and limitations like these is said to manifest "soft signs."[2] Soft signs would have been long discarded if not for the fact that they are suggestive of developmental deficits and often appear together with some benign forms of cranial deformities, as revealed in the asymmetrical placement of the external auditory canals, with the ears displaced low and forward more distinctly than in a patient with positional molding, abnormally sized and shaped skull, "bat ears," and "harlequin eyes."[3] The most consistent facial asymmetry is a prominence of the brow and vertical misalignment of orbits that give the child a peculiar look, dubbed "Mephisto's face."[4] The odd-looking faces, and the malformed ears and palate, are likely to be associated with deformed crania, such as plagiocephaly, a slant head (*plagios* means oblique in Greek), indicating deformity along the sagittal suture. In many cases the deformity originates either prenatally, when the infant's head is rigidly fixed against the uterine wall,[5] or unwittingly produced by parental postural preferences, as well as by socially or culturally-biased practices of child rearing. Various visual abnormalities that follow changes of the orbital and maxillary anatomy in plagiocephaly are exophthalmos, strabismus, reduced visual acuity, drooping lids, oculomotor cranial nerve palsies and nasolacrimal obstruction. This list depicts an individual with a somewhat unusual face. Wender[6] must have been impressed with these features when he wrote that his typical patient with minimal brain damage is a "funny looking kid" (p. 29). The popular notion that every child is born perfect is a mirage, because the period of gestation and the proceedings of birth are the most hazardous events to which an individual will ever be exposed.[7] In a way, a postnatal diagnosis becomes a snapshot of the present that began in the past and continues into the future, so that geriatric psychiatry might be said to begin in the womb.

Health practitioners may look at these children from diverse perspectives: psychological, socioeconomic, developmental and neurological. The primary purpose of this section is to shift the emphasis from adulthood to prenatal and perinatal periods of life, since some unfavorable events in pregnancy, delivery, and the neonatal phase leave persistent and apparently lifelong marks on the person. This shift was spurred by the studies of David Barker[8] and associates, who introduced, in the late 1980s, the concept that maternal malnutrition is at the source of the 20th century epidemic of cardiovascular morbidity and mortality of the next generation in adult life. It has come to be known as the "fetal origins hypothesis." The allusion to 'fetal' injury was a metaphor, unjustifiably limiting the notion of 'programming' to the fetal period[9] since more recent epidemiologic studies of humans and experimental studies using animals suggest that chronic disease may have its origins before, during, or even a short period after the fetal period.[10,11] Also, placental insufficiency may cause inadequate delivery of nutrients to the fetus, masquerading as maternal malnutrition. On the other hand, the 'critical period of vulnerability' may extend to a few postnatal years. Today, numerous disorders that are often labeled as disorders of civilization are believed to be *programmed* due to compromised intrauterine development or, to use a more obsolete term, *preformed* prenatally. Consequently, in this chapter we have two broad objectives: to review risk factors associated with prenatal injury and prematurity, and to outline their influence on morbidity in adulthood.

Preterm and Low Birthweight Infant

One infant in 14 that survives the neonatal period bears an abnormality of some kind and degree, and half of these babies have more than one abnormality. Neonates' abnormal birthweight and size are the most detectable harbingers of motor and cognitive dysfunction in adulthood. In developed countries, most low-birthweight infants are by and large preterm. The different fetal phenotypes are better distinguished by their ponderal index (weight/height^3), which characterizes body proportionality and potentially reflects the severity of the intrauterine insult.[12] Mental retardation, epilepsy, cerebral palsy and behavioral disorders appear among many others, in a longer list of low birthweight and the 'diseases of prematurity.'[7] Hypertension, and possibly even some aspects of Alzheimer's disease (see Chap. 4), are seemingly nurtured by prenatal aberrations. Obesity, too, may be determined by nutrition early in life. Obese people have more fat in each adipose cell, but their large fat deposits were predestined by the fact that they have three times as many fat cells in the body. It was shown in the 60s that the number of fat cells cannot be reduced by dieting; only the amount of fat they accumulated goes down even with a heroic effort to reduce food intake.

Normal birthweight in developed countries ranges between 2,500 and 4,000 g. Low birthweight is subdivided into three categories: extremely low (ELBW, <500 g), very low (VLBW, 500–1,499 g), and moderately low (MLBW, 1,500–2,499 g). These are only approximations since they do not take into account maternal weight and height. Also, a variation by 200–300 g may well be momentous in pregnancy-related deaths, and in future chronic diseases.[9] For the present discussion, it is not crucial to distinguish between very low and moderately low birthweight, even though some risk factors for the two categories may differ. Suffice it to say that 50 years ago, a neonate's chance of survival, particularly for a boy, depended on weight. One kilogram too light was a promise of a reduced chance of survival. The future cognitive and behavioral health of surviving low birthweight, or intrauterine growth-restricted babies, was also grim.[8] On the whole, the most unfavorable growth pattern is seen in smallness and thinness at birth, and continued slow growth in early childhood followed by accelerated growth, such that height and weight approached the population average. Very low birthweight, as well as injury during the first three years of life, might adversely affect the development of language, social-behavioral functioning, motor skills, as well as auditory visual and respiratory functions.[13] The adverse consequences of low birthweight will continue throughout the life cycle. A study of full scale IQ at age 7 years in 3,484 children born to 1,683 mothers during the years 1959–1966 with birthweights of 1,500–3,999 g showed that in both sexes, mean IQ increased monotonically with birthweight.[14]

Teratogenesis

Long-term disorders of developmental programming that appear as low birthweight may also show as gross anatomical distortions, often defined as *teratogenic* (from Greek *teratos* for a wonder or monster). Teratogenic insults are chiefly attributed to infections, malnutrition, and drugs ingested by mothers during the period of early organogenesis. They result in inadequate cell numbers, aberrant connections between cells, or a deletion of tissues. The latter is commonly considered a cause of serious disease or functional limitations that are immediately noticed by obstetricians and child neurologists.

Some insight into the nature of drug effects administered to or self-administered by pregnant mothers has come from environmental pollutants or recreational drugs. Teratogenesis caused by thalidomide was mentioned in Chap. 1. Fetal alcohol syndrome is another example. Infants born to chronic alcoholic mothers, or to women who are self-described infrequent drinkers, may manifest a variety of CNS abnormalities, small head size, along with low IQ scores. The teratogenic effect of alcohol is attributed to aberrations of the developing nervous system during the first trimester of development, as is evidenced by abnormal cell migration with misplaced (*ectopic*) gray matter. The minimal dose of alcohol needed to produce harm to the brain is unknown.

Maternal infections are frequent causes of prematurity, stunted growth and teratogenic effects, but they are particularly harmful when combined with the ingestion of neurotoxins (e.g. cocaine) and malnutrition, which facilitate the transmission of infectious diseases to the developing fetus. Most common infections are the herpes virus, toxoplasma, or even bacteria *E. coli*. Even when the combined (chemical or viral/immunological) assault on the embryo is insufficient to compromise its anatomical integrity and the maintenance of pregnancy, it can still leave a lasting trace in the form of dysregulation of immune parameters of the newborn, or behavioral and cognitive deficits in the child. That will hinder a smooth interaction of the new organism with its environment, physical or social. A person will acquire mild behavioral pathology designated as *behavioral teratogenesis*. Although a teratogen is defined as virtually any factor capable of adversely affecting progeny over the whole trajectory of development from conception to the fetal period and birth, timing is of crucial importance in determining the severity and anatomical location of a reproductive outcome.

One aspect of behavioral teratogenesis is associated with heterochronicity. The term is different from the well-known classical definition of 'heterochrony' by Ernst Haeckel (1834–1919). In the present context it was used just as a technical reference to a dissimilar timetable for the departure and migration rates of young neurons (neuroblasts) from the place of their origin in the ventricular plate to their destined sites. Heterochonicity determines the gradients of neuronal vulnerability during that journey and the final spatial map (heterotopy). Therefore, intrauterine insults affect some structures or functions they control without directly damaging other tissues. There are several experimentally reproduced phenocopies of psychopathology (e.g. those of heightened vulnerability to stress, epilepsy, hyperactivity and schizophrenia) that can be achieved by disrupting intrauterine development (for further details, see Refs. 10 and 11). Abnormalities may not necessarily be noticeable at birth, save for weight abnormality, but of course the experimental or clinical instruments that establish the presence of behavioral teratogenesis are much too limited to be sensitive perinatally. Although birthweight is a stable and convenient marker of injury it is mostly a stand-in for a process or processes that have affected events in intrauterine life and that are largely unknown.[11] Likewise, very few studies of neonates provide the full range of neurological or developmental outcomes, since so far the primary emphasis of comparative analyses of neonatal outcomes has been on mortality and major neonatal morbidities, rather than on neurodevelopmental, anthropometrical, and behavioral outcomes that are followed up into the school years.[15]

Experimental studies in laboratory animals provide some insight as to why prenatal care is so important. Ionizing radiation administered prenatally provides an interesting example. Radiation is a somewhat exotic stressor that is seldom relevant under normal circumstances. It is chosen not to demonstrate its harm in embryogenesis (adult animals would not be injured by doses that are deleterious to developing organism), but *why* a stressor in this period is particularly harmful.

Almost 40 years ago in a study with Yu. Geinisman, we exposed rabbits at Day 15 or Day 23 of embryogenesis to filtered X-rays (400 r; dose rate 20 r/min). Both groups showed significant damage of the cortex. While certainly no revelation, one aspect of injury was, however, quite intriguing. The cortex (only visual areas were studied), although inferior in its stratification, cell density and cell orientation, seemed more mature in both groups of exposed animals as compared to sham irradiated controls. Geinisman then subdivided cellular maturity into three arbitrary stages, and then tallied the cells of each stage in each of the cortical layers II–VI separately. As shown in Fig. 2.1, his quantitative analysis found significantly more mature (Stages 2 and 3) pyramidal and granule cells in both groups of prenatally exposed rabbits when they were examined eight days after birth. The meaning of this 'accelerated aging' was not immediately understood inasmuch as the pups were only slightly more advanced in some observable sensory-motor characteristics as compared to controls. We felt, though, that their praecox state shifted the development of the neuronal system to a juncture where plasticity might be deficient.

Consider the fact — actively discussed in the 80s — that early in ontogeny, the neuronal system is relatively insensitive to the neurotoxic effect

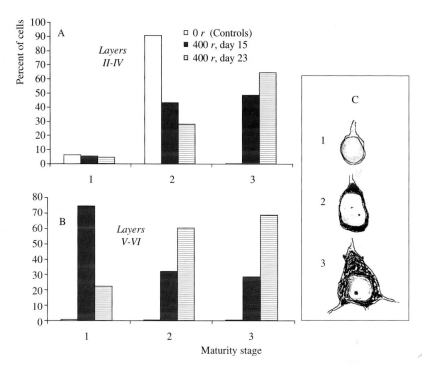

Fig. 2.1 Cell counts (in percent of cells) as a function of their maturity (Stages 1, 2, and 3) in 8-day-old rabbits exposed to filtered X-rays (400 r, 20 r/min) during prenatal Day 15 or Day 23 (see figure labels). Control rabbits were sham irradiated (0 r) prenatally on the same days. (C) Schematic of maturation stages as seen in Nissl staining is shown for pyramidal cells. It illustrates an evolution of neuroblasts (1, 2) into mature cells (3). The staging of granule cells development (not shown) follows the same logic. Only postnatal Day 8 is illustrated since it permits one to better visualize the disparity in cell maturation between exposed groups and controls. Data for layers II–IV and IV–VI of the visual cortex are collapsed for separate graphs ((A) and (B), respectively). (Geinisman & Myslobodsky, unpublished.)

of glutamate and kainite. During this brief period of life, an organism is thus spared from neurotoxic events that otherwise could have fueled a continuing process of cellular injury or, perhaps, epileptogenicity. Would then praecox maturation be considered a marker of an enhanced susceptibility to a neurotoxic attack? Further, given the recognized ability of posttraumatic recovery in infancy, one very speculative reading of these observations is that they signal a diminished capacity to utilize environmental or internal cues for repair of existing neuronal damage. Likewise, given that plasticity can be manifested long after infancy, prenatally injured animals would be inferior in terms of self-repair following any disease-allied or age-related eventuality throughout their lifetimes. Such subclinical damage may be caused by environmental pollutants, which would be followed over some time by age-related attrition of neurons. Although this hypothesis has yet to be examined, one indication of its likelihood comes from the recent findings[11] in γ-irradiated rats that showed virtually normal response to auditory stimuli in the early postnatal period, but manifested an exaggerated startle response in adulthood. Their startle responses appear to be enhanced such that these animals were proposed to model the brain excitability seen in posttraumatic stress disorder (PTSD). In normally responding 'adolescent' γ-irradiated rats, enhanced startle can also be elicited following *d*-amphetamine or even saline challenges.[11] Put differently, anxiety and hypervigilance suggestive of PTSD but caused by primary prenatal injury could appear as though triggered in adulthood by mild stressors. The meaning of such a mechanism will be illustrated by a case report in the next chapter.

A hypothesis such as that above, if generalized to other structures, may indicate the presence of aberrant plasticity in other systems, tissues or organs that respond maladaptively to stressors of life in adulthood. A structure pulled out of its ensemble of development introduces a note of dissonance in many other remote assemblies that we may not recognize as related. Such effects have been shown in the past in the example of malnutrition whereby some organs would grow slowly while others would go on growing.

In sum, embryological data provide a practical metric for making long-term comparisons between different species in experimental studies and individual organisms. A key objective of such research is to document in the future unambiguous 'embryo-signatures' (before their molecular signatures are obtained) that have predictive significance for various segments of postnatal development of the organisms and their interaction with environmental stressors.

Why Does Prematurity Happen? Role of Socioeconomic Disadvantage and Emotional Stress

In reviewing the findings and methodologies of studies devoted to the sociodemographic factors of prematurity, one may be struck with the popularity of the theme of psychosocial stress, particularly in the context of poverty. The idea is as old as the hills. Hippocrates is said to have deemed emotional states so potent as to affect the color of skin of unborn children if a pregnant woman were impressed by the look of her slave. That is somewhat more remarkable than attributing preterm birth to emotional stress. The majority of studies published 40–50 years ago were concerned with complicated deliveries, habitual abortions and prematurity, and 'morning sickness' in mothers who had greater than normal anxiety scores. This association enjoyed good historical mileage due to Menninger's[16] influential view that prematurity is a result of psychological and pathologic organismal rejection caused by the mother's disturbed emotions. This attitude was based on the assumption, as was ironically observed by Meehl,[17] that "any kind of unpleasant fact about the person's concerns or deprivations, present or historical, as *of course* playing an etiological role" (Italics in orig., p. 247).

Mothers' 'disturbed emotions' may not be surprising, since as many as 40% of pregnancies are believed to be unplanned. Even planned pregnancies may be unwanted, and a physician's advice is not sought by at least 50% of women until they are already pregnant. Admittedly, there is a complex relationship between mothers' stress and later abnormalities in their babies. Some mothers are anxious because they are much too young to have babies, and may also be poor, single, divorced, or have had a history of previous abortions. But the real reason for the stress of expectant mothers may be that they have undisclosed complicating factors, such as drug abuse, sexually transmitted diseases or attempted abortions.

The link between social class and successful pregnancy is evident in the higher rate of unsuccessful pregnancies among uneducated, poor and socially deprived people. Radical social scientists are still eager to embrace the notion of psychological distress of the oppressed as an important factor in prematurity. When the term 'low birthweight' was meshed with the term 'socioeconomic factors,' PubMed search revealed 997 studies published in the period between 1967 and 2001. Researchers churned out almost 50% (552) of such studies during the last decade. One of the greatest ironies is the continuous interest in the effect of psychosocial stress of the disadvantaged population on prematurity and even teratology, despite the fact that the teratogenetic role of emotional stressors has never been verified, and has therefore acquired the tenuous status of folklore. Likewise, the claim that stress is harmful in pregnancy by reducing its length and contributing to low birthweight, has so far gained remarkably little empirical support. Nor have the components of 'socioeconomic disadvantage' ever been spelled out. A study, conducted at the University of California in San Francisco, revealed *no* significant relationships among stress, self-esteem and race with newborn birthweight or gestational age.[18]

The fallacy of the psychological stress-harm factor is illustrated by a study of babies born to mothers who were displaced (internally within their own countries or externally) as refugees. Having the status of a migrant might be considered highly traumatic since exiles experience undeniable psychosocial burden, loss of social status and self-esteem, harassment, banishment, as well as lasting housing and financial problems. Yet, again, no overall influence of these factors has been found on the incidence of preterm delivery or low birthweight among the refugees coming from Eastern European countries, the Middle East, Africa and the Pontus region.[19] The foregoing results notwithstanding, a strong emphasis on stress and the locus of control as independent predictors of preterm delivery in low-income black women remains appealing.[20] For those who are interested in looking for the nature of preterm birth, targeting young black women without prenatal care is very pertinent. Much grief can result from racial hatred, social inequality and perceived unfairness. However, "*most black people are neither poor nor close to it,*" asserts John H. McWhorter[21] in his recent book (p. 9, ital. in orig.); the allusion to the crippling poverty of Black America remains a recognizable cliché. It is still used habitually regardless of the fact that it cannot explain *ipso facto* why nearly a quarter of black women deliver preterm. With the reduction of poverty, some preterm-related complications would have been expected to go away, yet the contrary is true.*

A tradition of scholarship in epidemiology recommends looking for the "root cause" or most proximal factors of the pathogenicity impact, since some potentially relevant but distant factors may not belong to a system whose manipulations are sufficient to affect health outcome. Scientists who behave as though such numerous peripheral lifestyle factors are relevant make an unfortunate error of attribution. The study mentioned above,[20] is an example of one that overemphasized the role of stress, and underestimated

---

*In labeling people as either white, 'Anglo,' Latino, 'African American' or 'black,' the text follows original studies or regards 'African American' or 'black' as corresponding terms. That does not mean I am sure of what is right. In different studies people self-designate themselves differently. That is, they could be "African Americans" or "Asian" by being biased by pride, attitudes, group sensitivities or politics or by a conviction of where their skin and hair color, or shape of the eyes might have originated from. Alternatively, they may be self-defined 'black' or 'white' in trust that such labels might matter more for some biological comparisons.

most proximal biomedical factors, in bringing about premature pregnancies, because it included a "high proportion of women without prenatal care." For example, a number of these young women could harbor infections or possibly engage in behaviors that place them at high risk of infection (e.g. unprotected sexual intercourse, multiple sex partners, unwanted previous pregnancies or substance abuse).[22] The etiological relevance of any putative risk factor is always determined by the choice of other factors marshaled as a yardstick of reference. As the methodological standard of studies have improved, the effects of stress on prematurity have proved to be particularly tentative. In research, like in a game of bridge, one may be wasting time and money, hoping for a 'decent hand' when a shuffle is crude. We shall see below why an emphasis on psychological helplessness is not a trivial oversight, for it implies the need to take public health efforts farther 'upstream' in the realm of peripheral (marginal) factors of pathological pregnancy.[23]

Allergic Disorders and Their Players

Clemens von Pirquet (1874–1929) coined the term 'allergy,' defining it in 1906 as the state of altered reactivity, which follows initial exposure to a foreign protein or any innocuous agent. It is a corollary of the fundamental principle of immunology that the immune system acts as a sensory organ educated to discriminate between 'foreign' (non-self) and 'not foreign' (self) materials, and reacts accordingly. Unlike the hardwired nervous system, it works as an endocrine gland with spatially distributed hardware (morphological components) that evolved to destroy the invaders of different tissues. Its software is an elaborate, parallel and redundant code based on short-lived molecules and macromolecules driven by chemical signals that secure a lasting effect.

Immune Machinery

The immune response to a bacterial or viral invasion is directed at the development of inflammatory response by increasing blood flow to the invaded area, raising vascular permeability and mounting of migration of immune cells across the local endothelium. There are two lines of cells organized in immune response. One of them can move, intercept foreign or undesirable particles and engulf them. A Nobel laureate of 1908, Elie Metchnikoff (1845–1916) was the first to call attention to the role of these phagocytosing cells in the body's defense against invasion. These are leukocytes (e.g. macrophages and natural killer cells) in the blood, glial cells in the brain, and astrocytes in the lung. Given that some of them do not require a prior exposure to infectious agents to be armed (e.g. neutrophils, macrophages, and natural killer cells) they are called *natural, innate* or *non-specific* immunity. Their action is often compared to that carried out by a sort of primitive 'parasitic' organism, which invaded a multicellular body for their own good and were subsequently adopted in order to attack, kill and digest any intruder, thereby guarding the health of a host organism.

The other group of cells is capable of flooding the pathogens with special damaging molecules (also previously called antibody-mediated or 'humoral immunity' cells). As soon as they learn to identify pathogens, they are assigned specific defense roles. They are said to belong to the *acquired* or *specific* type of immunity. Both branches of immunity are myopic, so to speak, in that they react to the presence of antigens only when the macrophage presents the trespasser to other cells (the macrophage that does this job is therefore designated as an 'antigen-presenting cell'). The immune system's response looks formidably complex and is schematically described in Box 2.1.

Understandably, that faulty recognition of some harmless substances as dangerous intruders or taking a 'self-antigen' for 'non-self' and mounting a blown up response might be compared to illusion or even a delusional phenomenon in the domain of the immune system. Admittedly, analogies are not to be taken literally, but even so, the beneficial effect of using them appears in their ability to pose significant biological questions. Symptoms of allergic disease are presumably determined by the host, chiefly at *points of antigen entry*. That is why allergic diseases are usually closely associated with the names of affected organs, such as the skin (dermatitis, eczema), lungs (bronchial asthma), gut (nausea, diarrhea, or other gastrointestinal disorders), and eyes (conjunctivitis) or nose (rhinitis and sneezing). The unambiguous response to potential antigens is an essential feature of the clinical profile of allergies and it is commonly assumed that the outcome can easily be traced to the cause. That is not necessarily the case. In keeping with the psychopathological metaphor, one might wonder whether the delusional response begins with the ways the immune system identifies the intruder, or rather the problem begins with the system of representation or the profiling the outside world, so that the 'imaginary helminthes' are fought on a mucosal surface of the nose or eyes rather than in the gut, where such a response would make better sense.

Box 2.1   Immune machinery.

The macrophage is the major arbiter of tissue match, its 'friendliness' or 'histocompatibility.' This is a relatively large cell that digests the pathogens and then transports their components through their cytosol to a genetic region on the outer membrane surface that is central to immune recognition and function, the so-called major histocompatibility complex (MHC). The latter presents the bound antigenic fragments to other more specialized cells of the immune system. In addition, the MHC molecules determine the overall pattern of the subsequent response since they can present either an unmodified antigen molecule or its fragments. MHC molecules exist in two forms (class 1 and class 2) that are sensitive to the size of the 'non-self' elements. Class-1 molecules capture peptide fragments that were produced within the cell in response to viral or bacterial infection. In contrast, class-2 molecules are sensitive to a variety of exogenous materials.

B-cells are a class of lymphocytes that originate from hematopoetic cells of bone marrow and are in charge of secreting soluble antibodies (immunoglobulins, *Ig*) to every conceivable antigen. They multiply and begin to produce Ig**M** in response to any novel antigen. By contrast, Ig**G** is synthesized after repeated exposures to a recognized antigen, and is the only class of antibodies which is capable of traversing the placenta, thereby protecting the fetus before its own IgG is produced. The scenario of allergy also includes Ig**E** molecules that contribute to immunologic memory and accelerate a response to future antigen trespassers, thereby causing a 'reactivity-on' state. They command the cells to release the content of intracellular granules (i.e. to 'deregulate') to affect intruders which are so large that cannot be engulfed (e.g. as big as worms). Once synthesized and released by B-cells, IgE antibodies briefly circulate in the blood before binding to high-affinity IgE receptors on the surface of mast cells in tissue or peripheral-blood basophils, and low-affinity IgE receptors on the surface of lymphocytes, eosinophils, platelets, and macrophages.[24] These antibodies are numerous and the list is likely being updated as the reader examines this chapter.

B-cells do not act unless they are actuated ('helped') by the thymus-derived cells (T helper, **Th**-cells). The latter have been extensively studied for their capacity to produce a variety of chemicals and chemoattractants known as 'cytokines.' These are small protein molecules (~150 amino acids, molecular weight <80 kDa) that mediate in local and distant immune reactions and synchronize the steps of metabolic and physiological responses to pathogens in various tissues including the central nervous system. Over the past few years, it has become evident that an exchange of information between cells of the immune system takes place at specialized regions of membrane contact that share many features with *neuronal synapses*. It is a dynamic mechanism that allows T-cells to discriminate among antigens from infectious and noninfectious agents,[25] and was therefore designated as the *immunologic synapse*.

A predisposition to allergic reactions to otherwise innocuous substances (low molecular weight substances such as antibiotics, metalloproteins, and perfumes) is called *atopy*. In 1819, when hey fever was first described, allergic diseases were relatively uncommon. Today, allergies in their various disguises can be diagnosed in almost every third individual. The number of the afflicted keeps increasing, particularly in industrialized countries, where 10% to 15% of all children can be considered to suffer from clinical allergy. In 0.24% of the cases, an allergy may develop into a severe systemic and potentially life-threatening generalized affliction called *anaphylactic shock*. Among the host of allergic conditions, asthma is the sixth-ranked chronic disease in children, with an estimated national cost in the US of over $12 billion. The prevalence of asthma, including pediatric asthma, has increased in the last decade by more than 70%. The worldwide economic cost of bronchial asthma is estimated to exceed the combined cost of AIDS/HIV infection and tuberculosis (*www.who.int/inf-fs/en/fact206.html*). Although recorded asthma-related deaths amount to 25,000 per year worldwide, the major harm caused by the various allergies (rhinitis, hay fever, sinusitis, eczema, and allergic cough) is in their contribution to morbidity and preventable mortality from other diseases, such as viral respiratory tract infections, and cardiovascular disorders as well as those we cannot yet identify (Chap. 3). This conclusion is based on the data collected from 7,556 middle-aged individuals with an allergy defined as eosinophilia (greater than or equal to 275 cells/mm^3).[26] The major reason for discussing allergies in a book intended for health psychologists is that allergic reactions might underlie a host of unrecognized symptoms in children and then later reappear in adults as gastrointestinal, eye and skin disorders that correlate with atopic symptoms and could be allergy related even if atopy is not identified.

Metamorphosis of Allergic Response in Ontogeny

Immunity develops relatively slowly and in a programmed fashion. Its various components are not complete until the child is two years old. However, the fetus is capable of a limited production of immunoglobulin and of responding to some *in utero* infections and antigens. One of the riddles of pregnancy (and allergy) is the mechanism whereby the maternal immune system becomes 'switched off' (and thus tolerant) in the presence of the fetus, which carries paternal antigens, and which a Nobel Prize winning British immunologist Peter Medawar (1915–1987) designated as an equivalent of a

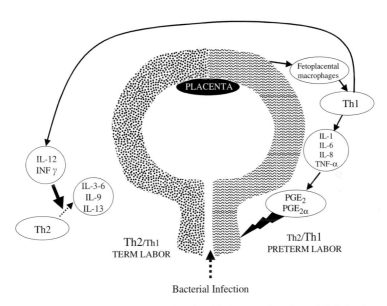

Fig. 2.2 Schematic of pathways associated with intrauterine bacterial infection that is believed to contribute to spontaneous preterm delivery. A prolonged Th1 response to intrauterine bacterial infection may induce tissue damage and inflammation. As might be expected from a specific set of cytokines involved in Th1 differentiation, the latter have particular functional activity in terms of promotion of prostaglandins synthesis. An important function of Th2 responses is in their ability to play an anti-inflammatory role. The Th1 response is associated with Th2 inhibition via IL-12 and Interferon γ.

foreign tissue graft that should have been rejected. Fetal cells are known to appear in the mother's circulation and alien molecules are likely to be identified by the mothers' antigen surveillance system. Nevertheless, genetic, environmental, nutritional, and immunologic factors all act to secure the success of pregnancy. The maintenance of pregnancy and the timing of delivery are controlled by among other things a lengthy dialogue between the maternal immune system and cells of fetal origin. This dialogue has yet to be made out. One of its themes, in particular, appears to be relevant for fetal security as it tends to suppress cell-mediated immune functions and Th1 cytokine production (e.g. IL-12, Interferon γ).

The current view is that decreased Th1 cytokines tip the balance of immunity towards Th2 cytokine production (Fig. 2.2). Ironically, thalidomide mentioned earlier (Chap. 1) is known to enhance IL-4 and IL-5, in effect promoting a desirable shift from a Th1 to Th2 response pattern. An important adaptive value of a decreased production of Th1 cytokines is in that they have been linked to spontaneous abortion and small-for-date babies. Perhaps the evolutionary pressure to preserve the fetus has adopted this weak weapon as a major guardian of pregnancy. In the final analysis, though, no matter how useful Th2 immunity in early pregnancy, it makes the fetus vulnerable to pathogens, inasmuch as the Th2 bias may persist into infancy. It may leave an organism open to infections that are resisted by Th1-dependent machinery. In virtually all infants, atopic and normal alike, the IgE response to environmental allergens is high, but it declines with continued exposure to ingested or inhaled allergens to the point of an anergic or tolerant ('off') state during the first year of life. Unless the pregnancy-protective Th2 > Th1 immune profile is reversed, an infant might remain atopic with allergic responses continuing well beyond early childhood.[27,28] The Th1 and Th2 immune responses are often portrayed as a kind of seesaw mechanism. The least expensive way to achieve an acceleration of Th1 cell maturation and postnatal reversal of the immunity profile is to foster closer physical contact between mother and a newborn by curbing the use of gowns by healthy mothers, and extend breast contact with the baby for a period longer than a year.[29] This process curtails the Th2-initiated production of IgE antibodies.

High Rates of Asthma in African-Americans: Nature or Nurture?

The elevated risk of asthma morbidity among people of African descent remains a mystery. Do blacks suffer more because of environmental factors, such as pollutants or poor living conditions, or the stress of dealing with racism in their everyday lives? Or is the difference contributed by discriminatory practices in medical treatment? Or is it genetic deficiency in blacks that makes them react to antigens in a dissimilar way to whites? Assuming that blacks are more likely to be poorer than whites, racial disparity in asthma rates might simply reflect socioeconomic dissimilarity between groups. Yet after controlling for socioeconomic status, level of crime, illicit drug use, family dysfunction, as well as insurance category, the disparity in the rates of asthma hospitalization by race and ethnicity persist.[30] Furthermore, asthma incidence, hospitalization, and emergency room use has declined with increasing incomes for families of non-blacks but not for black children.[31] What can this drawback be and how can we hope to find out the reasons for it?

The role of genes in allergies of the black population was a launching pad for the hypothesis by Peter N. Le Souëf and associates[32] attributing atopy among African-Americans to genetic adaptation needed to survive in the hostile, humid and hot tropical environment of West Africa. It consists of a proinflammatory profile (Th2) as a surplus of the resistance mechanism needed to fight parasite infections, even at a price of suffering from diarrhea in getting rid of the parasite. They predict that proinflammatory alleles will be more prevalent in populations of a tropical origin than in those of a temperate origin. True or not, one thing about this theory that makes it attractive is that it suggests how evolutionary development built on those who were capable of surviving. Having an intestinal parasite in a hunter-gatherer or subsistence-farming culture was akin to sharing scarce food with a younger kin. Such an imposed chronic 'altruism' could be mortal in bad times, as for example in famine. This presumably explains why those who have remained in the human genetic pool must have benefited from inheriting a Th2 immunity profile.

In a similar model, it has been established that there is a close relation in African populations between the intensity of endemic malarial infection and the frequency of hemoglobin S, or sickle-cell hemoglobin (normal hemoglobin is labeled hemoglobin A). In malarial-infested areas, homozygous AA individuals die of malaria in infancy; and SS babies die of sickle-cell anemia. However, AS heterozygotes are resistant to both diseases and pass both genes on to the next generation. Presumably, as the natives of Africa started migrating to more temperate zones, or were forcibly brought as slaves to Europe, or what is now the US, such a protective device has become progressively less relevant.[32,33] By contrast, in a world where the threat of *trypanosomes, leishmania, theilerial* and *filarial* worms was reduced, overly vigorous responses to harmless environmental agents have become a liability that is manifested as atopy. By the same logic, this inherited trait of a suppressed Th1 would increase morbidity and consequently Th2 immunity would be passed on to fewer and fewer future generations.

Although allergies have an undeniable though poorly understood genetic basis, this hypothesis has many moot points. Are Africans living in their ancestral countries uniquely resistant to parasite infections compared with other populations? There are no hard data. We do not know how long this migration took place to account for genetic drift. One might guess that — as in any relocation — it was compelled by the scarcity of food. But then malnutrition would work in the direction of suppressing immune response, atopy included.[34] Even when this poser is resolved, another question arises as to whether natural selection could sustain this advantage in the gene pool for any length of time, considering the fact that the bacterial threat in Africa is no less significant than the danger of flatworms. Still another controversy has been brewing in the portrayal of a Th2 profile as indispensable for asthma. That idea was recently contested by the fact that the presence of Th2 immunity does not herald *ipso facto* the presence of atopy.[35] In fact, many parasites, particularly helminth (worm) infections may vigorously dampen atopic reactivity, suggesting the possibility that the prominent anti-inflammatory networks associated with chronic helminth invasion might keep in check the progression to atopic reactions. Thus, it would be wise to keep looking elsewhere for an explanation of allergy prevalence among black Americans.

A baffling incursion of allergy into Eastern and Western Europe, whose population had neither the long-term tropical ancestry nor higher genetic liability, provides a possible clue. Such an accelerated, almost epidemic tempo of allergy within the span of a single generation is certainly inconsistent with the slower pace needed for genetic changes.[36] One is almost forced to conclude that if some sort of archaic Th2 type immunity was preserved by black Americans, it ought to have some simple environmental explanation. At first glance, excessive adiposity may certainly count as a contributing factor. It could predispose blacks to the accumulation of lipophilic organochlorine pollutants, which build up in the human body. They may reach the fetus via transplacental passage. A group of Slovak researchers has been able to collect placentas from term deliveries in two Slovak regions and conducted their analysis on 21 selected organochlorine compounds. For 16 of 21 organochlorine compounds, the placental contamination was higher in industrial regions as compared with rural regions. Their levels correlated with the cord serum IgE levels gathered from 2,050 neonates. This association was supported by the higher rates of atopic eczema in the populations registered in the industrial regions.[37] This bias has yet to be shown in black women but it might conceivably account for the stimulation of Th2 cells and elevated rates of atopy in industrial cities with a destitute black population. A population-based study in North Carolina showed that black women have higher plasma levels of lipophilic substances, such as organochlorine compounds, than white women. Predictably, body mass index was an independent predictor of organochlorine plasma levels,[38] but the circulating levels of such contaminants have yet to be examined for their role in allergy. In the future, blacks need to be oversampled in order to allow for a more reliable comparison by race and adiposity, since commonly, the sample sizes are too small to draw any real conclusions.

Sickle cell disease is another suspect. There is no statistical difference between the prevalence of atopic disorders (asthma, hay fever, and atopic dermatitis) in patients with and without sickle-cell anemia, even if their reproductive performance may be impaired.[39] Suggestively, however, sickle cell hemoglobin doubles the risk of bacteriuria. Given that bacteriuria is a common urinary tract infection in pregnant women and some find an increased risk of low birthweight and preterm delivery in women with asymptomatic bacteriuria (see, Ref. 40 for a review), the role of anemia in preterm delivery cannot be ruled out. Yet, a prospective study carried out to determine the outcome of pregnancy in mothers with a sickle-cell trait, did not support previous reports of low birthweights of infants born to women with sickle-cell anemia.[41]

Role of Bacterial Infections: The Silent Epidemic?

Bacterial vaginosis appears to be associated with preterm delivery of low-birthweight infants independently of other recognized risk factors.[42] Intrauterine infection is present in approximately 25% of all preterm births and the higher the frequency of intra-amniotic infection, the earlier the gestational age at delivery.[43,44] Females are constantly threatened by alien bacterial invasion. The most common microorganisms involved in intrauterine infections (bacterial vaginosis) are *Ureaplasma urealyticum, Chlamydia trachomatis, Fusobacterium species* and *Mycoplasma hominis*. It appeared that women who are afflicted with bacterial vaginosis, or are colonized with specific pathogens such as *Trichomonas vaginalis, Mycoplasma hominis*, are at particular risk of preterm delivery if they engage in frequent sexual intercourse (more than once per week) at 23 to 26 weeks of pregnancy.[45] That means that regardless of the presence of an 'enriched maternal microbial environment' bacterial vaginosis cannot accelerate postnatal development of immune competence. It may even delay it in prematurely delivered babies, because the role of infectious agents is thought to be less important than a favorable composition of the bacterial 'cocktail.' Also, bacterial vaginosis is a synergistic effect of multiple genital infections, some of which might potentiate allergic response, although this differential effect has yet to be clearly established. The shift of immune profile to that of Th2 in pregnancy further opens the mother to bacterial infections, and makes her less protected if such infections were latent before pregnancy. Even the presence of an intermediate form of vaginal flora disturbance at the first prenatal visit, rather than a full-blown bacterial vaginosis, appears to be associated with low birthweight and preterm birth.[46]

It remains to be elucidated how the temporary dominance of Th2 immunity is subverted by infections, so as to contribute to abortion or to preterm delivery. One of the explanations shown in Fig. 2.2 suggests that the Th1-dependent cytokines (e.g. IL-1, IL-6, IL-8, and TNFα), released in response to bacterial infection are potent inducers of genes that code for an enzyme called cyclooxygenase (COX). One of the cyclooxygenases, the COX-2 gene that codes for cyclooxygenase-2, is particularly relevant. That enzyme converts a long-chained fatty acid called arachidonic acid to prostaglandins (PGE_2 and $PGE_{2\alpha}$). The prostaglandins are among most potent hormone-like substances yet found. Among their numerous functions are the ability to stimulate intestinal and uterine contractions, thereby accelerating birth as soon as they reach the myometrium.[42,46] That might be why a Th1-type immunity is linked to spontaneous abortion.[47] Preterm labor was successfully reproduced in animal models by bacteria, bacterial cell wall products and inflammatory cytokines, such as IL-1 and tumor necrosis factor (TNFα). In view of this evidence one might ask whether the advantage of atopy among the early dwellers of the tropical forest was associated with a chronic malnutrition that protected the progeny at a high price for the mother. A slight change in mortality of offspring in those who were able to continue pregnancy to term in such precarious conditions must have made Th2 responses in the population more prevalent.

The role of infection in premature delivery was recognized in 1950, but abortion due to Chlamydial infection was considered as early as 1936.[48] It was implicated in the enzootic abortion of ewes, and the responsibility of the organism for ovine abortion has been attached to its name (*C. abortus*). It mainly afflicts sheep and goats that may harbor a latent infection, and contaminate the environment during lambing. Although human infections with *C. abortus* are infrequent, when they occur in the first trimester of pregnancy, spontaneous abortion is likely, whereas later infection causes preterm labor.[49] Once *C. abortus* was established as a cause of abortion of ewes, veterinarians knew that the only way to survive economically was to employ antibiotics in order to reduce the severity of placental infection, use Chlamydial vaccines, or DNA vaccination, which induce both cellular and humoral immune responses.[49]

The irony of this well-known fact was not immediately appreciated by neonatologists. Later, when the socio-demographic profile of women with bacterial vaginosis and preterm babies was examined, it was immediately apparent that they are likely to be unmarried and black, and to have previously delivered low birthweight infants.[50] Insofar as bacterial vaginosis could be sexually transmitted,[51] one might wonder whether or not other factors implicated in low birthweight, such as low social class, income and educational level, single marital status, trouble with 'nerves' and depression, reliance on help from professional agencies, and little contact with neighbors[52] are just proxies for the age and phenotype prone to harboring vaginal infection or sexually transmittable disease that collectively masquerade as "socioeconomic stress." Tellingly, only a dozen papers, all published during the last ten years, have been directly devoted to the study of the role of bacterial vaginosis in preterm labor and low birthweight. This is a peculiar phenomenon in biomedical research, when distant, low impact factors are favored over more proximal, pathophysiologically relevant "root factors" (see Chap. 7 for a general discussion).

All told, why dramatize bacterial infections of expectant mothers by calling it the *Silent Epidemic*? According to an Institute of Medicine report, the most common sexually transmitted diseases in the United States are infections with *Chlamydia trachomatis* and *Neisseria gonorrhoeae*.[44] Not only do gonorrhea and possibly chlamydial infection contribute to prematurity, but they are suspected to provide a favorable background to and catalyze HIV transmission. The other problem is that large proportions of infected persons may never have symptoms or have very mild and passing symptoms. This state of uncontrollable sexually transmitted diseases is better dubbed, in an effort to stop whispering about it, the *Asymptomatic Epidemic*.[53] Its cost is already loud enough, with US$10 billion per year on a par with the estimated costs for HIV infection. Apparently, only antibiotic administration to patients with asymptomatic bacteriuria would cause a significant reduction in the rate of preterm birth for the majority of women.

It is increasingly obvious that a greater death rate among US black men and women under 75 years of age as compared to their white counterparts does not disappear even after adjustment for income.[54] For some specific causes of death, such as prostate cancer, myeloma, and hypertensive heart disease, the relatively higher death rates among black men do not seem to reflect differences in income.[55] Despite increasing availability of prenatal care, nutrition supplementation programs, and drugs to stop preterm contractions, the preterm birth rate increased in the US from 9.5% in 1980 to 11% in 1998. Symptomatically, an increasing number of studies carried out with samples of adequate statistical power has arrived at the conclusion that preterm birth, but not growth retardation, predisposes the child to the development of subsequent asthma.[56–60] Obstetric, perinatal, and pediatric records have shown that afflicted black children had significantly lower birthweights and gestational ages than non-allergic children and more often required oxygen supplementation and positive pressure ventilation after birth than normal babies.[61] The only hope of handling these cases is by shifting the priorities of health care to prenatal preventive measures (broadly defined as the hygiene of pregnancy) and perinatal care (birth and early infancy) and away from the traditional emphasis on socioeconomic factors and lifestyle of adults who have a hard time sacrificing their favorable habits (Box 2.2). Both medicine and health psychology cannot wait until inequalities among races and classes will be eradicated sufficiently to impact on health.

Box 2.2   To screen or not to screen: The Chlamydia question.*

What would the benefit be?
- Women of child-bearing age would be free of sexually transmitted infections during pregnancy
- Identification of women with bacterial vaginosis could decrease the risk of numerous diseases of adulthood

What would the risk be?
- Young women would be overtreated with antibiotics consequent to an equivocal or false positive test result
- Potential consequences to the client's social and sexual life due to the need to examine and possibly co-treat their partners
- Anticipated psychological problems due to mislabeling of patients as having sexually transmitted infections
- Cost of retesting to assure whether the patients are clear of infection

www.chlamydiae.com
'Planned Parenthood' provides user-friendly information
(*www.plannedparenthood.org/STI-SAFESEX/chlamydia.htm*).

Somatic Disorders and Prematurity

A fetus depends on the mother for a continuing allotment of oxygen, removal of CO_2 and the waste materials of protein metabolism, and for suppressing the potentially damaging immunity shield mentioned above. On the other hand, a number of processes that secure the viability of the fetus may affect maternal systems, and in turn, damage the offending fetus. Molecular antigens from the fetus may cross the placental barrier, get into the mother's bloodstream and stimulate the formation of antibodies. Then they might proceed in the opposite direction, and injure the cells producing the antigens. Viral infections can also cross the barrier and damage the fetus (rubella is a case in point), while some vital vitamins and antibodies remain undelivered. Some bacterial infections, ascending through the amnion, can, as shown above, stimulate processes that may threaten pregnancy. The maternal-placental transfer system is a finely balanced process with a narrow margin of safety, so that either collectively or individually, these factors might handicap further development of the fetus. An apparently healthy infant may be moribund since a host of prenatal abnormalities might have programmed a disease that would emerge in the remote future.

David Barker's group[8] mentioned above pioneered the idea that the contemporary epidemic of coronary heart disease and diabetes in Western countries might have originated in fetal life. A strong argument in favor of Barker's concept is that low birthweight is associated with high risks for later ischemic heart disease, high blood pressure in childhood and adulthood, as well as impaired glucose tolerance. According to these studies, children who developed both hypertension and diabetes type 2 in adulthood had small placental size, as well as small body size at birth, and their accelerated postnatal growth continued beyond seven years. The effects of impaired fetal growth are modified by subsequent growth: the highest risks of heart disease and type 2 diabetes, insulin resistance syndrome, or impaired glucose tolerance (collectively referred to as impaired glucose tolerance), are found in those who were small at birth but became overweight as adults. This finding led to the second part of the hypothesis, that of the "thrifty phenotype." The gist of it is that a suboptimal intrauterine environment leads to physiological programming of the metabolic profile, which may increase the chance of survival during periods of starvation.

The long-time impact of both fetal growth and early postnatal growth on blood pressure at adulthood was supported by findings in the politically and economically diverse, but racially and socio-economically rather homogenous environments, such as in people born in Hong Kong[62] or Finland.[63] Almost counterintuitively, such an adjustment to malnutrition in fetal life, and permanent metabolic and endocrine changes, might be beneficial if sustenance remained scarce after birth. However, if nutrition becomes plentiful, this 'program' might predispose persons to obesity and impaired glucose tolerance, cardiovascular pathology, hypertension and diabetes. Can similar results be anticipated in other cultural groups or other countries? This question needs to be addressed by research studies in varied populations. Still, the appeal of the programming hypothesis is in its attempt to account for the social paradox that improved living conditions contribute to, rather than eliminate manifestations of the deficit. Since the kidney, like some other organs, has only a limited ability to replicate its cells after birth, the spur of postnatal body growth creates an excessive metabolic demand on the reduced mass of cells. The reduced number of nephrons leads to their hyperperfusion, glomerular sclerosis and nephron death. That establishes the vicious cycle of increasing blood pressure and further nephron death. Consequently, those who develop rapidly in childhood, as is the case for an increasing number of well-off families, are at risk for high blood pressure in adulthood. There are numerous other possible mechanisms of 'hypertension programming,' such as maternal factors, early effects of the fetal rennin-angiotensin system, impaired elasticity of the vascular beds, rarefaction, and aberrations of the sympathetic system (which will be discussed in a different context in Chap. 7).

Ethical and Social Issues

Latina Paradox

Mothers' roles are commonly seen from a psychological and sociological perspective, and both are essential. Socioeconomic status does determine to some extent behavioral choices and environmental exposures as well as access to medical care, but it is not a fundamental cause of illness. By overemphasizing economic drawbacks and ethnicity one may overlook other factors of morbidity. One reason for caution was provided by the observations that Latina and white 'anglo' women have similar rates of low birthweight infants,[64] despite their dissimilar socioeconomic profiles. This phenomenon was even dubbed the 'epidemiological paradox,'[65] since Latinos constitute the second largest ethnic minority group in the USA who are economically needy and overworked. One might suggest, as some do, that immigrants have certain health advantages over poor non-immigrants, since they retain traditional values or attitudes of the "old country" that are associated with good health. That "healthy immigrant" hypothesis is in itself a proxy for numerous factors,[64] none of which have been tested. Those "traditional values or attitudes" of immigrants have to be explicitly spelled out, so as to be available for emulation by young mothers of the host country and to improve reproduction and infant health.

After considering other recognized risk factors, including co-infections, the attributable risk of *Trichomonas vaginalis* infection associated with low birthweight was 11% in African Americans, as compared with 1.6% in Hispanics and 1.5% in Whites.[66] Not only might the low rate of bacterial vaginosis explain the "epidemiological paradox" of the Latina healthy progeny, but it also reemphasizes the relatively low weight of economic variables. Thus, vaginal pathogens might be a kind of environment that accounts for the increased rate of preterm birth, as well as much of the black-white-Latina difference in infant mortality. Further research is needed in order to identify the biological factors involved in pregnancy loss, so that effective therapies can be designed and their efficacy properly studied. An extra bonus of fighting bacterial vaginosis lies in reducing the rates of cardiovascular and metabolic disorders among black adults, since these conditions are associated with prematurity,[67,68] as well as with behavioral problems that aggravate prematurity in the presence of poor socioeconomic conditions.[69] Knowles[70] maintains that 99% of the entire population are born healthy, but get sick as a result of 'personal misbehavior.' The truth is that a great number of babies are born with latent disease due to the misbehavior of their mothers. Only mothers can alter the circumstances of their pregnancies and determine the fate of their progeny.

The agenda of public health disease prevention programs relies heavily on education of the populations at risk. These are the majority of young females who contract disease through unprotected heterosexual relations, the young men who take special pride in multiple sex partners and sexual activity at an early age, and teenagers (and even pre-adolescents) who flaunt an early debut of sexual intercourse[71–74] which may begin as early as at 11 years of age.[75] Of such sexually active youths, only 62% used a condom during their last episode of coitus. A significant number of boys and girls had had anal intercourse.[76] Not surprisingly, teen pregnancies are high on the list of risk factors for prematurity.

The fates of teen pregnancies vary. Some end in miscarriages. In a few young teens, first pregnancy is likely to be medically terminated unless it is discovered too late for abortion, but some older teenagers go ahead and have a baby. Interestingly, adolescent mothers in Sweden who experienced adverse perinatal events (including pre-eclampsia, preterm delivery, or intrauterine growth retardation manifested by small size for gestational age at birth) had early menarche.[77] Given that early sexual maturity is likely to promote early sexual experience and consequently, out-of-wedlock preterm births, a new round of somatic, cardiovascular, neurological, and allergic disorders might be launched. Those who have a baby are usually pregnant again within two years. Amazed health practitioners are wondering whether recurrent teenage pregnancies in adolescence are a random episode or a "planned" affair.[78] Very little is known about those who are at risk for the first or repeated teenage pregnancies other than their presumably low socioeconomic status. The studies of the Latina paradox suggest that 'psychosocial' pointers (family wealth, adequacy of educational and community facilities, low educational achievements, dysfunctional families, and attitudes of caregivers) do not provide an honest answer either.

On the Gamble of Tarnier and Budin

Almost to the end of the 19th century, Western society was not adequately equipped to rescue low birthweight neonates. In complicated deliveries, midwives used special intrauterine baptismal syringes to baptize unborn babies in order to save their souls rather than their lives. The shift to modernity and the resurgence of interest in securing fetal and neonatal survival was rooted in a military interest in the populational health.

After the Franco–Prussian War of 1870–1871, the Germans defeated the French and emotions in the French capital ran high. Louis Pasteur refused an honorary degree bestowed on him by a German university. Two patriotic Parisian obstetricians, Stéphane Tarnier (1828–1897) and Pierre Budin (1846–1907) were so alarmed that the falling birth rate following the war would make France vulnerable to future German invasions, that they organized an artificial system for saving the lives of bad neonates that were similar to contemporary incubators. Such an artificial environment, they believed, would save unviable babies and thus provide cannon fodder for the French army when their time to serve arrived. As Lewis Thomas once said, "New technology, for better or for worse, will be used, as that is our nature." The French gamble must have produced many survivors with cerebral palsy, mental retardation, blindness, deafness, and other long-term somatic and neurological symptoms. In wars, medical standards of any nation are not so much lowered for the recruits as altogether dropped.[79] The public has not been informed as to whether or not these French recruits were able to adapt to social demands, had cognitive flexibility and insights needed for planning and encoding contextual information about environmental cues, memory, abstract thought, and goal-directed behaviors. Patriotic French obstetricians confused achievability with feasibility but they won. As their goal was gradually forgotten, incubators evolved into an item of moral medicine despite the fact that substantial economic wealth was needed to achieve the contemporary low rates of infant and neonatal mortality. Quite naturally for physicians in charge, obstetricians were not bothered by questions such as whose welfare they were protecting by saving impaired babies: that of the parents who are eager to have children and always hope for a miracle, or that of the children who might have an uncertain chance to survive and cope, albeit only with a help of society or family wealth? An obligation to save has become an ethical code of Western society, so that today fetuses are kept in neonatal intensive care regardless of cost and irrespective of whether or not the future citizen will acquire the wisdom needed for social functioning, and the somatic and neurological competence needed for very survival.

Nowadays, the decision to adopt an alternative policy is not easy. The fulfillment of a programmed potential notwithstanding, one might notice that sometimes, sick people accomplish more than their healthy counterparts. Illness sometimes makes ordinary individuals more ambitious, successful and spirited. Patients, who have gross, permanent disabilities, observed McDonald Critchley,[80] often adjust better than those with minor dysfunctions. Among the famous early examples is that of Demosthenes who, born with a speech impediment, rose to be one of the greatest speakers of ancient Greece. Another one is the case of Blaise Pascal (1623–1662), a man with supernormal intellect, philosopher, master of language and style, scientist and theologian, who struggled with his lifelong bouts of sickness and even composed *Prayer for the Good Use of Sickness* in order to show that the terror of pain can be channeled into creativity. It is impossible to know, however, if they would not have topped their achievements had they been healthy.

Samuel Johnson (mentioned above), a writer whose fame is commonly compared with that of Shakespeare, makes this suggestion doubtful. He was one of the sickliest people known, almost blind and deaf. He was defiantly independent, an avid sportsman and fearless fighter. Although these examples do make a point arguing against the 20th century pathological eugenics ('good birth'), there are countless people who did not achieve adequate cognitive or physical potential. They tell us that the expansion of the relative size of the dependent population would exacerbate limited economical resources and increase inequality within our society.

Ultimately, advances in medical technology, such as ventilation techniques, surfactant therapy and glucocorticoids, have made it possible to save even extremely low birthweight (under 1000 g) infants, who in the past had no chance to survive. While society does everything in its power to reduce the death of preterm babies, the upbringing of such babies is left to the discretion and complete responsibility of the family. In its moral righteousness, medicine immorally overlooks establishing the medico-biological margin between salvaging life and delivering a baby into an individual and family tragedy. "What is the price of this extraordinary uncoupling of our species from millions of years of natural selection?" asks Silverman.[81] His alarmingly stark reflection was that such "skillfully executed intricate medical action is a prescription for social disaster in the immediately foreseeable future" (p. 76). It is hard to doubt that the artificially increased longevity that follows such obstetric success entails years of increased debility and an increased need for institutionalization and dependency.

A Glance at the Future

> 'Show me your face before your parents conceived you.'
>
> (An impossible Zen problem)

Romulus, the legendary founder of the city of Rome, and his twin brother, Remus were orphaned and nursed by a she-wolf and then raised by the herdsman. Having a wolf for a caregiver was probably better than none, but she was hardly an adequate substitute for a functional human family. As the legend goes, the orphans grew up as cruel and violent kids. Romulus was said to be a rapist and a killer, who made Rome into a place for outcasts and fugitives. The brothers often fought over trivial issues, and in one such argument over the place to build Rome, Romulus killed his twin brother. That legend might illustrate the value of a stimulating environment for brain maturation during early prenatal period. Not denying the role of the family, one is reminded of the twins' lineage: their father was Mars, the god of War whereas their princess-mother spent some time in jail (perhaps unjustly). Thus, an alternative moral for the myth suggests that the twins must have had some genetic liability, too. Most effective environmental stimuli are those initially provided during the fetal period by the mother through regulation across the placenta and, to a lesser extent by milk supply and sensory stimulation after birth. After weaning, control over development is shifted to the genetically regulated machinery of the infant. So far, medicine has learned enough to be able to disrupt pregnancy and to create experimentally a fetal environment that causes some phenocopies, including those of psychopathology. However, very little is known of how to put forward either a credible shield to protect a fetus against environmental hazards, or to use environmental or lifestyle factors as remedies. Likewise, molecular biologists have yet to learn to block a genetic predisposition for an impending disorder. The success of transduction procedures is not ripe for everyday practice. Therefore, in some cases, medical termination of pregnancy might be advised (e.g. in sickle-cell disease, Duchenne muscular dystrophy, or cystic fibrosis or numerous types of disorders that are only associated with mental retardation, *www.ncbi.nlm.nih.gov/omim*). An impossible Zen request, 'Show me your face before your parents conceived you' is about to be answered by examining the genetic profile of parents rather than by taking with amniocentesis a fluid specimen from the amniotic sac. Still, social attitudes to genetic screening range from acceptance to hostility.[82] The major reason for the rejection of screening is a worrisome practice of infanticide in some ancient societies (e.g. Sparta), which presumed to eliminate impaired genes from circulation by discarding the babies, or the more recent eugenic practices of Nazi Germany. Ironically, the increasing competence of medicine has reintroduced the question of when and whether to extend life if its quality for the patients and their families would be dreadful.

To appreciate the tenor of the current debates one might mention that a common problem is, who should be selected for *in utero* gene therapy? What degree of accuracy of molecular genetic diagnoses is currently available to direct correction procedures? How can we predict with confidence the genotype-phenotype relationship? Would a fetus with a chance of partial correction be an acceptable target to obtain the missing advantage for survival in a hostile environment, or should prenatal intervention be reserved only for a complete cure of defective somatic genes (those which control molecules making up human tissues)? Should a fetus with a genetic disorder that can be handled postnatally be rejected for prenatal treatment? How should we avoid risk to a pregnant mother, e.g. emotional risk, the risk of intrauterine infections, and ability of the mother to reproduce in the future? The real problem is that professional efforts are likely to be determined by the endless advances of technology, much as they were since the time of the incubators of Tarnier and Budin. In the meantime, those who object to screening of genetically imperfect babies, as well as those who insist on their survival at all costs, are blamed for investing into a 'biologically defective underclass.'[83]

Dealing with genetically determined disease is in itself a daunting task, yet it is further complicated by the fact that some disordered states or tissues lack distinctive features and their description has yet to be matched by the sophistication of molecular analytic devices. Even if they were available to clinicians, molecular biology does not have the tools to overwrite the genetic language of complex deficiencies. In a brief comment, captivatingly titled *What is the right way to fight the tragedy of genetic disease?* James Watson,[84] co-discoverer of the molecular structure of DNA in 1953, reflected:

There are three ways to interfere which gene-phenotype relations. One concerns the change of participating genes, another involves specific conditions for interactions, and still another concerns the timing of

> *"There is, of course, nothing pleasant about terminating the existence of a genetically disabled fetus. But doing so is incomparably more compassionate than allowing an infant to come into the world tragically impaired."*

the processes that are controlled by each gene. A given defect in the wiring of the developing system is difficult to locate, let alone repair, because of the multiplicity of interacting genes that are imbedded in a network of feedback loops on several levels of control. Morbidity is generated by a mix of genetic and catalytic environmental factors that makes our diversity. We are often cautioned that rigid, genetically programmed events are only a part of organismal adaptations. In most cases the phenotype is influenced by numerous genes and environmental factors. All individuals having "rank 1" mutations, such as those with a single mutated gene will exhibit the abnormality. But these are very few candidates. By contrast, "rank 2" and "rank 3" mutations appear in the phenotype of only some individuals who carry the mutation. An individual's health potential of the latter mutants is at the mercy of the bodily responsiveness to an unpredictable number of capricious environmental factors, such as nutrition, xenobiotics, infections, or exercise, which influence the expression of genes and membrane proteins and protein-protein interactions needed to rebuild ion channels, recycle receptors and neurotransmitters that govern signaling and excitability and ultimately translate ongoing stimuli into new experience. Most of these processes, however complex, are also genetically regulated even though the presence of widespread pleiotropy (the presence of multiple phenotypic expressions) in people with identical genetic programs makes genetic determinism rather fragile.

What then can be done with 'rank 1' genetically impaired children? Plainly speaking, the question is this: Should an infant be treated or allowed to die? Parents' ignorance and emotions can easily be exploited to convince them that making demands on the environment would correct the fetal program written in the language of genes. "There is, of course, the question of who should have the authority," pondered Watson, "to make decisions of this kind?" How far should one go to socially and cognitively test an individual in order to determine a potential inadequacy in the future? Should the risk of developing 'genetically programmed' disease be compared with the probability of other hazards, such as car accidents, Salmonella poisoning, or being struck by lightning? Steiner and colleagues[85] questioned parents and health practitioners about the "power to choose" with regard to preterm infants. Answers were rated on a four-point scale, ranging from strongly agree through strongly disagree, with no neutral option allowed. The overwhelming majority of the participants held that parents should have the final say. The difference between parents and health practitioners was in their attitude toward saving *all children*, irrespective of weight or physical condition at birth. Parents were overwhelmingly in favor of saving all. Their pro-save attitude was expected. In 1950 mortality rate of infants born under 1,500 grams was 70%. For somewhat heavier infants of fewer than 2,500 grams mortality rate was still 18%. Today, the risk of long-term complications in cases like these is much lower. With the advent of special ventilators and artificial surfactants, an infant born in 1990 had a life expectancy that was seven years greater than that of one born in 1950. That means that although the cost of medical innovation was considerable, the potential benefits of longer life and better health could be decisive in justifying the efforts.

Some parents do not deny that the costs to society should be considered in making decisions on saving underweight babies. By contrast, health practitioners were more cost-conscious; over two thirds of them believed that the impact of life saving of these babies on society should be a consideration. The problem is that almost everybody who is in a position to decide tends to skulk to avoid the guilt and anguish of ultimate moral responsibility of deciding in matters of life and death. Montello and Lantos[86] designated this tendency of diffusing individual authority by doctors, parents, and families as the *Karamazov Complex* (after Dostoevsky's *The Brothers Karamazov*). Unsurprisingly, in Steiner's study,[85] in a unity of mistrust, neither parents nor health professionals were prepared to relinquish authority to the government or other social institutions, such as ethics committees or law courts. James Watson voiced the same sentiment regarding genetically impaired infants. For him, only potential mothers should be given ultimate authority over the lives of their newborns. Regrettably, neither Watson nor Steiner and colleagues explicitly tell us who would guide the parents through the difficult choices that sometimes must be made about neonate survival; who would instruct them regarding risk assessment and uncertainty about cognitive development. "I am aware that some will argue that the fetus has an inalienable right to life," says Watson, treading carefully, "But the process of evolution never regards any form of life, be it adult or fetal, as inalienable

> Disease is reminiscent of a spectacle. When the curtains are drawn and the actors emerge on the stage, the viewer may not like what takes place there, but the play will last as planned. It was rehearsed for many months prior to the show. That is why the wish to diagnose latent disorders is as old as medicine itself.

right ... Working intelligently and wisely to see that good genes — not bad ones — dominate as many lives as possible is the truly moral way for us to proceed" (p. 62).

Coda

If you are reading these lines, rest assured that your mother is proud of *her* achievements, since she must be convinced that "there are millions of less fortunate children in this world who don't have wonderful parents like you do!" However, if your birthweight was low, her anxieties about your health were translated into *your* achievements by obstetricians and neonatologists.

Fetal and infant programming of metabolism and immunity are recognized as a crucial area of public health that has yet to be addressed in the future. Disease is reminiscent of a spectacle. When the curtains are drawn and the actors emerge on the stage, the viewer may not like what takes place there, but the play will last as planned. It was rehearsed for many months prior to the show. That is why the wish to diagnose latent disorders is as old as medicine itself. It rests on the sentiment that early detection is surely a better investment for an individual than waiting until symptoms appear. Only questions of the optimal level of prevention, its cost, and the menu of preventive measures are debated. A fair example is that of automobile accidents, over 40,000 of which in the US end up in death annually. Should we just put in airbags or invest in improving our roads or would averting human error be an adequate deterrence measure?

There may be more problems than malnutrition and prenatal injuries to influence adulthood morbidity. It was thought not too long ago that the placenta is a relatively impregnable barrier for almost anything in the maternal bloodstream other than nutrients of the embryo, or drugs and viral-size pathogens. Scientists recently discovered yet another phenomenon designated as microchimerism of fetal cells. The term describes the harboring of cells from another individual at low levels, commonly when maternally derived cells cross the placenta and settle in the fetus.[87] It is now recognized to occur due to bidirectional cell traffic across the placenta during most pregnancies. That means that the same passage may deliver cells via the placenta in the opposite direction so that fetal cells become maternal residents years or decades after delivery. Persistence of maternal microchimerism into adult life may contribute to disorders that are designated as "autoimmune." Microchimerism also implies that even after a short residence *in utero*, an embryo may flag a message that will be 'read' by all subsequent pregnancies, even if they were caused by different partners. In the absence of hard data, this hunch will remain tentative.

Rasmussen[9] argues that regardless of the excitement generated by Barker's hypothesis, it would be inadvisable for policy makers to organize preventive measures to help expectant mothers. Although not everybody is swayed, a number of studies examining diverse population groups have contributed findings that validate Barker's claims across countries and cultures. In many regards, the effects of programming determines whether the baby will be wanted, born, loved and then academically successful in adolescence and healthy in adulthood. In recognition of this fact, Russia has inaugurated a health movement, dubbed the "New Camelot," that rewards special certificates named after the Countess E.P. Dashkova (the first President of the Russian Academy of Sciences) for health achievements relevant for both expectant mothers and infants. In January 2000, the University of Southampton set up a *Centre for Fetal Origins of Adult Disease*. Its more broad-spectrum goals are to conduct epidemiological observations linking fetal health and nutrition with coronary heart disease, obesity, hypertension and stroke, non insulin-dependent diabetes and osteoporosis as well as certain forms of cancer, immunological and neurological diseases; to explore the underlying physiological processes of diseases that have fetal origins, as well as to outline new strategies for their prevention. Hence, this remains a priority area for health psychology that cannot be viewed as a discipline only focused on the enormous range of conditions leading to sickness, associated with sickness or caused by sickness through rational eating habits and lifestyle changes in adults. Organizations for pre- and perinatal counseling and help might be a cheaper and infinitely more effective investment in public health.

SO WHAT?

There is a gradual realization of the possibility that the seeds of diseases of adulthood may be planted early in ontogeny. In many cases, malfunctioning in adults is contributed to by 'bad genes.' In others, 'bad' infants result from maternal pathology, unfavorable events during pregnancy, delivery or the neonatal period. Either of these events might leave lasting, often lifelong, adjustments of metabolism, inadequate hormonal profile, abnormalities of vascular structure and blood flow, and ultimately to permanent somatic, neurological and psychological disabilities.

Specific clinical manifestations reflecting these changes, such as hypertension, stroke, chronic obstructive lung disease, renal failure, ovarian cancer, allergies and other disorders are commonly delayed into adulthood. It is impossible to be comprehensive, because so many different avenues are being pursued by various directions of practice.

In a way, a postnatal diagnosis becomes a snapshot of the present that began in the past and continues into the future, so that geriatric medicine and psychiatry might be said to begin in the womb.

If these assertions hold true, they will provide a compelling rationale for considering prenatal counseling and gynecological advice as a major focus of health psychology prevention programs. The arrangement for pre- and perinatal counseling will be a cheaper and infinitely more effective investment in public health than marketing rational eating habits and changing lifestyles that have a tendency to reach asymptomatic individuals. Health promotion researchers might want to examine the effectiveness of such early interventions.

3

---•---

Between Psychiatry and Medicine: Illness in Search of a Place

> "There is nothing more satisfactory in medicine than to be able to describe a collection of symptoms as belonging to an organic lesion of the kind which one may demonstrate in a glass jar — as one may describe the symptoms of appendicitis or coronary occlusion."
>
> *C.P. Symonds*[1] (p. 463)

Virtually any emotional symptomatology or distress associated with somatic symptoms is likely to be suspected for being responsible for an abnormal physical condition. Since the 60s, this attribution evolved from a psychosomatic to a biopsychosocial construct, which would be widely repeated in psychological and medical literature.[2] In an effort to amalgamate traditional and contemporary, the biopsychosocial model *"views health and illness as the product of a combination of factors including biological characteristics (e.g. genetic predisposition), behavioral factors (e.g. lifestyle, stress, health beliefs), and social conditions (e.g. cultural influences, family relationships, social support)"* (*www.health-psych.org/whatis.html*). Regardless of its enduring popularity and therapeutic elasticity, the model remains the same evasive Janus as its forerunner was. Its imperialistic comprehensiveness has become its liability, in particular with patients with *no* detectable organic disease who represent upwards of 70–89% of primary care practice.[3] These patients report numerous health problems, often in trying conditions, but seek to reduce their bodily pains rather than to mitigate the pains of life. Despite the lack of major physical signs, this condition could be associated with serious, even life-threatening psychosocial problems. Physicians usually fail in an effort to standardize treatment of this group and are uncertain whether the help is necessarily useful. Psychologists are less bothered with the unified approach and diagnostic difficulties for they are trained to think 'dimensionally.' But given that these dimensions are seldom ascertained operationally that simply means the necessity to customize the treatment for John, since quite sensibly his sickness is different from that for Jane and then dissimilar from that for Nick or Miriam and so on, rather than dealing with groups. It is fair to admit that this attitude has not been profoundly helpful. This chapter wrestles with the question of why.

Is There a Patient?

Bad practices begin with bad labeling. The search for a correct (or rather, politically correct) term for the sick provoked an ironic observation: "Just as language grotesquely inflates in attack, so it timidly shrinks in approbation, seeking words that cannot possibly give any offense, however notational. We do not fail, we underachieve. We are not junkies, but substance abusers; not handicapped but differently abled."[4] We are also not psychiatrists or psychologists, one might suitably add, but 'medical health providers' who do not treat patients, but accommodate the whims of clients and customers. These two terms are relatively recent additions to this balancing act. Although there is no harm in using them interchangeably, the practice reveals a medico-sociological divide in the approach to health care, as well as some confusion as to whether or not they apply to the same individuals. Merriam-Webster's dictionary gives away the difference: *Patient* (from Latin *pati* — 'I suffer') is someone able to bear or willing to bear; one that suffers, endures, or is victimized; sick individual, particularly when under care. In the latter meaning, a 'patient' is a subject of a socially and professionally sanctioned authority of a physician who is qualified to pronounce a person ill, and is entitled to provide professional help. *Patientia* (patience, forbearance) is an allegorical image of a protector from despair and anger. A patient is thus an individual who needs help in a *clinical* setting (from Gr. *kline* = bed or *klinein* = to lean, recline). An insight of one's state as opposed to that of others establishes the sense of a patient's identity and this awareness defines the name. The same insight formulated as a diagnosis also signals a degree of readiness to be the recipient and executioner of doctors' decisions and obeying the binding prescriptive regulation.

Occasionally, telling apart patients from non-patients can be problematic. McWhinney's[5] *bona fide* patients are individuals who achieved or exceeded a personal level of tolerance of pain, anxiety, fear and suffering. Still another kind is commonly misunderstood because of heterothetic presentations (from Gr. *heteros* — different; and *theticos* — laid down). These individuals are either unable to capture the essence of their distress or, more often, subsume real disorder under other more socially acceptable complaints. The body is a smorgasbord of practically all complaints, but some complainers jealously guard their personal anatomy from the 'self' and others, as socially sanctified dress code. They do wish to have their health restored, but are not at all straightforward about being completely deprived of the sick role. Also, the terms used for the description of complaints, and the importance attached to them, differs substantially across cultures. McWhinney's other two categories of consumers of medical assistance are individuals, apparently with no illness, who visit doctors for preventive reasons (e.g. regular checkups or vaccinations), and those who have administrative motives (e.g. seekers of approval for a specific occupation or for immigration documents). The latter are certainly neither patients nor 'help-seekers,' other than in a bureaucratic sense.

The term *'client'* is an old etymological relative of the 'kline' (from Latin *clinare* = to lean). But it is hardly ever used in this meaning. The words 'client' and 'patient' are considered only partially synonymous. If the term *patient* refers to a person who is confronted by a subjectively inscrutable force, or by an unforeseeable event, a client is a person who is at the liberty of 'purchasing' bonds for protection. The term 'client' prompts the listeners to invest some extra processing effort of whether or not therapeutic intervention is really needed. For medical professionals, the term 'client' communicates a narrower scope of services with a lower degree of responsibility than afforded by medicine. It does not include the concept of *'pati,'* even though the pain of loss, bereavement, or depression is something that both professions need to deal with. While being a patient is quite standard, the name of client is not a popular one in the world of medicine where all help-seekers are patients. That is why according to the analysis of the language of health through etymologies suggests that anybody on the threshold of a doctor's office might qualify for being called a patient. That does not mean that one looks at the crystal ball when applying these yardsticks. A difficult and potentially important decision is in distinguishing whether the person is a 'patient,' a 'client,' or both. In most cases the dividing line is fuzzy since some maintain that having a disease is a way of "shrinking one's world so that, with lessened responsibility and concerns, the person has a better chance of coping successfully."[6] (p. 75)

Those who object to heaping all the sick as a single entity of 'patienthood' opt for a more liberal name, that of a 'customer.' Presumably, dealing with a client requires understanding, empathy, recognition of pain and suffering, negotiations around a common ground of scientific and etiologic beliefs, non-labeling of the person, and work toward recovery in the absence of clear etiologic answers. The goal of the customer (client)–doctor partnership is simple, at least in theory: Give the customers what they want; most of it is your time, inasmuch as this remedy is seldom harmful in an overdose. Yet, defining an individual in anguish as a customer, strikes one as well outside the realm of medicine. It describes an informal visitor driven by a habit or whim, or rather 'one that purchases' services, such as we all do in a barbershop or a restaurant. It reminds one of the euphemistic term *guest* for a phthysic dying in a sanatorium (*'giving health'*) that was meant to boost the image of the institution rather than to sweeten the last minutes of life of the patient. There are other cases when the term is applied to a group, such as "consumer-survivors," that is, "psychiatric survivors" who may or may not be symptomatic, but collectively, they define themselves as victims of psychiatry. Should such patients be in charge of treatment, i.e. recognized as the customers? The answers differ widely. This section is devoted to some of the puzzles of *medically unexplained symptoms* since clients, customers, and certainly, patients are recruited from this group of individuals.

Medically Unexplained Symptoms and Misunderstood Patients

An English naturalist, renowned for his documentation of evolution, Charles Darwin (1809–1882) developed a peculiar incapacitating disease. Its symptoms, which waxed and waned through almost four decades, were comprised of disabling fatigue, abdominal cramp and flatulence, recurrent vomiting, hand trembling, fear, palpitation, and periodic facial skin eruptions of 'eczema'. This basket of symptoms and signs did not converge on a specific disability and was therefore a subject of acute interest and lively speculations by his physicians and biographers. As eloquently reported by Goldstein,[7] the tentative diagnoses ranged from organic etiology to psychogenic explanations and even malingering. Darwin was prescribed the common 'cures' of his time, such as good air, water cures, and a special diet, albeit with no substantial benefit for his state.

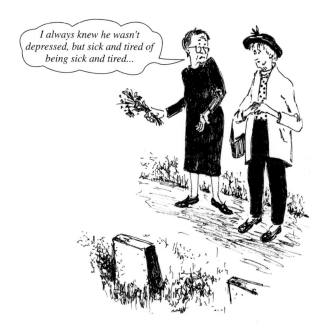

Merriam-Webster's dictionary defines a symptom as something that indicates the presence of something else. So, what happens when the mandatory 'something else' cannot be found? Is it proper to categorize that individual as physically fit, but having 'something else' just in the head? Such a dilemma frequently arises in emergency rooms when a visitor complains of suffering from a variety of diffuse somatic or neurological symptoms which either do not cluster into a recognizable syndrome, or are within the range of symptoms obtained from the general population. Almost all doctors soon learn to recognize patients with medically unexplained symptoms. The knack of acknowledging ignorance, or diagnostic and therapeutic helplessness when symptoms are 'medically unexplainable' is a signpost in the history of medicine, fundamentally associated with the development of laboratory-based medicine.

These unexplainable symptoms raise professional and ethical questions: Does this peculiar sickness intensify the patient's appeal for help? Do health providers respond to such complaints in proportion to the distress intensity? Finally, what is the cost of those complaints to the complainers and to the health practitioners? The answers to these questions are revealing. A chief source of exasperation for physicians is an excessive agony of these patients, their dissatisfaction with care, and their persistent attendance.[8, 9] Usually, they are not helped by pharmacotherapy. If anything, the latter is actually said to facilitate the chronification process.[10] For example, the differences between chronic pain patients and persons with chronic pain lasting less than one year who refuse to consult a doctor is in that the latter show relatively lower levels of distorted cognition, less pain-related upset, and higher levels of activity and self-control. Consequently, the 'stoics' who resist seeking help for pain appear happier *with pain* than do chronic pain patients who wish to lead a life without it.[11]

Due to functional limitations and occupational disability, patients tend to demand more and more medical assistance, and in the end they become 'veterans,' high-utilizers of health-care resources. Considering the fact that at least 36% of the patients with hypertension have panic attacks, such 'veterans' may create a major problem,[12] since the sufferer does not gain peace of mind by simple counseling. The low sensitivity of doctors to the presence of real bodily harm is associated with the fact that many such individuals manifest a degree of neuroticism, personality problems, or outright psychopathology. Although the rates of panic attacks may be inflated, because physicians tend to err on the side of diagnosing unexplainable symptoms as medically explainable ('hyperdiagnosing'), it is established that one third of new referrals to cardiology, gastroenterology and neurology clinics have symptoms that are either poorly explained, or completely unexplained, by identifiable organic causes.[13] Occasionally, such patients propose a firm diagnosis of their own. Depending upon their leading symptoms they self-refer to a specialist. Due to the bad relationships that they have developed with their original doctors, they tend to shop for other doctors. Some of them skip a visit to their family doctor altogether and shop instead for a specialist. Each medical specialty thus faces problems of this kind.

Some symptoms may have a character of catastrophic attacks, as in patients with nonischemic chest pain, that appear along with a variety of psychotic symptoms, most commonly, hypochondriasis, anxiety, and depression. Patients may experience vertigo, postural tachycardia syndrome, lightheadedness or syncope — all without relevant falls in blood pressure or evidence of cardiac, vestibular, or metabolic abnormalities.[14] These attacks of pain dominated by neuropsychiatric symptoms that persist despite treatment, tax the therapeutic capabilities of the physician to the limit. Some physicians are so convinced about the psychogenic origin of such somatic complains that they argue that somatic symptoms are incorrectly attributed to serious abnormality.[15] Treating them as such, they maintain, can reinforce the disorder due to symptom amplification, i.e. the idea that one has a serious disease which is likely to worsen. Patients then play the "sick role," which is facilitated by hopes of compensation; and an alarming portrayal of the condition as catastrophic and disabling.[16] An added psychological burden on the practitioner is the need to deal with the relatives of hypochondriacal patients who often are defensive, hostile, and dissatisfied with the medical care provided.

There seems to be a significant relationship between medically unexplained symptoms and prior experience of illness in the family, as well as previous unexplained symptoms in the individual's childhood. It is well established that personality variables affect disease manifestations and one's lifestyle. In addition, it is possible that, behind the façade of disturbed complainer, a real illness exists. In the late 70s, general practitioners recognized the problem of increasing numbers of dysphoric, unhappy, depressed, or plainly psychotic patients. They were overwhelmed by the fact that 30% of their patients manifest 100% of all theoretically possible complains and spend a great deal of time screening those who were 'worried well' with 'functional somatic syndromes.' As Hadler[8] observed in regard to fibromyalgia, "if you have to prove you are ill, you can't get well." Because of such patients, general practitioners became engaged in the "de facto mental health services system."[17]

Still more problems are accumulated due to an ethnic mismatch of patients and therapists; social and cultural distance between patients and doctors; stereotypes of psychopathology in blacks; and biased diagnostic instruments. Although physicians are educated to be tolerant of patients' personalities, in the real world of emergency rooms, underpaid, fatigued staff yield to an acute sense of mistrust and dislike by labeling such patients as "difficult," "noncompliant," "manipulative," "demanding," "clingers," "help rejecters," "hateful," "crocks," "hysterics," a "royal pain," or "GOMERs" (Get Out of My Emergency Room).[9] Such antipathy shown to a difficult patient is a thinly veiled irritation for the inability to effect a cure of what the individual believes *is* his or her somatic problem in the face of the physician's conviction that the problem is actually psychopathological. Thus, an effort to solve one's health problem might effectively put one on a collision course with the health providers. Anne Fademan,[18] who described the plight of the Hmong people of Laos, tells us that some exasperated doctors mused that the preferred treatment of choice for the uncooperative Hmong patients should be the "high-velocity transcortical lead therapy." When asked what that meant, her friend explained, "The patient should be shot in the head" (p. 63). These competent doctors, she writes, could at a glance tell apart "the ligament of Hesselbach from the ligament of Treitz." However, they were unable to understand the taboos of the Hmong against blood tests, surgery and anesthesia; "what the doctors viewed as clinical efficiency, the Hmong viewed as frosty arrogance." Doctors often cope with difficulties by using flippant and sardonic language. Notwithstanding, her objections, she does not say how much cross-cultural literacy might be helpful since many well-educated patients exhibit the same profile of 'difficult' behaviors while sharing with their doctors the same cultural, racial or ethnic backgrounds.

Patients with medically unexplained symptoms were expected to be best handled by psychologists who were ready to offer sympathy and bonds driven by the implicit assumption that patients are happier with a compassionate and trusting companion than a knowledgeable, but cold practitioner, and thus forgo medical care. However, this approach is not profoundly compelling. Patients would probably find it more comforting to be assured that their pain is attributed to somatic problems rather than perceive their emotional makeup as its cause. They do not care much about the name for therapy offered to cure their sickness as long as they appreciate that the physicians do not economize on their time. (More about this later, in Chap. 6.)

Boundaries of Discussion and Relevant Terminology

One of the functions of a scientific medical discipline is to develop a vocabulary whereby all disorders can be adequately described, so as to facilitate generalizations regarding their similarities and differences. This vocabulary helps recognize the factors that distinguish disorders of given persons from their preceding normal states, and from those of other persons. The term 'medically unexplained symptoms' has proven to be difficult to embrace in the charted territory. It reminds one of common taunts which evolved from medical jargon, such as 'idiot,' 'imbecile' or 'moron,' which were used to describe mentally deficient persons. In many cases, such labels simply reflect a degree of exasperation of physicians. When some Western clinicians saw patients with kuru for the first time, they felt that the disease is some sort of hysteria, simply because its peculiar symptoms were prevalent among women and children. Hysteria is an example of those diseases whose boundaries have been gradually blurred by the panoply of symptoms purged from other diseases. With time, the affliction has evolved into a group portrait, cutting across several recognizable disorders, and has become a chimera of dubious clinical relevance. When a subjective sensation of edginess, emotional numbness, and re-experience of past traumas graduated into Posttraumatic Stress Disorder, patients also felt like evolving into a new ontological state. The tendency to classify illness within labels of the common lore of physician's taxonomic culture is a historically justifiable practice. That does not mean that the taxonomic fences are not stressed or that they should be trusted as an immutable truth. Setting borders between different nosological entities is always an arbitrary affair. Even a border between perfect morphological entities, such as the cell surface and its environment, becomes capricious when the cells are seen under high magnification. A future goal for medicine in general and psychiatry in particular is to replace the phenomenological taxonomy with one based on etiology or pathophysiology.

Who Owns the Sickness, Americans or Russians?

In the late 1860s, American neurologist George Miller Beard (1839–1883) introduced the term 'neurasthenia,' which was further discussed in his book of 1881, *American Nervousness, Its Causes and Consequences*, which made the disease a feature of American culture and was designated as Beard's disease. Consider a patient complaining of stomach awareness, salivation, and nausea and vomiting, accompanied by pallor, sweating, dizziness, palpitations, paresthesias, headaches, anxiety, distress, muscular weakness, apathy and gait abnormalities. The syndrome may appear spontaneously, but can be provoked by a loud noise, riding a bike, or reading. There are many of these patients. They are exhausted and distressed, show heightened alarm, excessive emotionality, irritability, psychomotor agitation, readiness for anger display, and if the foregoing symptoms are not enough they might manifest a range of other symptoms from rheumatic, allergic, gastrointestinal, to neuralgic and neurological.

One might be tempted to file this entire catalogue with hysteria and that earned it an unforgiving reputation of a 'wastebasket'. An influential essay by Lewis[19] reminds us that hysteria is not a syndrome but a special form of mental disposition. Although some were clearly 'broadcasting' on the hysteria wavelength, "American nervousness refers only to a fraction of American society," Beard maintained, those who are "striving for honor, or expecting eminence or wealth." By contrast, hysterics have always been described as melodramatic, hyperemotional and theatrical. Less charitably, they have been characterized as manipulative, sexually inappropriate, deceitful, disloyal, devious, unreliable, and plainly dangerous; particularly when they were perceived as alien elements, unbalanced degenerates and vagabonds. In his historical essay, Mark S. Micale[20] recalls a rhetorical question, posed by J.M. Charcot during one of his clinical lessons: 'Where does hysteria hide?' Charcot's answer was, "in the gutter, among the beggars, the vagabonds, and the dispossessed, in the poor houses and even perhaps the jails and penitentiaries." One might mention parenthetically that in the early 1860s, the *Ostjuden*, the Jews from Hungary, Galicia and the rest of Eastern Europe, who had immigrated to Austria, Germany and France, scored high on the scale of 'otherness' due to features such as language incompetence, distinct apparel and unique religious practices which made them easily identified and stereotyped as degenerates and deviant eccentrics, distinguished from others to the point of incompatibility. French sociopolitical sensibilities and Charcot's diagnostic wisdom notwithstanding, Hassidic Jews were diagnosed as hysterics (cited after Janet Beizer[21]).

Clearly, neurasthenia was different. The marketability of Beard's idea proved exceptional, inasmuch as in his view the diagnosis of neurasthenia had to be made by elimination of the 'any organic cause.' A long list of permissible symptoms of a new disease and the dearth of infallible lab tests during his time provided a comfortable face-saving escape routes for both patients and their doctors; it became the main non-psychotic diagnosis of 19th century and remained popular until the beginning of the 20th century. It was devoid of the connotation of a 'shameful disease,' such as hysteria would be for a man, and men gratefully embraced the diagnosis by contributing from 33 to 50% of neurasthenia cases. Freud was comfortable in self-reporting himself as neurasthenic. It was a sign of an advanced civilization stripped of its untoward side effects attributable to polluted cities like cancer, suicide, traffic accidents, "French disease," and other communicable infections. Laura Goering[22] perceptively observed that the adoption of "neurasthenic Gestalt" in Russia, by showing high rates of the disorder, was a cheap way out of a cultural and political backwater and proof of their fitting in with Western civilization. Not surprisingly, between the 1930s and 1960s when neurasthenia was no longer a stylish diagnosis, much symptomatology evolved into psychasthenia, a diagnosis that contributed to its own demise. And yet, 'nervous exhaustion' was still very much an urban Russian disease that mandated a change of lifestyle, low-tech medication, some vitamins, sanatoria, balneological treatment, and country life, along with a hefty dose of ridicule for being confirmed by the disorder itself as someone of the petty bourgeoisie 'intelligentsia' stock. It remains a convenient bridge between psychopathology and a somatic disease. In the 1980s, an interest in neurasthenia was reawakened due to a number of conditions when the question of organicity could not be decisively answered regardless of the increased sophistication of scientific medicine. Like the immortal Phoenix, neurasthenia bounced to life to become chronic fatigue syndrome.

Coenestopathic States: A Tribute to Ernst Dupré (1862–1921)

"Nothing dies so hard as a word — particularly a word nobody understands." So began Laura Goering[22] in her essay on "Russian Nervousness." Well, some words are not as sticky as neurasthenia. The tongue twister, *coenestopathic states*, coined by Ernst Dupré,[23] was so conceited that it is now hardly recalled by historians of medicine. It was meant to portray "an aggregate of general sensations, as opposed to the more specific sensations of sensory or genital origin." Dupré modestly acknowledged that all psychiatrists see these patients, even though many coenestopathic patients consult their general practitioners rather than psychiatrists, or seek a reference to the appropriate specialist, "*according to the apparent site of the disorder*," ophthalmologist, urologist, gynecologist and other specialists. These symptoms comprised, as they do today, headaches, impaired ocular accommodation, spasms, cramps, tremors, myoclonic jerks, vertigo, and rigidity. Visceral coenestopathies gravitated towards such symptoms as palpitations, genital sensations, coughing, and dyspepsia.

Contemporary nosology decomposed hysteria into less pejorative components, such as somatization disorder, conversion disorder, hypochondriasis, body dysmorphic disorder, somatiform pain disorder, and dissociative disorders. So, one might wonder whether neurasthenia is any of those recent components of hysteria. Dupré admitted that some complaints sound a little strained. Yet, he doggedly emphasized their veracity as distinct from those made by hysterical patients. He reiterated that *rarely* do these patients manifest any signs of hysteria, neurasthenia, or hypochondriasis, regardless of the fact that their physicians arrange for a neurological consultation after they fail to find anything wrong with the "sites" of patients' complaints. Yet, a limited range of standard, cross-culturally accepted anatomical descriptors, and the presence of psychological aberrations in many patients, made it easy to pigeonhole patients into the semi-psychiatric trashcan, and then completely disregard them as medically incomprehensible. The coenestopathic state is a construct which is not directly observable, but is suggested by some manifestations and symptoms. In the majority of cases, it was the *diversity* of symptoms and signs that was required for diagnosis. With it, coenestopathic patients have been monopolized by the psychosocial model that shifted the emphasis from the medico-biological perspective to personality related maladaptive responses to environmental 'challenges' or psychosomatic disorders. The term 'coenestopathic' was an excellent amnestic package for the unexplained. Consequently, it was quietly abandoned and then gradually replaced by the term *medically unexplained disorders* or mutated together with neurasthenia or psychasthenia into several overlapping more specific afflictions or diagnostic suggestions that codified the range of physicians' 'understanding' or rather their tolerance to patients' symptoms. Several of these mutants are given below.

'Mutants' of Neurasthenia

Chronic Fatigue Syndrome

This is a perplexing disorder with an estimated prevalence of between 0.1% and 2.6% in the USA. It is synonymous with antiquated labels, such as 'neuromyasthenia' — a diagnosis that originated in North America, but found a second home in Europe, where it is still legitimate in spite of its 'neuromythological' status. Similarly to neurasthenia, chronic fatigue manifests persistent, relapsing bouts of fatigue, cognitive difficulties, memory decline, and poor sleep. Patients' common turn of phrase when admitting their underachievement, "*If not for* ..." (... chronic state of disability), reminds one of the temptation to designate this illness as *nisity* or *nisitism* (from Latin *nisi* for "If not ...").[24]

Irritable Bowel Syndrome and Dyspepsia

For a century, the syndrome has been diagnosed under such names as colonic neurosis, colonospasm, spastic colitis and the like. King James I of England apparently suffered from diarrhea whenever the matters of state upset him. In the past, neuroses were tied to specific organs, so that an 'unhappy' colon was fixed with gastric neurosis, very much like the 'soldier's heart' was a part of battle fatigue. At the turn of the 19th century, physicians were preoccupied with interventions in bowel functions. Enema parlors and colonic irrigations were common therapies to improve the 'nerves' and well-being of patients.

For doctors, these terms are just a collection of diffuse symptoms, perhaps suggesting the presence of uncertain intestinal motility abnormalities for which no pathophysiological mechanisms is available. Their exasperation might seem disproportionate to any psychiatrist who is perpetually confronted with the same problem. Gastroenterologists are uncertain about the reality of irritable bowel syndrome and functional dyspepsia, other than the nagging presence of demanding patients who expect their physicians to do something for them. In the US alone, there are upwards of 3.5 million annual physician visits by patients with complaints suggestive of this benign or 'functional' gastrointestinal disorder, and one-quarter of the US population is said to be afflicted with it. It remains a "name for the unknown."[25]

Despite historical mutability of the syndrome, symptoms like nausea, gurgling, excessive flatus, and constipation were noticed early on to cluster with frequent headaches, fatigue, and various 'nervous' manifestations (emotional instability and palpitations). Among the trigger factors were marital dissonance, anxiety over career or finances, and obsessional worrying. The illness thus showed typical 'functional' features, which are believed to require specific personalities rather than specific states of the colon.

Dyspepsia is an old kin of irritable bowel syndrome. It is an antiquated diagnosis that apparently originated in the 4th century B.C. in Aristotle's notion of the 'primary' reaction in the body designated as '*pepsis*.' Aristotle thought that pepsis is responsible for the normal digestion when bodily fluids are thick. Correspondingly, dyspepsia (watery stool) was conceived of as a deficient process of innate heat that thickens these fluids. A little more than a century ago, however, stomach upset and peptic ulcers were attributed to masturbation. In a patient diagnosed with dyspepsia, the gratification of the first bites of food is experienced at the price of the revulsion of nausea, epigastric pain, and the expectation of intolerable abdominal tension of bloating some time later.[26] Vomiting and/or diarrhea are associated with a tendency for the gut to respond to infections, toxins, inflammation, allergens, as well as overeating by secretomotor reactions that induce a hurried evacuation of its content. One contentious possibility is a local inflammatory change induced by chronic infection by *H. pylori*.[27] Parenthetically, one should mention that bacterial enterotoxins may not be all that bad. A bacterial heat-stable enterotoxin was demonstrated to suppress colon cancer cell proliferation. Apparently, this antiproliferative effect associated with diarrhea is behind unusually high resistance to primary and metastatic colorectal malignancies in under-developed countries with poor sanitation.[28]

Premenstrual Syndrome

The label is akin to 'womb complaints' of old doctors, i.e. aches and bloating, weight gain, fatigue, moods swings, headaches and food cravings around the menstrual cycle. No single causative factor of the premenstrual syndrome has been firmly identified. The diagnosis seemed useless and, until very recently, worth discarding altogether, inasmuch as its dominant symptom is that of "[feeling] more emotional," so that it is often called premenstrual dysphoric disorder, and handled as mild depression. This obstetric enigma may be associated with disturbances in the metabolism of tryptophan, as it is responsible for depression, anxiety and impairments of glucose tolerance occurring in some users of oral contraceptive agents and individuals with pyridoxine (vitamin B6) deficiency.[29] Another explanation of premenstrual syndrome is as an exaggerated host response to otherwise asymptomatic intrauterine bacterial toxins.[30]

Catamenial Seizure

Premenstrual syndrome should not be confused with epileptiform disorders in women occurring exclusively in the perimenstrual period. One third to one half of epileptic women have *catamenial* seizure patterns, with seizures most likely to occur in the perimenstrual period and during ovulation.[31] Occasionally, catamenial fits are accompanied by anxiety, autonomic symptoms, such as sweating, piloerection, paresthesias, as well as cardiovascular symptoms (tachycardia and hypertension) when it is difficult to discern the picture of epilepsy without special laboratory and neurological analysis. A biological basis for this fluctuation is in the ability of ovarian steroid hormones, particularly estradiol, to alter neuronal excitability, thereby predisposing the women to seizures.

Fibromyalgia

This chronic musculoskeletal pain syndrome that combines with complaints of fatigue, anxiety, sleep disorder, headaches, and gastrointestinal discomfort is difficult to distinguish from other 'functional' somatic syndromes (chronic fatigue syndrome and irritable bowel syndrome) and psychiatric disorders (depression and anxiety), with which a striking comorbidity is documented. Thirty-three of 60 patients with fibromyalgia studied by Slotkoff[32] met the criteria for *multiple chemical sensitivity*. Eleven of these patients also fulfilled more restrictive criteria of a "higher degree" of chemical sensitivity. Up to 20% of rheumatology outpatients present complaints consistent with fibromyalgia.[33] Likewise, chronic fatigue syndrome is characterized by persistent fatigue, musculoskeletal pain, sleep disturbance, and subjective cognitive impairment.[34] Mercifully, it is encountered in a mere 2% of the population, particularly in women.

There are numerous pathophysiological hypotheses for fibromyalgia, none of which are fully satisfying. Most commonly, it is conceived of as a multifactorial syndrome where all factors lock into a vicious cycle leading to global hyperalgesia. Recent studies implicate the development of immune hyper-responsiveness, at least in a subgroup of patients with fibromyalgia,[35] but fibromyalgia may be a case of a complex pain disorder debuting in early childhood or adolescence and then resurfacing as a new illness in adulthood. The fact that patients who seek assistance from a general practitioner about their widespread pain are diagnosed with a mental disorder does not tell the whole story, and can be very disturbing for a patient. Multiple sensory points of pain might suggest the presence of 'sensory polyneurities' akin to nearly forgotten Wartenberg's *migrant sensory neuritis*[36] whose reality is hardly in doubt. This disorder has been called abortive, incomplete, interrupted, broken up, split, and blown-to-pieces polyneuritis. It was long attributed to 'neurasthenic breakdown,' and rather dismissively, the Rorschach test was recommended for its diagnosis. As Wartenberg[36] mused, "It can hardly be assumed that Rorschach would lead anywhere."

Another perspective on fibromyalgia was provided by the notion of referred pain to various trigger zones, discussed by Ronald Melzack in his seminal book, *The Puzzle of Pain* of 1973. Such trigger zones are easily pointed out by cardiac patients, but pressure applied on virtually the same points is frequently somewhat painful even for presumed normal individuals. Pathophysiologically, painful responses in these patients might be the opposite of the tenderness associated with conversive anesthesia with or without pain. The mechanisms possibly comprise alterations of processing within the somatosensory system, as well as allied cortical (frontal/cingulate) and subcortical circuits (basal ganglia).

The Stiff-Person Syndrome

This is another elusive and disabling condition with uncertain prevalence. In a typical presentation, it is comprised of muscular stiffness and episodic spasms (occasionally asymmetric) superimposed on rigidity that involve axial and limb musculature.[37] Except for this global inflexibility, results of neurological examination are usually normal. The outcomes of conventional computed tomography and magnetic resonance imaging of the brain are also normal. The syndrome may emulate dystonias and extrapyramidal syndromes. Given that it is difficult to document axial stiffness objectively, conversion symptoms may be suspected albeit when other disorders are ruled out. Lately, however, an impaired γ-aminobutyric acid (GABA)-ergic neurotransmission has been implicated in the disorder. Also, an autoimmune pathogenesis is suspected, based on the presence of antibodies against glutamic acid decarboxylase (GAD), the rate-limiting enzyme for the synthesis of the inhibitory neurotransmitter GABA; the association of the disease with other autoimmune conditions; and the presence of various autoantibodies that interfere with the synthesis of GABA. Drugs that enhance GABA neurotransmission, such as diazepam, vigabatrin, and baclofen, provide mild to modest relief of clinical symptoms. Immunomodulatory agents, such as steroids, and immunoglobulin also seem to offer substantial improvement.[38]

Low Back Pain

About 20% of those who report for medical help also complain of low back pain. It is estimated to cost US $60 billion/year to the US taxpayer, which makes its treatment more expensive than AIDS, cancer and heart disease.[39] Low back pain might also originate in infancy, particularly in infants who have signs of plagiocephaly. This oblique calvarial deformity is associated with a persistent tilting of the pelvis, and lateral curvature of the trunk.[40] The alarming increase in the incidence of low back pain in adolescents drew attention to the prevalence of infant ('idiopathic') scoliosis. Screening for scoliosis may not only reduce unnecessary suffering but also save up to US \$50 billion, which the economy of the US loses to this disorder every year.

Low back pain is mentioned in the context of medically unexplained syndromes because it is often suspected to be a variant of depressive syndrome, pain behavior, or even a state akin to frank fibromyalgia. Given that most patients do not mind having access to most of the diagnostic and treatment techniques, in a good number of cases this barrage of tests plays a role of deluxe "placebo" given solely in order to reassure them that they are in 'good hands.'[41] Therefore, doctors are prepared to buy time by recommending alternative therapies for low back pain, such as those offered by chiropractic, acupuncture, and massage (Chap. 6). The latter may reduce anxiety and delay costly imaging procedures in the hope that nature will run its therapeutic course, which it often does. As a postscript to this section one should add that the deep-seated low-grade infections caused by low virulent microorganisms, such as *propionibacteria*, might also cause low back pain. Over 50% of patients appear to have positive cultures after long-term incubation.[42]

Sick Building Syndrome

This is a name for aberrant responses elicited by a variety of unrelated chemicals at very low levels of exposure that is commonly termed *multiple chemical sensitivity*. Epidemiological data from three American states puts the prevalence of chemical sensitivity at 16% to 33% of the general population, 2% to 6% of which have already been diagnosed with the disorder. More than 80% of such patients are women who also report symptoms centered on different organs, mood disorders, irritability, anxiety, sleep disturbances, stress and depression. Thus, this is a truly hidden epidemic that deserves notice of public health researchers and policy makers.[43] Clinically, the affliction may look like an allergy, and often as an asthmatic attack. Patients' history may include additional complaints, such as fever, hepatic reactions, arthritis, gastrointestinal problems and CNS abnormalities.

Hypotheses regarding the origin of multiple chemical sensitivity range from direct toxicological effects, a sort of neural sensitization phenomenon, akin to limbic kindling, 'toxicant-induced loss of tolerance,' allergy through the notion that it is purely a psychological (doctor-induced) effect, and a post-traumatic (hysterical?) phenomenon. It is often described as a curious phenomenon spurred by "belief system" that accounts for a significant 'borrowing' from other diseases. The ambivalence in its nature is reflected in the fact that it has appeared in the past under various names, such as 'chemical hypersensitivity syndrome,' 'universal allergy,' 'cerebral allergy,' 'total allergy syndrome,' 'environmental illness,' 'environmental maladaptive syndrome,' 'food and chemical sensitivity,' '20th-century syndrome,' and even dubbed a 'chemical AIDS.'[44] The syndrome has a tendency to cause panic and as such it is also described in Chap. 5.

This syndrome validates an ancient attribution of disease to fetid smells ('corruption of the air') emanating from dead animals, sewage, and stagnant waters that was meant to justify street cleaning, sewage disposal, delivery of fresh water, and later, zoning of industries in the Western world for disease prevention.[45] The concept of "chemical sensitivities" has evolved into a political campaign under the banner of ecologic medicine[46] that struggles to eliminate "active hazardous waste sites" and represent such organizations as "Chemical Victims" and "National Foundation for the Chemically Hypersensitive."

Veteran Claims Syndromes

This is a disorder with complex manifestations, and whose 'group portraits' widely vary. Gulf War Syndrome was exhibited by at least 12% of the veterans of the war in the Persian Gulf in 1991. They received some form of disability payment from the Department of Veterans Affairs due to complaints of weakness, hypersomnia or even lethargy, psychomotor retardation, eczema, fatigue, muscle and joint pain, anorexia and general anhedonia with diminished curiosity, reduced libido, as well as deficient social and cognitive functioning. Some of the symptoms were consistent with chronic fatigue syndrome, fever, fibromyalgia, depression, eating disorders, and multiple chemical sensitivities. Given that no organic signs of disease were found, these veterans were unceremoniously dumped on the medical bureaucrats who suspected the presence of psychosomatic syndrome or malingering (see Ref. 47 for a review).

A turn in the understanding of the syndrome was made after it was shown that some clusters of symptoms in Gulf War veterans hint at their neurological impairment.[48] Principal factor analysis yielded six syndrome factors, explaining 71% of the variance. Most significant among them were three that appear to reflect neurological injuries involving the central, peripheral, and autonomic nervous systems:

- Syndrome 1 — "impaired cognition," characterized by problems with attention, memory, and reasoning, as well as insomnia, depression, daytime sleepiness, and headaches;
- Syndrome 2 — "confusion-ataxia," characterized by problems with thinking, disorientation, balance disturbances, vertigo, and impotence. Veterans showing these symptoms were 12.5 times as likely to be unemployed as those without them;
- Syndrome 3 — "arthro-myo-neuropathy," characterized by joint and muscle pains, muscle fatigue, difficulty lifting, and extremity paresthesias.

Gulf War syndrome thus looked guardedly organic, possibly associated with a shift in the cytokine profiles from Th1 to the grossly immunosuppressive Th2 response. Factors that could have led to the shift might include exposure to multiple Th2-inducing vaccines against possible natural diseases and biological warfare agents, as well as the taxing circumstances in which these vaccinations were administered that might have maximized Th2 immunogenicity.[49] This hypothesis was carefully considered, but no shift in cytokine balance toward a Th2 profile in soldiers with symptoms similar to those of Gulf War syndrome was obtained.[50] There might have been, however, an interaction between the vaccine regimen, stress, and pesticide — especially organophosphate pesticides that were used in the Gulf to cause a Th2 promoting effect.[49] For example, the servicemen afflicted with chronic fatigue syndrome could have been more sensitive than others to stress or organophosphate agents. This guess proved to be somewhat more rewarding. It appears that all veterans with the neurologic symptoms were more likely to have the R allele (heterozygous QR or homozygous R) than to be homozygous Q for the paraoxonase/arylesterase-1 (PON1) gene. PON-Q is a genetically controlled isoenzyme that hydrolyzes organophosphate agents, such as warfare nerve agents and some pesticides (including sarin, soman, and diazinon). PON1 type Q, formerly designated as type A, distinguished ill veterans from controls better than just the PON1 genotype or the activity levels of the type R, formerly designated as type B.

Intriguingly, the cocktail of protective vaccines was given chiefly to the US and British soldiers. The French troops were not exposed to so many preventive antibacterial measures, and the sickness was not recorded among the French. The possible role played by vaccinations in producing this syndrome was somewhat strengthened by the fact that aluminum, which is used as an adjuvant in many vaccines, is also one of the potent triggers of IgE antibodies, and thus a potential allergen. Hotopf and colleagues[51] explored the relation between ill health after the Gulf War and vaccines received before or during the conflict. They conducted a large survey of Gulf War veterans of the UK armed forces who still had their vaccine records for six to eight years after deployment. Their findings were puzzling. Of all servicemen who received multiple vaccines before deployment, only one of the six health outcomes was obtained, that of post-traumatic stress reaction. By contrast, multiple vaccines received *during* deployment were associated with a variety of 'medically unexplained' conditions, such as fatigue, poor health perception, and decrements in physical functioning. It therefore appears as though multiple vaccinations are not harmful, unless combined with stressors. A list of potentially detrimental encounters is sufficiently long in any war. The Gulf War added to it the fumes and smoke from burning Kuwaiti oil wells, expectations of deadly harm following the destruction of facilities that might have housed chemical and/or biological weapons, and ingestion of drugs against possible organophosphate-based nerve agents.

Also, these findings seemed to support the proposal that neurologic symptoms were caused by low-level exposure to environmental chemicals in some genetically predisposed Gulf War veterans.[52] Together, they justified a probe for possible intracellular biochemical signs of damage in the basal ganglia and brainstem in Gulf War veterans matched for age, sex, and education level with well veterans. Haley and colleagues[53] used magnetic resonance hydrogen (^{1}H MR) spectroscopy. They found that N-acetylaspartate-to-creatine (NAA/Cr) ratio, which reflects functional neuronal mass, was significantly lower in the basal ganglia and brainstem of Gulf War veterans showing three of the syndromes mentioned above than in the corresponding anatomical structures of the control veterans.

Veterans with "confusion-ataxia" (Syndrome 2) who were most severely affected showed decreased NAA/Cr in both the basal ganglia and the brainstem. Those with Syndrome 1 showed effects only in the basal ganglia whereas those with Syndrome 3, were only affected in the brainstem. That was the first demonstration that Gulf War syndromes have biochemical evidence of neuronal damage in the absence of any other alternative causes, such as demyelinating, inflammatory infections, or neoplastic processes.

Mild Head Injury Syndrome

According to some estimates, patients with mild head injury (MHI) represent over 80% of all admitted to the hospital for head injury.[54] In fact, a cardinal worldwide burden of head injuries is not mortality, but disabilities following mild trauma that has long been pronounced a 'silent epidemic'[55] since any concussion, however mild, is likely to produce a persistent deficit. The polychrome of clinical symptoms of MHI includes[56–58]:

- Fatigue, confusion, disorientation, poor memory;
- Loss of interest, reduced volition and initiative withdrawal, isolation;
- Excessive concern, anxiety, worries and complaints about health;
- Lack of concern, anosognosia, indifference;
- Hypervigilance, edginess, impatience, excessive demands;
- Compensation tendencies;
- Inappropriate approach, violation of interpersonal boundaries.

Consequently, a number of patients with 'mild' trauma cannot achieve premorbid interpersonal and occupational goals. Furthermore, one might notice that the whole spectrum of symptoms rests almost at opposite ends of the continuum, and thus as useful as describing someone as wasteful, frugal, stingy, and generous.

Batia Stern (unpublished), in my program, confirmed that MHI leaves a lasting disability with diverse symptoms that varied widely in patients with presumably similar severities of head injury. She noticed, however, that patients vary in terms of the number of complaints and an impatience with which these complaints were reported. Based on personality profiles, she found that it was possible to subdivide — aided by Joseph Glicksohn — the latter into two subgroups, characterized as "introverted-withdrawn" and "extroverted-aggressive."

Their veracity was supported by the fact that in Stern's study, the profiles of symptoms were sampled in the course of psychiatric interviews, general neuropsychological and personality evaluations, which unlike a checklist of symptoms is less liable to channel specific responses. It has yet to be ascertained whether they represent two dissimilar features of post-concussive syndrome or an aggravation of premorbid disposition sharpened by traumatic experience and expectations of compensation. Given that psychosocial and physical functioning following mild head injury varies as a function of its severity and time, numerous manifestations such as irritability, anxiety, fatigue and headache may be unrelated to trauma. Such trauma-independence of the clinical presentation and the puzzling persistence of symptoms in some individuals is in keeping with the doubts voiced by Symonds[1] as to whether the effects of concussion, however slight, are ever completely reversible:

"... the symptoms of mental disorder at the highest levels are determined to a large extent by the mental constitution of the individual. *The symptom picture depends not only upon the kind of injury, but upon the kind of brain*" (p. 464, ital. added).

Symonds' allusion to "the kind of brain" de-emphasizes the role that traumatic history, family background, socioeconomic variables and learning play in the outcome of minimal head injury. Rather it posits that similarly to medically unexplained symptoms, premorbid innate susceptibility sets off the major somatic or psychopathological event in response to minor environmental stimuli. Such an episode may be so unexpected and painful in its impact that it is perceived as almost cataclysmic. In mathematics, such cases are designated as a 'catastrophe' and illustrate one of the most interesting theories of the 70s, *catastrophe theory*. Here, the term is used only as a metaphor since in the majority of cases we cannot quantify the magnitude of psychological stress nor can we often determine the kind of neurodevelopmental abnormality on the basis of brain anatomy.

A case in point is a healthy and successful (before trauma) 45-year-old man, father of four children, who developed a psychotic episode following mild head trauma with no loss of consciousness or physical injuries, and then remained apathetic and depressed for many months. His brain imaging demonstrated intracranial (quadrigeminal plate) lipoma and a somewhat hypoplastic vermis (see Fig. 3.1, also for further description). The latter two findings are typical neurodevelopmental aberrations originating in embryogenesis, which one may term 'dissipative' systems, again metaphorically, but consistent with the terminology of catastrophe theory. Admittedly, both are represented by numerous internal variables that cannot be specified because either lipoma or mild anatomical abnormalities of the vermis were found incidentally. These are conceived of as markers representing "the kind of brain" that may not be able to cope with stressful or effort-demanding situations, as long postulated by C.P. Symonds. They could be on occasion associated with a variety of psychopathological abnormalities and neurological signs. Of course, such 'harmless' injuries are very frequent, but for

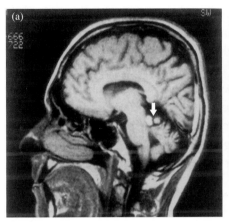 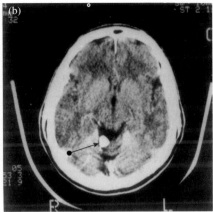

Fig. 3.1 Brain images of a patient with a history of mild head injury. This 45-year-old man emerged perplexed after a car accident and gradually become apathetic, depressed and withdrawn. A mental state examination revealed a fatigued or sedate patient with constricted range of affect. He repeated a story of having no energy, and of being a burden and a disgrace to his family for several months. He remained cognitively adequate, but depressed and passive. The foregoing picture was difficult to attribute to the impact of the car accident. Physical examination, serum chemistries, urine analysis and EEG were all normal. Two years later, the patient's state was dominated by depression, loss of interest and energy. Verbal contact was formal, meandering and frequently irrelevant. He denied auditory or visual hallucinations. There was no evidence of delusions. The MRI (conducted on a referral from Dr. Max Stern) showed (a) quadrigeminal plate lipoma and a somewhat hypoplastic vermis (MRI, TR — 600 msec; TE — 24 msec). The findings illustrated on a parasagittal cut show that lipoma was not large enough to put pressure on the ventricular system; (b) an axial view in a CT study shows the presence of a heavily calcified structure within the lipoma (regions of lucency on the anterior and posterior edges of the calcified mass) as well as a small *cavum septi pellucidi*. The latter might be a marker of enhanced vulnerability to stress.[59] With findings of this kind, which are often incidental, one is in a quandary: how abnormal is the test? Are there molecular (genetic) markers that correlate with these findings to signal enhanced susceptibility to environmental stressors? If it is a marker of risk, could a risk for developing disease be given on a numeric scale, for example, as an "*n* in 100,000" of having, say, depression? Would people be better served if risks were conveyed in qualitative terms (as possible or probable, high or low)? Could this finding become clinically troublesome in the patient's lifetime? And then, if the answer is affirmative, when is one to expect diseases to develop? What is his chance of living a normal life (or his risk of dying) if the patient chooses to remove the lipoma?

social and procedural reasons, they are also hard to track locally. Their 'invisibility' makes them seem trivial. For one thing, health care providers do not even discuss them as a matter of policy. In addition, the absence of gross anatomical brain abnormalities does not rule out microscopic abnormalities that lie below the resolution of current imaging modalities. Thus, although anecdotal reports have to be considered with a degree of caution, there are numerous data to suggest that the association of such incidentally discovered minor aberrations with psychopathology is more dependable than previously thought. Admittedly, the allusion to the "kind of brain" ceased to be a reference to brain anatomy since the latter may not explain *ipso facto* how psychological stress produces lasting psychopathology. Organic brain lesion therefore evolved into the 'kind of gene' notion that determines *when* troubling stimuli would trigger a production of some molecules that affect memory or mood.

The Q Syndromes?

The *coenestopathic states* of Dupré[23] were conceived of as a single systemic disorder with diverse end-organ manifestations. Together with neurasthenia they gradually filled in the territory between frank psychoses and normalcy. However, the 'end-organ manifestations' left an impression that *coenestopathies* are also somatic disorders, inasmuch — as Dupré himself observed — that *coenestopathic* patients tend to maintain their symptomatology over time. However, the criteria for the existence of subtypes on etiological and pathophysiological levels have not been successfully demonstrated. All what these patients presented, remained for the better part of 20th century just a story, or using Reiser's[60] line written in a somewhat different context, a "tapestry woven of events subjectively experienced." Finding adequate terminology for the group posed a real problem. As a result, when the border between somatic and psychopathological was difficult to draw, a number of descriptive terms have been created with the understanding that mental aberrations were also a leading comorbidity.

A Case of Amy Tan: Lessons Learned

Imagine a patient who has experienced an assortment of seemingly unrelated symptoms, such as hair loss, sleep punctuated by sensations of constant vibration, fatigue, memory loss, vertigo, tinnitus (ringing in the ears), occasional numbness, aching muscles and joints, a sore neck, speech disorder (that looks like Wernicke-type aphasia), and olfactory hallucinations. Random testing and symptomatic treatment does not help. The patient is still sick. Now what? If a patient is a woman, a frequent flier, and about 50 years of age, her doctor would likely attribute all this to her age, fatigue and postmenopausal hormonal disturbances. Of course, there is no simple solution, but the simplest and most disturbing — when a patient insists on additional testing for fairly nonspecific symptoms — is that she might eventually be diagnosed (read 'accused') of hysteria. As portrayed, the picture eludes etiological classification. The diagnosis is largely determined by age, family history, psychopathology, and ethnicity.

At this point, let me complicate the scenario by adding that the woman is of Chinese extraction and that she began experiencing startling visual hallucinations. Such well-formed visual hallucinations might well be triggered by the epileptiform discharges that originate in the temporal lobe for a variety of reasons, including infections. But even without the latter possibility you have got the idea what a quandary her doctor(s) might have been in or rather what they imagined they were dealing with (see Chaps. 6 and 7 for further discussion). With this myriad of complaints she had to collect numerous medical opinions, but her doctors (now in plural, i.e. her primary care physician, an endocrinologist, a sleep-disorder specialist, two neurologists, a psychiatrist, a cardiologist and an orthopedic surgeon) quickly ran out of all unambiguous 'organic' possibilities. In fact, the symptoms described above were not synthesized for a fictitious patient. The patient was Amy Tan, a novelist, whose sickness was vividly described in her recent book of 2003 (*The Opposite of Fate: A Book of Musings*). Given years of delay, denial, and barking up the wrong tree her frustration should not be underestimated. "By having Lyme disease, I have automatically been drawn," she mused, "into the medical schism over both its diagnosis and treatment." Much earlier in her case, the major objective was to determine whether the disorders sampled in Table 3.1 are identical with slightly different manifestations, or etiologically distinct conditions with overlapping manifestations. This dilemma is that of pleiotropy. For example, dissimilar allergic, parasitical and microbial diseases may appear in similar phenotypic attires, but may have a range of phenotypic expressions handled at different times of sickness course by special medical professionals. Following the hunch of Dupré, the common conjecture was and remains today that "the existence of specific somatic syndromes is largely an artifact of medical specialization."[61] The problem is that with so many players in a diagnostic process, a referral for definitive diagnosis may not be made until years later simply on the model of 'delegated responsibility' (Chap. 7).

Delayed manifestations are more difficult to attribute to any specific cause. When they develop, commonly available tests may fail to identify the culprit. Given that diverse clinical manifestations of an unexplained origin

Table 3.1 Medically unexplained symptoms ('mutants' of neurasthenia) by medical specialties (modified after Refs. 61 and 63).

Cardiology	Psychoneurocardiologic syndromes (e.g. tachicardia, palpitations, atypical chest pain, and hyperventilation)
Dental	Atypical facial pain, temporomandibular joint syndrome
Endocrinology	Hypoglycemia, labile hypertension, X-syndrome
Gastroenterology	Functional dyspepsia, irritable bowel syndrome
Gynecology	Pelvic pain, premenstrual syndrome
Infectious diseases	Chronic fatigue syndrome, epidemic vertigo
Internal/Occupational medicine	Multiple chemical sensitivities
Neurology	Insomnia, spasmophilia, syncope, vestibular dysfunction, hyperventilation syndrome, minimal head injury, tension headaches/fibromyalgia, pseudoepilepsy
Orthopedics	Low back pain, stiff-man syndrome
Otorhinolaryngology	Vestibular dysfunction
Rheumatology	Fibromyalgia, stiff-man syndrome
Rehabilitation	Minimal head injury
Psychiatry	All of the above (such as hysteria, depression, anxiety)

still pose more questions than it is possible to answer — because doctors might be unfamiliar with the disease, or because they are unable to find a sensitive test for its unambiguous identification (as often is the case in Lyme disease) — it might be fitting to honestly acknowledge them to be, only if temporarily, as syndromes of questionable etiology (thus, Q syndromes). In fact, Amy Tan, although a best-selling novelist, was not in the league of Samuel Johnson in challenging her doctors, who *queried* her diagnoses to the point of guessing that she was afflicted by syphilis and Lou Gehrig's disease. They failed to entertain the possibility of Lyme disease, an illness that is increasingly prevalent in the US, and which is caused by *Borrelia burgdorferi*, a bacterium that enters the body via the bite of a deer tick. It might seem intellectually confusing to name disorders for what they are *not*, waiting until their true nature is understood. Yet, in point of fact, the letter 'Q' was used as a label for a febrile disease, first described by a public health official in Australia in 1937. Its nature was unknown, and no etiologic diagnosis was made.[62] The label *Q fever* has stuck and was used long after it was established that the disorder is a highly contagious infection caused by *Coxiella burnetti*. 'Q' is a better alternative than the dubious allusion to a psychiatric ('non-organic') obscurity. It has the virtue of being easier on the tongue than the more archaic terms of neurasthenia or coenestopathy, and devoid of patho-physiological undertones of a unified syndrome where the unity may not exist.

The inescapable conclusion of Amy Tan's case is that Q syndromes encourage one to treat medically unexplained disorders with the same caution as treating the so-called cryptogenic disorders. This is a long list of diseases in all divisions of medicine from cryptogenic chronic liver disease and crypto-genic retinal ischemia to chronic cryptogenic sensory polyneuropathy and cryptogenic fibrosing alveolitis. Neither of these disorders have a psychologi-cal connotation. By labeling them 'cryptogenic' one simply delegates their explanation to the future, and dispatches such diagnoses with a more cautious prognosis than usual. Likewise, the Q label merely requires returning the patients to where they belong to, the offices of medical practitioners rather than telling them that their disease is 'all in the head.' Hopefully, as for Q fever, a specific mechanism will eventually be implicated in Q syndromes that will then acquire a new, 'respectable' label, and be amenable to legitimate medical ('organic') diagnosis (e.g. nutritional, hormonal, infectious or autoimmune).

The history of Darwin's chronic illness mentioned above,[7] which actu-ally must have been Chagas' disease, makes an instructive supplement to Ami Tan's history. Chagas' disease is one of those asymptomatic infections caused by *Trypanosoma cruzi* that can linger for decades, while occasionally leaving behind cardiac autonomic impairment and digestive symptoms. One-third of all *Trypanosoma cruzi* infected patients eventually develop chronic Chagas' disease cardiomyopathy,[64] which is consistent with the ultimate cause of Darwin's death. Nevertheless, he was suspected to have developed chronic psychosomatic syndrome.* Ironically, an abnormally

---

*One might recall that muscular pains, headache, cardiac palpitations, anxiety, profuse perspiration, and fatigue comprised a syndrome of the much dreaded malady confined to medieval England, and therefore called *Sudor Anglicus* or the '*English sweate.*' There were five epidemics of the English sweating sickness in the 15th and 16th centuries. The first occurred during 1485 at around the time of Henry Tudor's (later known as Henry VII) victory over Richard III. The sickness was explosive and led to death within a few days. The last episode took place during the reign of Edward VI in 1551.[65] If not for the high mortality rates, these epidemics would have been forgotten by now. In 1840, Hecker, a German historian of medi-cine, described the sickness in his historical treatise. Perhaps, the 'cultural' coupling of the syndrome and its inexplicable disappearance from the world inspired Rudolph K. Virchow to make his infamous decla-ration that "epidemics appear, and often disappear without traces, when a new culture period has started; thus with leprosy, and the English sweate."[66]

drowsy infant, who is easily fatigued, refuses to eat, and occasionally vom-
its, would be suspected of having signs of neonatal infection. An adult with
similar symptoms has a better chance of being referred to a psychiatrist as
afflicted by 'a neurosis of choice.' The appropriate identification of patients
as victims of infectious disease is obvious. The problem is that establishing
an etiological diagnosis of viral infections might be tricky. Today, it might
be apparent that epidemiological features such as the season of the year,
recreational activities (e.g. hunting or hiking), animal contact and other factors may provide helpful clues to guessing the diagnosis as they might have
been during epidemics of '*English sweate.*' In Virchow's time, it was impossible to make epidemiological sense of the quasi-periodic changes in cli-
matic conditions (e.g. temperature), the level of immunity in the population,
and the cycle of expansion of the potential virus–host populations (e.g.
rodents), and thus to notice that some of these factors are also culture-bound.
In fact, the disease was prevalent among relatively insular and affluent male
adults (who were likely more susceptible due to a lack of prior exposure and
contact with the less fortunate folks?) and during the spring or early autumn
(during a hunting season coincident with rodent activity). The etiologic
agent of the '*English sweate*' is still unknown, although the possibility of a
viral disorder, similar to *Hanatvirus pulmonary syndrome* has been suggested.[67] The latter is an epidemic characterized by phases of sequential
fever, hypotension, and urinary disorders. *Hantaviruses* are life-long infections common to murine rodents in the region of the Hantaan River of Korea,
which shed infectious virus in urine and feces. The primary mode of infection among humans is by inhaling contaminated aerosols or soil particles,
for example, when soldiers dig the trenches. The disease is not limited to
Korea. It is a persistent problem in Asia, Russia, and northern Europe and
was also recorded in the south-west of the USA.[68] In 1950–1953 it was the
Korean War equivalent of the Gulf War syndrome, but its reality was not dis-
puted due to a 5–15% mortality rate worldwide.

This historical detour shows that old questions may reappear in entirely
new terms. Contemporary practitioners look at essentially the same patients
that their colleagues described over a century ago, but their way of thinking
about them has begun to change. Thus far, help has not come fast enough, as it
has not in the Ami Tan case. The discovery of new pathogens is, in a way, too
successful for comfort. A virus, causing maladies akin to the English sweating

sickness or Lyme disease, has apparently adapted to survive due to a buildup of immunity in the population and/or to a loss of lethal virulence. A pathogen in one condition may be an innocuous cohabitant in others, with the result that adding conditions sharpening its virulence has always specified the term 'pathogen.'[69] As mentioned above, children who grow up exposed to high rates of complaints about physical health and psychiatric disorders in the family are said to monitor their symptoms and respond with somatic symptoms in adulthood in the absence of defined organic disease.[70] However, such a 'family effect' may be easily contributed by common genes or a shared pathogen rather than by exposure to mentally subcompetent parents and their grousing. That is why an interest in latent infections is 'on' and 'off' the agenda of the neurobiological research.

Pathogen-related proinflammatory cytokines may conceivably contribute to a range of abnormalities. However, that variability has some heuristic advantages. The most important one is the lack of pathogenic specificity for each disorder of the spectrum of Q syndromes, as well as the possibility of several dissimilar combined syndromes that have yet to be teased apart (e.g. cognitive deficit, somatic syndrome, affective disorder, autonomic dysfunction). Peripheral and central injections of interleukin-1 (IL-1) is a key molecule in brain-immune interactions that induces the expression of proinflammatory cytokines in the brain and has profound depressing effects on spontaneous and learned behaviors, including social behavior.[71] Cytokines produced by leukocytes activated by pathogenic microorganisms on the periphery transmit messages to the brain using humoral and neural pathways. Subjectively, these messages are interpreted as sickness whose first objective sign is a reduction of motility. Any pet owner can tell apart a healthy, playful dog or a cat from an apathetic, lethargic animal that refuses to eat or fool around. With no intention of giving a more precise name for those conditions, veterinarians long designated them as *sickness behavior*. In humans, sickness behavior is a complex state with cognitive deficits, neuropsychiatric disorders, including disorders of mood, steady weight loss, sleep disorders, loss of appetite and libido, along with numerous somatic signs, such as fever, exhaustion, back pain, fibromyalgia, and asthenia that are collectively referred to as sickness behavior (Table 3.2).[72] In turn, sickness behavior syndrome modulates the immune system so as to enhance recovery.[73] The production of proinflammatory cytokines either in the context of therapeutic

Table 3.2 Symptoms of sickness behavior and cytokines. (Partial list based on Ref. 72.)

Symptoms	Cytokines
Fever	Interferon-1α; interferon-1β; interferon-1γ
Pain (headaches, myalgia, arthralgia)	TNF-α; interferon-1α; interferon-1β; interferon-1γ
Tachicardia	Interferon-1α; interferon-1β; interferon-1γ
Fatigue	Interferon-1α; interferon-1β; interferon-1γ; TNF-α
Somnolence	IL-1; TNF-α
Insomnia	IL-10?
Anorexia	IL-1, TNF-α; interferon-1α
Loss of energy, libido, and drive	TNF-α
Loss of attention, confusion	Interferon-1α; interferon-1β; interferon-1γ; Il-2
Suicidal ideation	Interferon-1α; interferon-1β; interferon-1γ
Total: "Sick behavior"	Interferon-1α; interferon-1β; interferon-1γ; TNF-α; IL-1; IL-2; IL-10

administration (e.g. interferon-alpha-2β for hepatitis C infection) or during medical illness, induces a state of sickness behavior that closely resembles major depression.[74] That may not be typical clinical depression, but antidepressants have been shown to attenuate cytokine-induced syndrome in laboratory animals and to protect against the development of major depression in the context of therapeutic cytokine administration in humans. Although major depression is accompanied by activation of the inflammatory response system, its cognitive and somatic components may not be contributed by the same machinery.[75] This range of individual variability of the syndrome might be associated with dissimilar involvements of the lateralized cerebral machinery inhibiting the secretion of cytokines or blocking or abrogating the behavioral responses induced by inflammatory stimuli. Using IL-1, Neveu[76,77] demonstrated that the severity of sickness behavior may differ as a function of brain lateralization. Using a robust paw preference in a food reaching task in adult C3H mice, he showed that intraperitoneally injected IL-1 induced more pronounced depression of social investigation in right-pawed mice than in left-pawed animals. Likewise, they were more visibly immobile and less interested in food. The role of brain laterality in IL-1, IL-6, and TNF-α induced sickness behavior in humans has yet to be elucidated. It is known, however, that conversion symptoms more often involve the left side of the body thereby implicating the right hemisphere.[78]

Although conversion reactions are commonly explained in psychodynamic terms as the symbolic expression of an unconscious conflict, one study[79] showed that they can be readily rephrased in neurobiological language. Using single photon emission computerized tomography, the study revealed a consistent decrease of regional cerebral blood flow in the thalamus and basal ganglia contralateral to the deficit shown in *each* of the seven patients with lasting unilateral 'hysterical' sensorimotor loss. Importantly, the activity abnormalities in the contralateral basal ganglia and the thalamus normalized after recovery. These data suggest that "hysterical conversion deficits" may be placed in quotes as they entail a disorder in the striato-thalamocortical circuits controlling sensorimotor function and voluntary motor behavior, much as they are deficient, say in Parkinson's patients. It is of interest that the latter patients, too, particularly women often debut abnormalities on the left side of the body,[80] and are less likely to be diagnosed with conversion hysteria simply because they occur in elderly women who would not be suspected to manifest 'a neurosis of choice.'

Generations of students heard from their professors that a reduction or loss of sensation with no organic explanation, e.g. when they do not conform to the borders of dermatomes, such as the classical 'gloves'- or 'stockings'-type distributions of loss, are rather pseudo-neurologic symptoms indicative of hysterical anesthesia. Such "non-dermatomal somatosensory deficits" were also recently submitted to high-resolution functional MRI (fMRI). It appeared that unperceived stimuli were associated with deactivations in the primary and secondary somatosensory cortex, posterior parietal cortex, and prefrontal cortex. They failed to activate the thalamus, anterior and posterior regions of the anterior cingulate cortex and Brodmann area 44/45, i.e. all those areas that were activated with perceived touch and pain.[81] Although these aberrations are functional (dynamic) and can be restored pharmacologically, they clearly show that 'pseudoneurologic' conversion disorders may be returned to neurology wards where they historically belong, after all.

Melzack (mentioned above) speculated that prolonged, intense, somatic input may produce long-term central neural changes that act as 'trigger points' within the central nervous system itself. They may not become a source of impulses with the strength sufficient to produce pain, but interacting with stimuli from other sources (e.g. caused by troubling emotional events) can produce persistent changes initiating pain. Enhanced psychological weakness is thus at risk for responding with sensory aberration, including nociceptive or neuropathic pain.[81] Whether there is a need for a 'specific kind of brain' or a fairly specific kind of liability for such summation to happen has yet to be elucidated.

Q Syndrome and Channelopathies

When repetitive yawning, fatigue, stiff neck, nausea, vomiting, photophobia or phonophobia are triggered by minute quantities of odorous substances, such as the smell of strong perfume, one is more likely to suspect an attack of atypical migraine than 'indiscriminate' sick behavior. Like migraine that other than 'hemicrania' has numerous autonomic and gastrointestinal symptoms, changes of thermal sensitivity, eating disorders, and mood changes, such attacks could be associated with a phenomenon of 'spreading depression.' The latter term refers to the waves of slowly (2 mm/min) propagating neuronal depolarization, so termed because it 'flattens' (depresses) the electroencephalographic (EEG) response on the brain surface. Such an electrographic event is well documented in the neocortex of lisenchephalic animals (mainly rabbit and rat), but it can be reproduced in other brain areas of other species, including subcortical regions (e.g. the hippocampus) and human neocortex. The wave of spreading depression engages large areas of the neuronal soma and dendrites into the depolarization or hyperpolarization electrogenesis determined by a collective action of the protein subunits forming aqueous-filled pores that span the lipid bilayer of the cell. These pores or 'channels' are 'gated' by particular physical conditions or chemical stimuli (e.g. acetylcholine, γ-Aminobutyric acid, glycine, glutamate), so that the channel may be traversed only by a particular class of ions (e.g. sodium, potassium, calcium or chloride). Migraines might thus be an example of deficient channels that account for the enhanced level of extracellular $[K^+]$ (along with the parallel $[Cl^-]$ and $[Na^+]$ level decrease), rapidly causing neuronal hyperdepolarization with a temporary inactivation of the mechanism of spike generation, followed by neurovascular changes and release of vasoactive intestinal polypeptides and inflammation. In Ptacek's[82] view, genetic mutations that cause specific changes in channel protein composition may lead to significant alterations of channel permeability, and a spectrum of diverse disorders designated as *channelopathies*. Such ion channel mutations cause a human hyperexcitability phenotype with diverse clinical manifestations in the skeletal muscle, heart, and brain.* The pathophysiology of the syndrome is unknown, yet symptomatically, antiepileptic drugs are occasionally helpful, as they are in migraine (e.g. sodium valproate, topiramate).

Epilepsy is a complex neuropsychiatric syndrome affecting about 1% of the population. Local electrographic seizures in the limbic-prefrontal and orbitofrontal areas, known as low-threshold epileptiform regions, have long been associated with emotional disorders, and periodic deficit of memory and cognitive functions. They may also underlie non-convulsive states that emulate bona fide ('functional') psychopathology. The presentation of epilepsy is often protean, and its manifestations can still easily be confused with a wide range of other conditions. Among its numerous 'façades' are almost any psychopathological syndrome, autonomic disorders, abnormalities of behavior and emotions, and sleep disorders. One third of epileptic patients have psychopathological signs (hostility, paranoia, emotional liability, obsessionality, hyposexuality, episodes of *déjà vu, jamais vu*) and occasionally frank psychoses (manic-depressive illness, paranoid states). A classical syndrome of intermittent affective-somatoform symptoms with irritability, depressive and euphoric moods, and anxiety, anergia, fatigue, insomnia, and stomach pains was presumably exhibited by Vincent van Gogh while in Arles. Some epileptiform abnormalities can be so camouflaged by autonomic or psychological aberrations that they are easily misdiagnosed. Emil Kraepelin (1856–1926) spoke of this group as of the "*epileptoid convulsive forms* of mental disorder." On the other hand, there are emotional states, paroxysmal movement disorders, self-induced syncope, startle disease (hyperekplexia) and many other states that are reminiscent of hysteric fits and whose relevance to epilepsy is still debated. The collective term for these impostures of epilepsy is *pseudoepileptic* seizures.

Pseudoseizures remind us of other look-alikes, such as pseudoparalysis, pseudosensory syndromes, psychogenic movement disorders, pseudoneuroophthalmologic syndromes, and pseudocoma or other unknown conditions

---

*They include paroxysmal choreoathetosis, exercise-induced paroxysmal dystonia, cyclic vomiting syndrome, and hypnogenic paroxysmal dystonia. Paroxysmal kinesiogenic dyskinesias, which appears in the form of episodic ataxias, dyskinesias, or paroxysmal nocturnal dystonias, are akin to epileptiform conditions, in that they may be heralded by infantile convulsions, and may have familial gravitation.

collectively termed "essential" (synonymous to congenital, deep-seated, elemental, inborn, and intrinsic). Gates[83] sensibly abstained from using the term *pseudo* in connection with psycho-neurological conditions. Given that *seizures* are not necessarily an exclusive sign of epilepsy, terms like 'non-epileptic states,' 'quasi-epileptic disorders' or 'epileptiform states' might be favored. Among quasi-epileptic disorders, most common are spasmophilia, sleep disorders, and syncope. *Syncope* is a transient loss of consciousness accompanied by a loss of postural tone.

Epilepsy has inspired countless pathophysiological insights by genera-tions of neuropsychiatrists and neuroscientists, which earned the affliction a respectful name of *The Great Teacher*.[84] It also provides a rationale for the development of novel calcium ion (Ca^{2+})- or potassium (Na^{+})-channels blockers that hopefully offer an opportunity to treat some 'coenestopathic conditions.' Zinc and calcium ions in particular play a central role in the nervous system, including action potential generation, neurotransmitter release, or neuronal plasticity. However, dysregulation of Ca^{2+} traffic into neurons leads to a cascade of events which causes cytotoxicity and neuronal death. The advantages of epilepsy as a paradigm is that unlike any other dis-order it permits modeling in experimental animals the acquisition of certain types of behaviors, and then allows one to explore treatment strategies for their prevention. Do channelopathies make pathophysiological sense in regard to Q syndromes? The answer is uncertain.

The gracious design of our neuronal machinery is that we are seldom bothered by the unremitting noise of mechanical action inside our bodies, in the gastrointestinal system, in the bladder or in the heart, since to be 'exces-sively conscious,' as Feodor Dostoevsky, incisively observed does not mean being 'excessively healthy.' Our obliviousness to the 'noise' does not mean that the visceral world is completely opaque to consciousness. Some people may have reduced thresholds for subliminal chemical or somatic (visceral, muscular and proprioceptive) sensations, and cannot filter them out from con-sciousness. In this regard it is important to point out that multiple-pain syn-drome is not a problem for anxious adults only. The cluster of complaints that include abdominal pain, headaches, back and leg pain, chest pain, and neck pain are more common in childhood and adolescence than is commonly thought.[85] A survey of pain complaints in 5336 Dutch children in Rotterdam showed that 54% of children 4 to 12 years of age had experienced pain prior to the survey. At least a quarter of the respondents (mostly girls, 12–14 years) reported recurrent or continuous chronic pain.[86] In the search for therapeutic targets that would control conditions where chronic diffuse pain is comorbid with immune and mood disorders, several new hopefuls are being explored. Among those relevant for Q syndromes, tryptophan metabolism via the 'kynurenine pathway'[87] is attracting particular attention. Fluctuations in the levels of neuroactive metabolites in that pathway and consequently, impaired regulation of neuronal excitability and deficient biosynthesis of serotonin were found in such diverse ailments as chronic infections, autoimmune diseases, hormonal dysregulation and in movement disorders.

The foregoing poses a question: Could clinically similar pain syndrome be an expression of mutations in different components of the same channel complex or by mutations in dissimilar channels that debut as migraine involving intracranial blood vessels, but later kindle the pain-processing machinery via the NMDA receptors in other brain sites? Given the difficulties in managing this syndrome by 'single-system' pharmacotherapy, it is hoped that a better understanding of disturbances in the wide variety of membrane channels involving endorphins, γ-Aminobutyric, monoaminergic and serotonin receptors will help to determine the limits of disease phenotypes. Some directions in which reclassification of classical disorders are based on genomics can implicate numerous other neurotransmitters. Such a search provides hope for successful therapy over the next decade.

SO WHAT?

Medically unexplained symptoms are a contemporary nemesis of medicine. Upward of 70–89% of primary care practice consists of patients with no detectable organic disease. Patients with such symptoms report fatigue, gastrointestinal and cardiovascular problems, multiple pains and headaches, particularly in trying conditions that are difficult to account for. Their persistence poses the question as to whether these individuals simply manifest "maladaptive reaction to a stressor" or "mental disorder due to a general medical condition" and thus could be better served by psychiatrists or clinical psychologists.

As the mystery of these states unfolds it becomes apparent that their theory has been hopelessly trailing behind advancements in scientific knowledge. These were thus noncommittally labeled in this book as Q syndrome (with 'Q' for question). These syndromes have created multiple treatment difficulties since physicians are taught to look for somatic causes of somatic complaints and label disease as sickness behavior when they find none. Accordingly, patients responded by 'shopping' for doctors who, they believe, might successfully locate the cause of their sickness. Given that doctors are champions of categorical labeling, these patients receive conflicting diagnoses from different specialists, and more than a regular load of palliative treatment with them, or worse still, inappropriate treatments for diseases that they do not have.

Ultimately, these Q syndromes are treatable. The responsibility of a physician overseeing a case of *medically unexplained symptoms* lies more in a familiarity with the conceptual context as it relates to allergic conditions, channelopathies and latent infections. The advent of treatment for this (mistakenly) perceived relatively trivial and low priority condition will have to wait until its theories are shared and successful techniques for their diagnoses become commonplace.

Medicine is on the verge of a substantial increase in the understanding of many or most obstinate disorders. Our students may anticipate in the next decade convincing progress in the development of therapeutic interventions for neurodegenerative disorders, psychopathology, malignancies, cardiovascular, and gastrointestinal disorders. As this goal is achieved, the population afflicted with Q syndromes will also diminish.

4

The Deadly Trio

Of all the diseases on the Western world, three have been assigned an epidemic status, deservedly or not. These are obesity, dementing disorders and suicide. Despite a prodigious effort to clarify other disorders, the progress in the understanding of this trio remains modest. Perhaps, the major reason is that only recently have they acquired the status of diseases. Due to the uncertainty arising from the mountain of contradictory data, they have been of greater interest to those in charge of setting public policy than to the scientific and medical community. In the following, we have two general objectives: to provide examples where health psychology seems to be more profitable in establishing the principles that can be put into practice to control these disorders (Sections 4a and 4b), and to suggest where the public and politicians have a better chance of making an impact (Section 4c).

4a

The Obesity Epidemic

What do I fear? Myself? There's none else by.
William Shakespeare (Richard III; 5.3)

Throughout the ages, obesity has been associated with social rejection and ridicule, setting an individual aside from the normal-size majority of the population. Of course, we approve of fat when it softens body configuration,

119

sculpts breasts, rounds buttocks or thighs, but chiefly in women, and to an extent such shapely forms were more in vogue a few centuries ago. Otherwise, fat is commonly kept in contempt as a rather unattractive if not outright revolting addition to the body, as well as a sign of weakness of the characters of people unable to live up to elementary standards of good looks. In men, the same buildup is rather seen as pathetic. Overweight people are reluctantly hired, usually earn smaller salaries than lean folks, and tend to marry down. They are still tacitly assumed to be indolent, sloppy, slobs, socially clumsy, foul, noncompetitive, plainly lethargic or leading intemperate lifestyles. In France, 'corpulence,' as the French euphemistically call obesity, carries with it the widely shared stereotype of indifference, reduced insight and gluttony. Even in the politically correct US, obese people are dismissively designated as 'horizontally challenged,' sort of afflicted by 'the hyperactive fork 'n hypoactive foot syndrome.' Well recognized in developed countries, the inverse association between socio-economic status and corpulence could only add more fuel to the idea that such invectives are some sort of 'sizeism' or 'weightism' intended to stigmatize more impoverished individuals. Given that a greater proportion of children, adolescents and adults become obese each year, society has a dilemma of either combating obesity or making it a national norm along with the diseases that go with it.

According to Merriam-Webster, the word 'obesity' originates from Latin (*obesus*) to eat more. Eating immoderately, made obesity a personal problem, one of the deadly sins that shared company with sloth. In order to divorce it from sinful behavior the U.S. Surgeon General's *Call to Action* classifies obesity as a disease that qualifies for reimbursement (U.S. Department of Health and Human Services, Rockville, MD, 2001; *www.surgeongeneral.gov/topics/obesity*). Perhaps, it would be even less stigmatizing to designate medically overweight as *generalized adipose tissue hypertrophy* (comfortably abbreviated to GATH). Direct health care costs for diseases that are attributed to being overweight (such as hypertension, heart attack, stroke, diabetes mellitus, spontaneous autoimmune thyroiditis and some forms of cancer), and indirect costs due to loss of productivity already costs the US about US$118 billion annually. It has an added cost to society in that boys at risk of delinquency with episodes of dyscontrol manifest signs of obesity and elevated blood pressure, with 30% of the children appearing clinically obese and 24% having blood pressures above the 90th percentile for national norms in their age cohort.[1] As adults, obese individuals spend more on health care and medication than lean individuals. If they made more visits to doctors and dietitians for being overweight and were prescribed more diet drugs, the cost would go up significantly. The conservative estimate is very simple: a single trip to the doctor a year (at US$60/visit) by 25% of the 54 million obese Americans would cost more than US$810 million. Nevertheless, the US keeps providing nearly twice as much energy as required for a normal adult (3800 kilocalories per person per day, which is nearly the maximum metabolic needs of highly active prehistoric cave dwellers) as well as more reliable cars, better quality television screens, more diversified cable TV, powerful computers and the World Wide Web, and invests more into technologies that promise to make us all happy with virtual activity.

Thus far, society has been seemingly helpless to overcome the rise of the expanding waistline, inasmuch as there are no miraculous remedies. To encourage slimming, some employers offer paid days of vacation to those

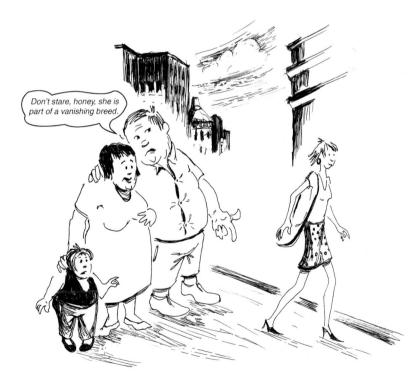

Thus far, society was seemingly helpless to overcome the rise of overweight, inasmuch as there are no miraculous remedies against it.

who meet fitness objectives that they set themselves. Although in some cases (e.g. military, police, fire service) it makes sense to establish such standards for hiring and promotion on the basis of body mass, the tendency to recruit legislators for writing slimming incentives into policy is likely to be defeated since the majority of those who are eligible to vote for such guidelines are now decisively overweight. Inspired by successful anti-tobacco laws, many health care professionals accept that the rate of obesity might be curtailed by restricting environmental temptations. Is this an act of faith or an etiologically justified conviction? And how is the term 'etiology' defined with respect to the epidemic? Do we look for etiology of individual 'high-risk' obesity cases or seek to identify the incidence rate? The two attitudes are not necessarily in rivalry, but neurobiologists and health psychologists are more interested in the former while epidemiologists tend to define the causes of incidence.[2] It is important to explore the possibility that in keeping with Shakespearian epigraph, we have to fear ourselves more than the 'noxious' food environment; that the weight-gain factors that are considered as 'extra-personal' belong in fact to the 'person-centered' domain. To paraphrase Raymond B. Cattell in 1950, it is not environment, but neuropsychological profile of an individual that enables us to predict his or her interest in food and ingestion behavior in a defined situation.

The question of 'why' obesity develops is answered in the language of either genetic predisposition, the effects of pre- or postnatal stressors, the role of early education and priming, and environmental forces to overeat, or obscure viral infection when the initial viral impact, say in the hypothalamus, triggers changes in later immunoneuroendocrine communication. This section will briefly consider the failure of obesity treatments and review the concept of obesity as reward deficiency and the environmental dependency syndrome that provides a hypothetical etiological dimension to obesity and returns the problem to the 'person-centered' or rather 'brain-centered' domain.

Gourmand Savants and Environmental Determinants of Obesity

Genes versus Environment

The role of genes in obesity is undeniable, but it is not certain what these genes are and what they are doing. Sociologists have gone far in showing that considerable cultural pressure upon children to act as their parents reduces genes to obscure regulators of bodily functions. Indeed, adiposity seems to begin with the parents who may imprint their weakness to ingest foods high in fat and energy density on their children, and then deprive them of adequate channels for energy expenditure. Likewise, children may acquire the same habits at a dinner table because of the coercive power of the roles in which their lives are cast. The generation of post-WWII kids grew up with their mothers' pledge, "you'll sit there till all that plate is clean!" So, are obesity and obesity-related disorders contributed to by early inactivity, postnatal overfeeding or parental genes?

In a paradigm that has become standard since Seymour Kety and colleagues, analyses of the Danish Adoption Studies of Schizophrenia, Thorkild Sørensen and Albert Stunkard[3] proposed a fast and elegant method to answer the question. Using a sample of 840 selected adoptees they operationalized obesity as a phenotype that was common in the genetic high-risk group (here adopted away offspring of the obese parents) and thus requested the parents and children to identify the degree of resemblance between them on silhouette templates, as shown in Fig. 4.1. There was a significant relationship in scores between the adult adoptees and their biological mothers and between the adoptees and their biological full siblings reared by the biological parents. Weaker and nonsignificant associations were found for the biological fathers and for the maternal and paternal half-siblings. There were no relationships in silhouette scoring between adoptees and adoptive parents. That led to the conclusion that human obesity is a disorder with complex genetic traits, whereas the family environment in childhood seemed to have little, if any, influence on obesity in adults. However, based on the findings by others, Sørensen and Stunkard grant that familial environment does have an effect while subjects are living together. A situation is reminiscent to that of allergy which has a strong genetic component and yet there are powerful prenatal and perinatal factors that determine whether the atopic genotype will be expressed. As a result, we are in the midst of an epidemic of allergies caused by an overwhelming environmental component.

Teleologically speaking, 'obesity genes' are said to be needed to secure individual survival when food was limited, such as during lasting famine, or arduous migrations of the population. Consequently, these genes might be thought to provide a strong defense against malnutrition and weight loss, but apply a much weaker resistance to overconsumption and weight gain,[4] since

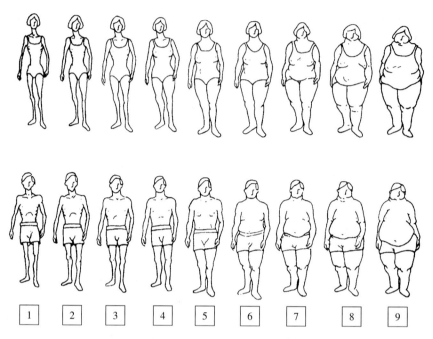

Fig. 4.1 Silhouettes from which the subjects picked the one that best represented themselves or their parents. After Sørensen & Stunkard[3] with permission.

in the short term, the capacity to stockpile fuel in the form of fat even in grotesque amounts does *not* lead to untoward events (well, not until we out-lived our procreational utility). Curiously, it was observed that body weight reduction in both normal and obese individuals by at least 10% is associated with metabolic adjustments to maintain body composition and a parallel decrease in energy expenditure. Therefore, metabolically, adiposity could be likened to the 'Plushkin syndrome,' after a miser and a squalid burger in the famed Russian novel, *Dead Souls*, by Nickolas Gogol. Obese individuals act like the misers who obsessively deposit into their banking accounts, which they practically cannot or are reluctant to access. Although immensely wealthy, they live with limited liquidity and thus behave as though they need to save more for a rainy day. Given that the heritability of obesity varies from 40% to 80%, one wonders, in the spirit of that metaphor, why our fat genes permit us to store fat regardless of energy requirements and make these adi-posity deposits energetically useless and so poorly accessible. Why is the sys-tem of consumption so uncoupled from the system of expenditure? Finally, if over 40% of the population still has an adequate body weight, one might wonder what distinguishes these people, their life-style, biochemical profile, behavior or personality from those who are overweight. Are they really 'normal' or do they have a somewhat higher metabolic bar and are thus destined in due course to gain weight unless a healthy lifestyle is institutionalized? If they differ psychologically, the question is: what is the nature of cognitive 'foraging' mechanisms that encourages everyone but them to overeat, regardless of the fact that the food is plentiful?

'Environmentalists' have long been in vogue in health psychology and the public debate for slimming is currently led by the wing of 'environmentalists,' so to speak. Preventing obesity, according to their view, "will not be forthcoming until the food industry is forced to lower production and change its marketing strategies, as the liquor and tobacco industries in the United States were compelled to do."[5] In the same summary, John G. Kral makes a surprisingly swift U-turn: "This cannot occur until the large and fast-growing populations of industrialized nations become educated in the *personal* implications of the energy principle" (ital. added). So, is it the food industry's or our fault? Convinced that personal problems are a leading cause of obesity, some theorists have long advocated the need to confront the current epidemic of obesity by building cognitive management skills into the educational curriculum so that everyone becomes equipped with the minimum capability needed to deal with the noxious gastronomic milieu that encourages overeating.[6]

Marion Nestle,[7] author of the popular book *Food Politics: How the Food Industry Influences Nutrition and Health* is less ambivalent regarding the source of obesity. In her view, there is an evil network premeditated by the food industry to make people eat more. How can one ask people, she protests, "to control what they eat when the food industry spends US$30 billion and more on marketing designed to make them eat more not less." Of course, we do not expect the food industry to advertise carrots any more than the tobacco industry to persuade us to abstain from tobacco in favor of chewing gum, or for liquor stores to post milk commercials. Many of those who commit sexual assault justify the crime by an irresistible temptation when they see overexposed shoulders (without going any further). Do we not, asked Murphy, after all have "brain and action systems which lead us to adapt not only to our whims but to our *environment*"[8] (p. 365, ital. in orig.).

Nestle's rhetorical question is a recognizable Machiavellian ploy squinting in the direction of litigation in order to save consumers who, she implies, have no self-control nor personal responsibilities; who but passively respond to the manipulative industry encouraging their self-gratification. This position does not take into account the fact that the food industry is only too sensitive in responding to public motivations, tastes and demands. According to the *US National Restaurant Association*, the restaurant industry alone will need to find two million people to fill its ranks by 2006. Its share of the food dollar today has increased by almost 200% compared to 1955 (from only 25% to 45.8%). Salespeople have long recognized that they could depend on the fact that the diners are driven by the things they like: taste, cost, and convenience. Responding to public lipophobia and fear of calories, they now market a variety of delicious fat-free products, which give people false confidence that by ingesting them they can respond to their whims and invest in their longevity at the same time.

The Obesity Bomb

In states like California or New York, an industrious lawyer can force food companies to disgorge all profits attributable to a zealous advertising that entices people to eat by employing product descriptions such as 'yummy,' 'scrumptious' and 'rich,' as though they are not fair descriptions of what we expect to enjoy. The January 2003 issue of *Fortune* magazine reported that after an overweight associate referred to a hamburger as a 'fat bomb,' the New York City attorney Sam Hirsch was inspired to file a suit against McDonald's (and thus, Burger King, KFC, and Wendy's) on behalf of obese and overweight children. Here is his argument. The fast-food chain "negligently, recklessly, carelessly and/or intentionally" markets to children their products failing to warn of the ingredients that are linked to "obesity, diabetes, coronary heart disease, high blood pressure, stroke, elevated cholesterol intake, related cancers," and other conditions. In the spirit of the 'bomb metaphor' of this section, it would be even more convincing to blame fast-food restaurants for collective terrorist warfare. Indeed, food as party fare, treats, snacks, prizes in games, rewarding relaxation is everywhere in our culture. It is therefore useless to blame commercial advertising and crave for the 'government to run the food police' when the family capitulates in establishing any discipline in food selection. Of course, it is desirable to reduce the size of the meal we are served and the amount of fat in it. But childhood obesity relentlessly goes up while the percentage of energy from fat in children's diets has been declining. Would it not be more prudent to reduce the size of the parking lots of many of our high schools to let the kids cycle or walk home thereby increasing energy expenditure?

Good tasting foods are not forced upon us. To be sure, they are aggressively advertised, but so are garments in department stores. Yet, it would be hopeless to fight shoplifting by banning commercials. Imagine a suit against Bloomingdales on behalf of individuals with self-image or body-image problems that the retailer markets to the young. Dressing in clothes from a Gucci boutique is a matter of personal taste, vanity, and fiscal responsibility (particularly for a shopper with limited means). Imagine if Bloomingdales, Neumann Marcus and Saks Firth Avenue stores agreed to pay individual 'victims' who were forced to rob a bank to buy Armani or Zegna because the retailers took advantage of the low level personal responsibility and narcissism of their customers. By the same token, it is our call to make a choice: either to ask for a 'doggie bag,' make a trip to the salad bar, request an extra helping or abstain from it.

A New York Judge, Robert Sweet, dismissed a lawsuit filed on behalf of obese children by Samuel Hirsch against "deceptive practices" in McDonald's promotion and distribution of its food. This ruling did not foreclose opportunities for individual plaintiffs to file more inventive claims. Consider the following scenario. Chocolate is one of the most desirable desserts among women (about 23% of women are said to crave for chocolate). The nature of this craving seems to be attributable to one of its biologically active ingredients, *anandamide* (N-arachidonylethanolamide), which appears to have affinity to *cannabinoid* receptors. Thus, by eating chocolate we legally activate the docking mechanisms for Δ-9-tetrahydrocannabinol (THC), an active ingredient of marijuana. Anandamide is unstable and is rapidly degraded in the body thereby limiting the socially untoward influence of craving, but pressing the need for another chocolate bite. In 2003 alone, the world ate US$42.2 billion worth of chocolate. The most avid consumers were Europeans, but the US was not far behind (*www.mindful-things.com/newsletter_archive/03-02-17*). The National House-hold Surveys on Drug Abuse conducted in 1999 and 2000 indicate that first-time marijuana use among the young is often a pathway to marijuana addiction or addiction to more potent drugs such as cocaine or heroin (*www.cannabisnews.com/news/thread13916.shtml*). Thus, a plaintiff might claim to have experienced social, economic, or emotional damage by developing an addiction to marijuana or other drugs consequent to chocoholism. What's more, normal young individuals might claim to be simply concerned for future personal addictions arising from the usage of, or a temptation to make use of, a substance known to be associated with latent addiction which they would be unable to control. Will we challenge the legal and moral astuteness of the Belgian "universal competence" law of 1993? Will chocoholics seek recourse in the International Criminal Court by filing lawsuits against Belgian chocolate magnates? Sounds sensational? No more than obesity lawsuits.

The American Secret

A heroine of Diane Johnson's novel, *Le Mariage*, Anne-Sophie, was shocked to discover that after only three days of her first visit to the US she gained weight: " 'It must be something they put in the food,' Anne-Sophie wailed. 'They are very fat, *Maman*. What shall I do?' "

Anne-Sophie's paranoia was explicable. There must be something in American food that made her more corpulent within a few days. Amusingly, Marc Kaufman (*Washington Post*, March 25, 2003) reports on the 18 ex-Taliban combatants being freed from detention at the U.S. military base at Guantanamo Bay. A young Afghan solider stared at the men as they passed by outside the run-down Kabul compound where he ate his dinner: "Very fat and in good spirits," he commented, "better than us here in Afghanistan." However, Anne-Sophie was not intimidated by animal fat consumption since it is a regular food component in France, where heart disease and obesity are on the decline. By contrast, total fat intake in the US has declined, while obesity has simultaneously gone up. The secret poison she was worried about must be high-carbohydrate meals of excessive volume, particularly the overwhelming presence of refined sugar.

We are all primed to like the sugary stuff and develop a 'sweet tooth' before our milk teeth erupt. Carbohydrates provide 250,000 kcal/yr to individuals in the developed countries. It is equivalent to the amount of energy needed to run three marathons a week, year round.[9] Such a therapeutic mission, none of us is capable of carrying out. Overall, up to 60% of the Western population is inadequately active and 25% are completely inactive. Only 1% of the US population cycles to work and just 9% walk. By comparison, in the Netherlands, almost half of the population tends to metabolize their energy intake while heading to the office, either by riding a bicycle (30%) or by walking (18%). A transition to a more active lifestyle is mandatory. Yet, even if commanded by a decree, a change will not happen overnight. It is more realistic to look at the reasons why people eat in excess of necessity, or using a banking metaphor, why they keep accumulating more deposits.

In sum, the deflation of the role of inheritance in weight gain, and the affront to the biological wisdom of the organism setting a point of optimal body weight, has shifted the focus of researchers to 'extra-physiological determinants' of adiposity,[10] such as environmental (cultural and socioeconomic) and cognitive (neuropsychological, personality) variables. However, these are dissimilar factors. Some are 'person-centered,' so to speak, in the sense that therapists are enlisted to deal with the individual psychological and medical problems contributing to obesity. Other recognized factors are considered to be 'extra-personal' since they deal with the environmental pressures that determine the population's feeding preferences and govern their practices.

Reward Deficiency Syndrome

Obesity has been designated an outcome of a "reward deficiency syndrome," akin to other reward disorders such as drug addiction or gambling that are thought to be due, in part, to a reduction in dopamine D_2 receptors.[11] Indeed, a deficient dopaminergic system may even contribute to an abnormally increased appetite that is reduced in Parkinson's patients with clinical improvement following L-Dopa medication. Bulimia was once proposed as a new autonomic sign in Parkinson's disease (PD).[12] It might well be informative to extend this work to carry out detailed comparisons of abnormalities between the cortico-striatal-thalamic-cortical-mediated "hypophrenic" disorders, such as PD patients who have difficulties in maintaining behavioral sets, and "hyperphrenic" disorders (such as obsessive-compulsive disorder), in which there are difficulties in relinquishing preferential sets of behavior.

Departing from this idea, as well as the psychopharmacological findings that drugs which block dopamine D_2 receptors increase appetite and result in a significant weight gain whereas drugs which increase brain dopamine release are anorexigenic, one group of researchers used positron emission tomography (PET) to assess whether there are differences in brain dopamine D_2 receptors in obese individuals.[13] The dopamine system was traced with [^{11}C] raclopride, a radiotracer that docks to dopamine D_2 receptors. As expected, they found that there was lower striatal dopamine D_2 receptor availability in obese individuals as compared to normal controls. They also showed that within the obese group, body mass index correlates negatively with the measures of D_2 receptors, such that the individuals with the lowest D_2 values had the largest body mass. Thus, dopamine D_2 receptor availability seemed to quantify, in a way, the severity of food addiction. This might possibly suggest why food, although the cheapest means of self-gratification, is not equally alluring to all. Given that a similar finding was reported in addicts to mind-altering drugs, such as cocaine, alcohol, or opiates, these findings suggest that obesity may be conceived of as a kind of addictive behavior as well as a sort of self-medication. However, although dopamine clearly plays an essential reward function, that function is a complex one. The work of Schultz and colleagues[14] showed that the dopamine system becomes increasingly responsive to reward predictors but seemingly unresponsive in the presence of the reward "itself." Overall, their work suggests that activity changes in a subset of dopamine neurons in the ventral tegmental area and substantia nigra represent prediction errors in the time and amount of future rewarding events; that is, changes in spike rate encode an ongoing difference between experienced rewards and long-term predicted reward. Thus, dopamine release does not equal pleasure and cannot be linearly related to changes in a radiotracer uptake to the same extent as it is not related to the rate of spiking.

The more modern terms for addiction are psychological dependence and physical dependence. Since all of us are physiologically dependent on food consumption, the question of why someone might become addicted to food as evidenced by excess weight is superfluous. Thus, the term 'addiction' in regard to food is used metaphorically as a case of overpowering 'wanting' to consume immoderately (in amount and/or frequency) something that is essential for survival. To a point, obesity — like addiction — is an affront to the notion that living systems are homeostatic, systems with self-correction, since a persistent ingestion of high energy foods is an example of a trend to maximize rather than optimize input. Getting overfull is like getting drunk — a temporary escape from the sovereignty of mind.

Although it has yet to be established whether all kinds of gratification trigger the same neurochemical machinery or its elements regardless of their object,[15] the fundamental insensitivity to reward in obese people is difficult to miss. Some of them are in a perpetual state of readiness to eat even when they are *not* particularly hungry. They habitually violate the dietetic norms set for them by their therapists as well as the self-imposed rules of common-sense reasoning. The history of dieting shows that a prolonged period of energy-restricted diet may be useless because, ironically, most dieters cannot remember what they eat, often have limited recollection of the taboo food items consumed, or even cheat on their food intake. Many dieters underreport the amount of food eaten, and underestimate their daily energy intake, particularly in foods that are both sweet and high in fat. This behavior is often rationalized as a reluctance to disclose the details of personal lives, even when disclosure is in the best interest of obese patients or when anonymity is assured. Why, indeed, would people seeking assistance and medical help behave dishonestly? Is it a problem of deficient working memory, repression, or self-deception? In his editorial for the *American Journal of Clinical Nutrition*, Blundell[16] mused that the inability to admit what was gobbled up seems counterintuitive:

"If humans represent the most intelligent form of life on this planet, why is it that they find it so difficult to make the apparently small adjustments in daily behavior that we calculate would halt the continuing raise in obesity? Is a highly developed intellect useless in the presence of a permissive biological system and a provocative environment structured on consumerism?" (p. 3).

Regardless of the explanations that might be offered, "reward deficiency syndrome" reminds one to a certain extent of "goal neglect" behaviors. This latter term is applied to frontal lobe patients who are aware of specific task goals, yet fail to activate the means of achieving them when circumstances demand.[17] Unlike in frontal patients, the conflict between motivated behavior and the need for its intentional inhibition in the obese may be psychologically costly by causing discomfort, emotional instability, and maladaptive social responses.

Signs of excessive interest in food usually begin in childhood or early adolescence, well before the onset of obesity for some individuals. In the 1960s, psychologists tested four-year-old children from a university community on a self-imposed delay situation.[18] They interviewed the children individually and, after briefly playing with them, explained that they needed to leave the room for a while. The children were told they could have one marshmallow as a reward immediately but would receive two if they waited until the tester had returned. Rash children would grab the marshmallow as soon as the experimenter had left the room. Others played, sang, or used other distractions to get the reward of two marshmallows 15–20 minutes later. It is of interest that there were statistically significant correlations between the tendency to tolerate a delay time in such conditions in preschool, and cognitive and academic competence and the ability to cope with frustration and stress in adolescence fourteen years later. Those who had resisted temptation were more confident and motivated and better able to cope with the frustrations of life. Regrettably, we do not know whether these two groups of children had different body weights in late adolescence.

Obesity and the 'White Bear' Effect

Many dieters who join 'self-help' dieting groups (e.g. 'Gourmand Anonymous' or 'Obese Anonymous') complain of feeling powerless to inhibit thought intrusions associated with foods. They slip back into thinking about food items they do not wish to think of. What conclusion should we derive from that? A learning theorist would say that they tend to react stronger to environmental and/or cognitively elicited food-related cues than to internal signals of satiety. Imagine a participant in a psychological study who is given a pre-trial instruction, such as: "Just relax, and don't let any bizarre images, like pictures of a juicy hamburger in your hands, enter your mind." Following these instructions, the participant will surely have an invasive image of the hamburger occupying their thoughts, and the cleverly designed study is ruined. Such intrusive items are reminiscent of the oft-cited 'white bear effect,' so named after Leo Tolstoy's portrayal of a child who was unable to stop thinking about a white bear (a punitive act of his older brother). A person who is preoccupied with thinking about proscribed behavior is said to experience a 'white bear effect' or the 'ironic effects' described by Wegner.[19] This phenomenon is part of the obsessive thought characteristics of depressed or traumatized individuals.

The white bear effect is also pervasive among the obese. W. Somerset Maugham's[20] character, Beatrice, is one of those 'white bear' victims as well as someone who was exceptionally dependent on food cues for she "knew what was good for her, and she could resist temptation well enough *if temptation was not put under her nose*" (emphasis added). Somerset Maugham, a doctor himself, must have entertained the possibility that behavioral phenotypes, in contemporary parlance, of some obese people include their inability to resist food stimuli 'under the nose.' Although firm results are still lacking, obese individuals share some aspects of personality, such as lack of self-control, impulsivity, along with an obsessively perfectionistic attitude.[21] These cognitive features persist across syndromes; none are really pathognomonic for obesity. Schacter and his colleagues[22] were apparently the first to emphasize the captivating character of external cues for obese individuals. They had long confirmed that, in overweight individuals, eating is guided by extracorporeal (environmental) cues whereas normal-weight individuals are influenced by internal cues. Even in the absence of the environmental cues, obese individuals are unable to suppress the 'white-bear' cognitive intrusions during dieting. The dependence on environmental cues causes a few lucky dieters who have been able to keep up with the demands of the dieting regimens to rebound into food hunting once the established weight objectives are met. It seems to elude them, as was pointed out by Hatter in *Alice in Wonderland*, that "I see what I eat" and "I eat what I see" are altogether different. Why do obese individuals show signs of the *environmental dependency* alluded to by Blundell?[16] What are the factors that contribute to the overwhelming motivational arousal, with enhanced hedonic impact of reward, or heightened vigilance and affective tension, in the presence of food?

Social psychologists tell us that people modify their self-presentations so as to match the expectations of others. Some are extremely labile in this regard (high self-monitoring people). These individuals manifest low behavioral consistency whenever others' expectations vary. Others are more independent of social expectations (low self-monitoring people). To an extent, resistance to healthy eating overlaps with the notions of behavioral consistency and self-monitoring. For example, when on a diet, high self-monitor (low consistency) people might readily respond to environmental stimuli during 'high-risk seasons' (e.g. holidays). Boutelle[23] randomly assigned 57 participants in a long-term cognitive-behavioral treatment program to either self-monitoring intervention or to a comparison group. During two holiday weeks (Christmas and New Year), the intervention group's treatment was supplemented with additional phone calls and daily mailings, all focused on self-monitoring. As expected, individuals in the intervention group self-monitored more consistently and better managed their weight than the comparison group during that period.

The Environmental Dependency Syndrome

We presume that healthy, well-adjusted individuals are self-directed and, insofar as food preferences and health habits are concerned, are behaviorally autonomous. That is not to say that some responses are predictably automatic. "The process," wrote Gardner Murphy[8] in 1947, "by which general motives (which are at first rather nonspecifically related to a class of stimuli) tend, upon repeated experience, to become more easily satisfied through the action of the specific satisfier than of others of the same general class, has been known so long that it would be impossible to name its discoverer." This tendency may become exaggerated so as to signal a loss of this autonomy that exposes the individual to irresistible environmental stimuli, including food. Under such conditions, spatial cues become not only relevant, but also excessively valued, instantly recognizable and thus capable of biasing ('canalizing' or 'channeling') behavioral responses. Once a food item has been handled, it reactivates another action, such that obese people have trouble inhibiting the tendency to continue eating until completely overstuffed. This pattern, too, is reminiscent of perseverative tendencies in frontal patients: once an action is carried out, a patient can have trouble inhibiting it.

Almost forty years ago, Russian neuropsychologist Alexander R. Luria,[24] pointed out that patients with anterior cortical lesions cannot intentionally suppress the execution of practiced motor and cognitive responses. They also act as though they are unable to plan ahead of time. The tradition of generalized models of cognitive deficit took a new direction when French neurologist Lhermitte and co-workers[25,26] began testing patients in the natural environment taxing their ability to implement a set of learned rules. Lhermitte was blazing a trail for future neurologists since his 'ecological' testing procedures are more appropriate for examining frontal lobe patients as opposed to tasks, such as the Wisconsin Card Sorting Test, originally developed for use with patients with frontal lesions. His studies described two forms of behavior, exhibited by frontal patients: *imitation* behavior and *utilization* behavior. The former consists of the tendency to copy gestures of the examiner. The latter "consumes" or makes use of any object in front of the patient (pick up a cup on the examiner's desk, reach for his eye glasses, or peel and eat an apple that was on the desk, but not offered, and so on) that are quiet irrelevant to the circumstances of examination. These patients provide a vivid example of dependence upon social and physical environmental prompts in that they tend to imitate gestures of the examiner, and manipulate any physical objects within their reach, regardless of their social relevance. Therefore, those two forms of responses were conceived as a part of a more complex behavior designated *environmental dependency syndrome*, in which patients behave as "though implicit in the environment was an order to respond to the situation in which they found themselves." Although the presence of utilization behavior in frontal patients has been repeatedly confirmed, not all fully agree. In one study, utilization behavior was quite infrequent while imitation behavior was observed in only 39% of cases (as compared with 97% in the French sample).[27] Also, imitation behavior was predominantly associated with damage to the upper medial and lateral frontal cortex, rather than with the mediobasal area of the frontal lobe. These and other differences notwithstanding, the effect of frontal lobe damage on environmental dependency syndrome remains unchallenged. Interpreting these findings into a theory, Lhermitte, proposed that a bizarre openness to the environment in frontal lobe patients might be a parietal response unopposed by the damaged prefrontal inhibitory circuits. It is of interest that patients with frontal lobe dementia and prefrontal atrophy frequently present with hyperphagia.[28] Hyperphagia and hyperorality were among other clinical features of nine British families with neuropathologically verified fronto-temporal dementia with tau-positive neuronal and glial inclusions.[29] Bilateral lesions of the orbitofrontal cortex and the mesial surface of the frontal lobe results in a syndrome of disorganized hyperactivity accompanied *inter alia* with impulsive overeating.[30] Given that the prefrontal cortex is part of a system that is responsible for planning, social conformity, and inhibition of socially improper impulses, one could ask: Might food dependency in normal obese individuals reflect an imbalance in the fronto-parietal function? The fact that people succeed better on diets with prescribed schedules with certain fixed characteristics and instructions for each step rather than on regimens allowing considerable flexibility in selection of food suggests that structure and plan might be factors that were missing in dieters' behavior and cognition. That does not mean that obesity is synonymous with cognitive deficit, let alone dementia and socially improper behaviors. Therefore, some aspect of normal variants of environmental dependency, if any, should be looked for in more subtle functional and morphological brain changes.

Only recently has functional brain imaging made it possible to examine the potential deviation of the functional anatomy of satiation and hunger in obesity and eating disorders. Gautier and colleagues,[31] who used PET to measure regional cerebral blood flow (rCBF) as a marker of neuronal activity, observed a significant flow decrease during satiation in a region of the parieto-temporal cortex (including Brodmann's areas 40, 21, and 22) of obese volunteers (BMI $\geq$ 35 kg/m^2) as compared to lean men (BMI $\leq$ 25 kg/m^2). Although the result is intriguing, it is unclear how it should be interpreted since parietal deactivation was recorded in obese as opposed to lean participants in response to drive reduction, i.e. satiation. One might wonder whether drive induction (hunger) would produce an opposite pattern of rCBF. Assuming that compared to lean individuals, obese people have more deeply modulated cycles of hunger and satiety — meaning that they enjoy more what they ate when they eat it — and suffer more than lean people when they are deprived of food, it is tempting to speculate that their hunger might actually be associated with greater frontal deactivation. One study of obesity,[13] assessed brain glucose metabolism with 2-deoxy-2[^{18}F]-D-glucose (FDG), but noticed no difference in the functional brain landscapes between lean and obese volunteers. Admittedly, however, such abnormality might have been revealed, had they studied regional brain glucose metabolism during stimulation by food rather than only at baseline. Interestingly, the profile most frequently attributed to anorexia nervosa is right posterior *hypo*metabolism, followed by right anterior *hyper*metabolism, both associated with right-sided abnormal electroencephalogram spiking.[32]

Stimulus-Bound Behavior

The role of the dorsolateral prefrontal cortex in interference control and inhibition of prepotent responses is widely recognized.[33] An individual with neurodevelopmental injury of prefrontal machinery finds it difficult to overcome prepotent response tendencies.[34] Thus, excessive psychomotor impulses created by a shift of the "fronto-parietal seesaw" may be especially compelling in the context of enhanced motivational arousal commonly experienced by obese individuals.

The ability of environmental cues to channel motivated behaviors has long been designated as 'canalization' (Gardner Murphy attributed the term to the French psychologist Pierre Janet). In neurosciences it is known as stimulus-biased or "stimulus-bound behavior." Elliot Valenstein[35] wondered whether the brain circuitry involved in making drive-related environmental selections in a rat settles on one, and only one, intrinsically predetermined choice or whether the system could be forced to commit a search of an infinite number of 'drive' alternatives. Valenstein used electrical stimulation delivered to a broad area of the hypothalamus (and even outside it) to bring about an 'interpretation' — so to speak — of a novel object in the cage as expressed by the rat's appetitive commitments. Valenstein knew upfront that the location of brain structures he was about to stimulate were involved in specific behavior since they had long been associated with specific drives. Normally, the association is accomplished by cueing an animal to biologically neutral objects. In the presence of objects to which the rat had previously been indifferent, an aroused animal used to respond in an object-specific way (feeding, gnawing, copulating, drinking, carrying objects, etc.) by selecting such an item from a display, thereby responding as if the neural circuitry was responsible for the consumption of goal-object available in the cage. The beauty of these stimulus-specific behavioral patterns is that it was a model of biological commitment that exhibited signs which Lhermitte much later labeled environmental dependency. Similarly, in the patterns exemplified by Lhermitte's cases, these behaviors can easily be switched from one type of response to another with no apparent aftereffect from the previous responses. Various features of environment dependency syndrome (such as seeing a gesture produced by the examiner or an object displayed in the doctor's office) are exhibited only during the period of "stimulation." From the fact that a patient exhibits a new, highly specific act, a learning theorist could have hypothesized that this act was a result of an enhanced arousal and anxiety that activated a motivational state and channeled behavior to a stimulus that otherwise would be less tempting.

Valenstein's theorizing may be applied to numerous findings indicating that the sight of food triggers ingestion not only in the presence of hunger, but also, for example when 'hunger behavior' is maintained by negative emotions and fear.[36] Comparing animals in their natural habitats with domesticated animals, ethologists have long realised that overeating, very much like excessive sexual activity, is a species-specific adaptation to the unmitigated stress of domestication, boredom, and space restriction. That is likely why we have a tendency to generalize anxiety and stress as though signaling that food may not be readily available, and that excess energy should better be stored in the body as a buffer against future food shortages.[37] Stressed animals eat more often and consume larger meals to maximize the storage of energy in situations of adversity. A decrease of glucose plasma levels prior to the onset of meals[38] might further enhance hunger and prompt feeding to reduce the pain of arousal thereby serving as some sort of a positive feedback that is activated in preparation for the meal. Changes in affect during eating revealed a significant decline in negative emotions such as tension and tiredness, and, in the heavier subjects, a trend was observed of an increased sense of well-being and happiness following eating.[39] "When in doubt, eat," pronounced Andrew Weil in his popular book, *Spontaneous Healing*, and anxious people do plot a course to grab food when they are uncertain, tense, and uneasy. The question is why such poor judgment is being made while they appreciate the likely outcome of their actions.

Gourmand Savants

"If you want to know the normal healthy body, study it when it is abnormal, when
it is ill. If you want to know functions, study their singularities."
Imre Lakatos, Proofs and Refutations (p. 23)

Occasionally, people with neurodevelopmental abnormality, overall cognitive
impairment with deficient social interaction and communication, display
exceptional skills, such as artistic, poetic, or computational talents at a level
superior to the general intellectual functioning. This paradoxical narrow
cognitive facilitation has long been recognized as the so-called "savant"
behavior or "savant syndrome."[40] A similar 'functional facilitation' was
described in patients with the temporal lobe variant of fronto-temporal
dementia, who acquired new artistic skills in the setting of devastated
language and social skills.[41] If loss of function in the *left* anterior temporal
lobe may lead to facilitation of artistic or musical skills, right hemisphere
damage might be expected to show 'functional facilitation' in adults in the
hedonic and motivational aspects of taste. Indeed, Regard & Landis[42]
described a preoccupation with food along with other impulse control disorders in two individuals who were otherwise indifferent to fine foods for most
of their lives, but developed an irresistible craving for fine-food eating after
sustaining brain damage. They also rescued the theme from the unfalsifiable
'just-so' stories by the analysis of clinical and anatomical data of 36 patients
who were reported in the literature. It appeared that in 34 of them there was
a strong association with lesion location in the right anterior part of the brain
involving cortical areas, basal ganglia, or limbic structures. This condition
was designated as gourmand syndrome.[42] According to Webster's Dictionary,
a *Gourmand* is someone who is very fond of eating and drinking or one who
is very interested in good food and drink (*epicure*). Some of these patients
appear to be attracted to fine foods as though brain lesions disinhibited a formerly concealed hedonic aspect of taste thereby opening a novel channel of
appreciation of the subtleties of cooking. It remains to be explored whether
or not this "gourmand syndrome" is also associated with abnormal sharpening of the sense of taste (*hypergeusia*), or whether right hemisphere damage
has lead to the enhancement of affective dimensions of hunger which
involves structures such as the hypothalamic nuclei, thalamic nuclei, and the
cingulate cortex in the left hemisphere. It has yet to be ascertained whether
these 'food-savants' begin to discern specific qualities of food that elude

other less savvy mortals rather than engage in ritualized compulsive food-seeking behavior. And what way are they different from normal stimulus-dependent obese people? How soon would they settle for the low quality ('unsatisfying') food items that otherwise would cause a dysphoric state akin to withdrawal when temporarily deprived of fine foods due to imposed hardships (e.g. traveling, incarceration, behavior-modification routine)? Do they change eating practices, driven by their newly discovered expertise? In short, are these individuals really finicky connoisseurs (gourmets) as opposed to gluttonous gourmands?

A Lesson of the Antiobesity Remedies

If the frontal cortex is involved in sustaining the normal flexibility of behavior by imposing volitional restrictions on cues selected by attention at each given moment, therapists or educators must realize that the loss of this flexibility may not necessarily be reinstated, as hoped,[6] just by providing nutritional guidance or a new set of coherent regulations. Thus far, the job of controlling the preoccupation or obsession with food said to characterize many dieters has required pharmacotherapy. That is not an easy task and never was. Even leeches have been tried to cure obesity (Fig. 4.2), but to no avail.

Operationally, the goal of treatment is to try to uncouple the pleasure of [over]eating from the gaining of a pouch of adipose tissue. This goal is deceptively simply since it has been attained in the realm of sexual behavior where 'recreational sex' is no longer threatened by the risk of procreation. Like contraceptives, an ideal antiobesity remedy should be full-proof, potent and show neither tolerance nor addictive potential. Given that obesity may be complicated by comorbidities, a perfect drug should also manifest no untoward interactions with other drugs used for other disorders. Finally, antiobesity drugs should be safe since obesity is handled as a chronic condition. Alas, a single drug with such characteristics does not exist.

Amphetamine-based anorexics with no undesirable side effects, which might help in a weight-reduction program, have yet to be designed. Williamson[43] shared with us an anecdote of his childhood experience: "In the summer of 1957," he summons up, "my pediatrician became so concerned about my weight that he convinced my mother that I should begin taking pills to curb my appetite. I was 7 years old and weighed 70 pounds with a goal of

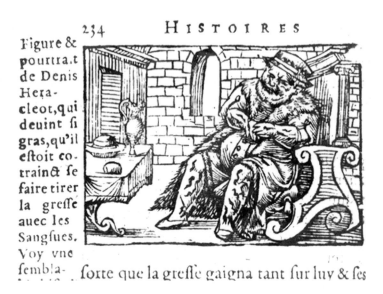

234   HISTOIRES

Figure &
pourtra.t
de Denis
Hera-
cleot,qui
deuint fi
gras,qu'il
eftoit co-
trainct fe
faire tirer
la greffe
auec les
Sangfues.
Voy vne
fembla-   forte que la greffe gaigna tant fur luy & fes

Fig. 4.2   This 16th century woodcut communicates some idea of the intense misery of an obese man (Denis Heracleot) who has placed many leeches on his arms and legs in an effort to reduce his weight. Pierre Boaistuau, *Histoires prodigiÈuses et memorables, extraictes de plusieurs fameux autheurs*, Grecs, & Latins. Pais 1598. Images from the History of Medicine, NLM (*http://wwwihm.nlm.nih.gov/ihm/images/A/29/360.jpg*).

reaching 60 pounds. I still remember how those pills made me feel; I had no appetite and felt chronically anxious. Most remarkable to me that summer was that my hands were always cold. I did not reach my target weight but the chronic anxiety continued and pills were stopped. I promptly regained all the weight that I had lost" (p. 278).

There are intriguing findings indicating that hypophagic effects in experimental animals require an increase of 5-HT at receptor sites. Such widely prescribed appetite suppressants as d-fenfluramine and its metabolite d-norfenfluramine cause hypophagia by acting at 5-HT and 5-HT$_{2C}$ receptors, respectively. Fluoxetine acts in a similar way, and in this regard differs from other antidepressants that cause weight gain in depressed patients. However, a combination of appetite suppressants, like phentermine and fenfluramine (phen-fen), has been associated with primary pulmonary hypertension and valvular heart disease. There are also reports of valvular disorders in persons taking fenfluramine or dexfenfluramine alone, especially when taken for more than three consecutive months. The mechanisms whereby these drugs caused valvular damage are poorly understood. Their side effects proved to be more deleterious than obesity. In mid-September of 1997, fenfluramine was removed from the market. By the time this decision was made, over 18 million people had already taken the drug.

The role of some brain monoamines and serotonin in the regulation of appetite is undeniable. Experimental studies in rats following experimental 5-HT depletion demonstrated their increased number of premature/anticipatory or impulsive responses, as well as a reduced capacity to work for larger but delayed rewards. The systemically administered D_1 receptor antagonist, SCH 23390, blocks this pattern of rash responding.[44] Serotonin (5-HT)-containing neurons make synaptic contacts with cells of the substantia nigra pars compacta (SN_c) and the substantia nigra pars reticulata (SN_r), so that serotonin deficit may reduce its inhibitory influence over dopamine neurotransmission thereby predisposing the animal to impulsiveness. The sympathetic activity and brain serotonin levels remain a major target in the search for a better understanding of obesity and the development of pharmacological paraphernalia for its treatment. Still, in view of their abysmal record thus far, drug interventions are commonly recommended in combination with diet and lifestyle changes so as to jumpstart the dieter's self-restraint. Given that much has already been tried with vanishingly small effect, an editorial in the *Annals of Internal Medicine* of January 2001 asked, "So what is to be done?" The answer was depressingly blunt: "Obesity is too big a problem to be left to the physicians." Who then should be in charge? The recommendation is predictably evasive:

"There is no simple solution to the problem of obesity. Dealing with it will require action at several levels: policy, education (or both the public and health care providers), and incorporating a team approach to patient care that involves dietitians and health educators" (p. 73).

Thus, we are told that we have a problem and propose a worn-out solution of 'science by committee' — to do what? Although health clinical psychologists were apparently not included in the team, unless they are disguised as health educators, they should not feel snubbed. It is not at all clear why this delegated responsibility assures any success or what this team mix would add to the obesity paradigm.

Molecular Jigsaw Puzzle

One of the reasons that pharmacotherapy of obesity was so ineffective might be explained by the fact that it is associated with multiple deficits in the cellular and molecular mechanisms of appetite control and energy homeostasis. There are several major peripheral players of the appetite regulation players. Most of them appear to be represented also on different levels of the telencephalon as part of the orexigenic or anorexigenic control system. Ghrelin is a recently described orexigenic hormone synthesized in the gastric epithelial cells and secreted into circulating blood. Its receptors (known as GHS-R) are expressed in peripheral organs as well as in the hypothalamus and pituitary gland. Ghrelin exerts powerful endocrine and non-endocrine activities and modulation of the endocrine and metabolic response to variations in energy balance. Its plasma levels are enhanced in fasting, hunger and anorexia, and reduced in obesity. 24-hour plasma ghrelin profiles in 13 obese subjects studied before and after a six-month dietary program for weight loss showed that plasma ghrelin levels rose sharply shortly before and fell soon after every meal.[45] The most radical treatment for morbid obesity, gastric-bypass surgery, seems to work by affecting plasma ghrelin levels. Not only does it reduce the amount of food ingested, but it also suppresses the appetite. Given that ghrelin is produced primarily by the stomach, Cummings[45] and his colleagues compared the 24-hour ghrelin profiles in five subjects who had lost weight after gastric bypass and ten normal-weight controls. Strikingly, the normal, meal-related fluctuations and diurnal rhythm of the ghrelin level were practically flattened after gastric bypass surgery, thereby suggesting that it might have contributed to the weight-reducing effect of the procedure. Ghrelin activates neurons in the arcuate nucleus of the hypothalamus that express neuropeptide Y (NPY), which is also widely distributed throughout the central nervous system, and agouti-related peptide (AGRP), as well as the orexins neuropeptides (also known as hypocretins). It is recognized that NPY along with corticotropin-releasing hormone exert a reciprocal regulation of responsiveness to stressful stimuli, possibly via an interaction of these two systems in the amygdala.

By contrast, Cholecystokinin is an example of those 'peripheral' satiety factors that apparently contribute to meal termination. Given intravenously prior to a test meal, it causes a significant reduction of meal size. Interestingly, cholecystokinin works better when the stomach is slightly distended by a preload.[46] Yet, cholecystokinin is increasingly recognized as an important 'top-down' signal that possibly communicates that food is not sufficiently rewarding, or associated with learned fears thereby precluding ingestion. It is implicated in attention and/or memory enhancement, anxiety-, panic- and stress-related behavior.

Hypocretins in the lateral hypothalamic and perifornical areas were shown to participate in the control of feeding. Yet, that is only part of their duties. Hypocretins are particularly interesting messengers because their neurons project throughout the central nervous system and have close anatomical connections with mesocorticolimbic dopaminergic neurons in the ventral tegmental area.[47] Ciriello and associates[48] identified two distinct clusters of neurons, one within the amygdaloid complex of the rat; another in the anterior lateral subnucleus of the bed nucleus of the stria terminalis and in an area just ventral to the lateral ventricle. The amygdala complex integrates stimuli of potential threats and thus is potentially implicated in overeating/anorexia following aversive stimuli, stress and anxiety. Injury to the amygdala has long been recognized to produce obesity. A common example of its role is the Klüver–Bucy syndrome following bilateral lesion of the amygdaloid nuclear complex in monkeys or surgical removal of the temporal lobes in man that are associated with bulimia, hypersexuality, and emotional placidity. The syndrome also includes compulsive exploration of environmental objects, dietary changes, and hyperorality. On the other hand, some 'stress-eaters' might also have a particular genetic liability of orexin circuitry that make them more responsive to specific contextual factors promoting food intake. It is recognized that some people are more sensitive than others to the variety/novelty of food-related stimuli, which may be described as something akin to 'the Coolidge effect' in the domain of feeding behavior.

Additionally, hypocretins may be intimately associated with many other aspects of wakefulness, motor activity, neuroendocrine homeostasis and autonomic regulation. Essentially, an organism may be 'programmed' by a redundant system of orexigenic networks of peptides to worry about potential danger of starvation and thus tend to grab-and-mouth regardless of how much energy was lost because the system was always in a higher energy expenditure ('hunting') mode.

That 'hunting mode' is paced by the circadian cycle or postprandial rest or sleep. Although drowsiness is a common experience following food ingestion, until very recently it was not known that satiety control and the mechanism of sleep regulation have a common neuronal territory. It appears though that a mysterious sleep disorder such as narcolepsy, characterized by cataplectic attacks of excessive daytime sleepiness, is associated with mutations in one of the hypocretin receptors, the hypocretin receptor 2 in the hypothalamus. The cerebrospinal fluid of narcoleptics shows no hypocretin. These findings are particularly exciting, because "a disease that not too long ago could find itself on the couch of psychoanalysis"[49] (p. 415) is now emerging onto the stage of the more common neurodegenerative diseases.[50] It is likely that hypocretin-containing neurons monitor the level of glucose. As mentioned above, under conditions of intermittent starvation and constant food shortage, a hypothetical paleolithic cave-dweller will hunt for fats and proteins, but perhaps more often being in a hypoglycemic state would settle for carbohydrates nibbling on ripe fruit and twigs. Metabolically, carbohydrates are not the same as fat, since a gram of the latter provides almost 9 kilocalories as compared to only 4 kilocalories per gram of the former. However, our cave-dweller was primed to seek carbohydrates and they do provide an instant reward, granting a short-term or between-meals effect to quench feelings of hunger, thereby signaling the need for terminated meal ingestion. The consumption of carbohydrates increases the production of insulin in order to keep blood sugars normal. A fall in glucose in the plasma inhibits its release.

Carbohydrates have some analgesic efficacy. Only 2 ml of oral sucrose was reported to reduce the duration of crying in newborn babies subjected to heel pricks or circumcision.[51] In the past, this effect was studied experimentally and ascribed to EEG synchronization caused by ingesting sweet liquid, designated as 'fragments of sleep' or as 'pleasure waves.'[52,]* Such a fast response to carbohydrates suggests that using sweeteners as appetite inhibitors is not at all irrational, albeit mostly for those who overeat because of a deficient short-term satiation feedback that maintains foraging ("orexigenic") cells in a hyperactive mode. Hunger for sweet rewards is also increased by a depressive mood, such as during premenstrual syndrome, mild depression, or seasonal affective disorder. Some sufferers of the latter more often report craving for carbohydrates and experience improvement in mood following carbohydrate-rich meals.

Searching for carbohydrates is thus a useful adaptation, and it might work perfectly well in early ontogeny. But organisms that live or die by predation

---

*Given that the activity of thalamo-cortical inhibitory circuits underlies the bursts of synchronous electrical activity in the posterior parietal cortex,[52] one might wonder whether the NPY/GABAergic mechanisms are also responsible for food reward or these EEG bursts are just a marker of an overall state of drive reduction consistent with unruffled ingestion.

and are constantly at the mercy of environmental hazards will evolve a life span commensurate with their particular environment. Let us assume that a cave dweller was born prematurely (Chap. 2), which makes her somewhat more resistant to insulin. Even with a nearly adequate load of glucose in her blood, she must have felt hungry. Since insulin is an important fat-building hormone of the body, extra insulin produced by the β-cells of the islets of Langerhans of the pancreas would add a little bit of fat to keep such children alive through the next food crisis. In turn, adiposity helps to promote insulin secretion. This is also an excellent adaptation because she would develop faster and would be able to procreate sooner. Insulin acts on this junction in tandem with ghrelin-pituitary connection by accelerating pubertal development. However, it has been shown that acute delivery of fatty acids to muscle results in insulin resistance. That sets in motion a potentially dangerous process. Studies in animals may underestimate the risks, because the time needed for the development of untoward effects may exceed the lifetime of the animal. Likewise, these processes were irrelevant to our remote ancestors since they made use of the benefits of adiposity but did not live long enough to harvest its drawbacks. If the cave-dweller in this scenario lived to a ripe old age, extra visceral adipose tissue would increase the level of neuropeptide resistin (a newly discovered hormone), raise insulin resistance and boost still greater insulin levels, thereby making her a bit more hungry and lethargic unless more food were consumed, and as a consequence more weight would be gained. The vicious circle thus established would ultimately lead to a depopulation of β-cells, uncontrolled blood sugar level, dyslipidemia, and systemic inflammation or what is known as full-scale type 2 diabetes. However, a primitive hunter's lifestyle necessitated sacrificing longevity for reproductive fitness. To conclude, this hypothetical example might point out that a sluggish insulin feedback to glucose ingestion would force one not only to eat more, but also to eat faster. There are many obese individuals among such fast eaters who clean up their dinner plates with embarrassing rapidity. These people might possibly reduce energy intake on a diet, in which the major meal is anticipated by a small starter, loaded with sucrose or low-calorie sweeteners.

Leptin, like resistin, is apparently the major circulating hormone secreted by fat cells. Its deficiency or defects in leptin receptors are associated with massive obesity similar to that produced by damage to the ventromedial or the paraventicular nucleus of the hypothalamus. In fact, metabolic effects of leptin are mediated through these medial hypothalamic centers. Discovered by

Jeffrey M. Friedman of the Rockefeller Universtiy at New York a decade ago, leptin is believed to be a crucial hormone in the regulation of body weight and energy homeostasis. However, unlike insulin that has a short plasma half-life of about 3 min, leptin has a half-life of about 45 min and provides a signal about the prospects of body fat stores. It has a two-prong action. One activates an appetite-suppressing ("anorexigenic") proopiomelanocortin (POMC) neuropeptide, with the adrenocorticotropic hormone (ACTH), α-melanocyte stimulating hormone (α-MSH), and β-endorphin polypeptide cleaved from that precursor. The other inhibits foraging ("orexigenic") neurons, producing appetite-stimulating neuropeptide (NPY and AGRP). Yet, it appears that obesity with high serum concentrations of leptin may exist without subsequent inhibition of food intake. Actually, the majority of humans with obesity are resistant to leptin. This is an interesting puzzle. Based on the evidence from baboons living in the wild, some authorities[53] suggested that during most of evolution serum leptin levels were much lower than those currently considered normal, and evolutionary pressures have not selected against levels that are commonly seen in Western society. This is another example, among many, that our supply system evolved at a time when men lived in uncertainty about the prospect of their next meal and so it is easily overwhelmed in the time of plenty. It also suggests that the leptin molecule does more than ensure the slow (long-term) feedback signal of weight gain. Leptin operates in a variety of reproductive processes in both animals and humans, acting as a primary pointer of puberty and as a permissive regulator of sexual maturation[53] that could interact in a complex way with food ingestion and the circadian cycle. Proposed physiological roles for leptin in pregnancy include the regulation fetal/placental angiogenesis, embryonic hematopoiesis, and hormone biosynthesis within the maternal-fetoplacental unit.[54] Leptin-treated prepubertal female mice reproduced at an earlier age than did non-medicated controls, indicating that leptin may help to trigger puberty.[55] Suggestively, peripheral leptin concentrations, adjusted for adiposity, are dramatically higher in females than in males throughout life.

In sum, our brains are no different from those of cave-dwellers who were eager to devour every extra bit of food. What evolved, however, are their inhibitory circuits, the ability to better handle delayed gratification and resist the temptations of appetite by cognitive effort. That means that we are expected *not* to overreact to oversized meals, tantalizing deserts, handsome packaging, creative commercials, and social vibes that collectively add to the long list of implicit reminders of food. So far, the major remedy in treating obesity is critically dependent on the volitional behaviors of dieters who need to impose self-restriction on food intake. This method is notorious for its inefficacy. Psychologically, restraint of motivated behaviors always involves a conflict between the desire to suppress an impulse and to execute a wanted behavior. And the craving is more often the winner. As the bank metaphor implies, our bodies zealously guard their fat deposits by a number of neuronal participants.* Yet, a review by Schwartz and associates[56] is still a useful guide to caution that "it is overly simplistic to reduce a behavior as complex as feeding to a series of molecular interactions."

Figure 4.3 implies that for the majority of the obese, an effort at losing weight focuses mostly on calorie restrictions, whereas the bypass of the stage of foraging (indicated by the dashed line) requires an added effort of hours of workout every week to maintain weight. Since we do not need to put our bodies into daily overdrive in a hunt for dinner, the only way to help in determined dieting is to start exercising — or else ...

Coda: Phenotypes of the 'Cookie Monsters'

A molecular description of each participant of the obesity machinery seems achievable in principle, but a complex model describing all of the metabolic, hypothalamic, pituitary and peripheral factors along with their direct and indirect short-term and long-term feedback loops, as well as interactions with intermediates in the casual pathway of appetite control system, is beyond our grasp. Therefore, although the new strides in describing the fundamental principles of obesity are gratifying, this molecular information will not be translated into a dream of health psychology — a drug for a specific person — any time soon. Obese people may look cosmetically similar, but morbid adiposity is probably comprised of a variety of somewhat dissimilar syndromes. Some could be caused by erroneous 'top-down' signals originating in higher brain centers that interact with the metabolic sensors in the hypothalamus; others are 'bottom-up' conditions that are determined by endocrine factors and receptors in the digestive tract mucosa, whose signals are then relayed into the brainstem and the hypothalamus. That is why an effort to prescribe a one-size-fits-all drug has failed thus far. The job of understanding this diversity should begin with identifying some basic phenotypes. This is an exciting area for applied psychology. A simple example is that of Schuman

---

*A review by Schwartz and associates,[56] which is still a useful guide to the ingestion-control system, cautions that "it is overly simplistic to reduce a behavior as complex as feeding to a series of molecular interactions."

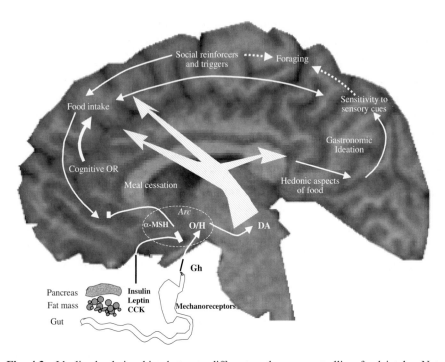

Fig. 4.3 Idealized relationships between different pathways controlling food intake. Note that the major emphasis in triggering food ingestion is given to the cognitive cues and sensitivity to environmental cues. Interrupted connections represent muscular efforts directed at obtaining food that are no longer required in civilized societies. Competing signals transmitted by the arcuate nucleus neurons, as well as the hypocretin terminals make sense of peripheral signals of energy deficiency as either the signals of hunger or satiation. The neocortical neurons presumably act to make these signals available to conscious experience, contribute incentives, cognitive appraisal and modulation of messages coming from the 'downstairs' sensors. A growing number of peptides and neurontransmitters are now being shown to be involved in the control of food intake and energy homeostasis along with the integration of behavior, learning, circadian rhythms, thermogenesis, pain modulation, and reproduction. Abbreviations: α-MSH — α-melanocyte stimulating hormone; CCK — cholecystokinin; DA — dopamine; Gh — ghrelin; OH — orexins/hypocretin. *Arc* — arcuate nucleus represented by inner ellipse. Note that the nucleus has two systems with opposite effects on food ingestion.

and colleagues,[57] who administered the Foods and Moods Inventory to a group of subjects with an identified interest in chocolate. It appeared that the tendency to eat compulsively and show enhanced appetite for sweets and chocolate, in particular, were significantly greater among women. Those who reported "self-medicating" with sweets or chocolate were more likely to have personality traits associated with hysteroid dysphoria, an atypical depressive syndrome, as compared to a comparison sample, and a sample of former alcoholics. Such uncontrollable movement of the cognitive processes in the direction of need satisfaction might be called autistic.[8]

Thus far, the term 'obesity phenotype' portrays a grossly overweight individual with hypotonia, small or missing teeth, genital hypoplasia, mental retardation, and cardiovascular disease (in different combinations) as seen in the Prader–Willi-type syndrome or Bardet–Biedl syndrome. The rationale for studying the latter as models of obesity is best defended by a dictum of Gamma in *Proofs and Refutations by Imre Lakatos*[58] cited above. Yet, however useful, their features do not define garden variety obesity when an uncertain genetic error is associated with mood changes, an enhanced search for novelty or pleasure-seeking behaviors, loss of restraint, and the persistence of hunger, disquietude, unease, and worry over an impending or anticipated illness, and many other features. Nor do they deal with impulsivity, deficient planning, self-deception and a low persistence in maintaining a new lifestyle. Only infrequently will this cognitive phenotype overlap with a psychiatric disorder (e.g. depression). It remains to be elucidated whether a unique action of neuropeptide Y as an endogenous anxiolytic, as suggested by the Koobs' group in La Jolla, may be associated with overeating in some individuals in clinical states of fear and anxiety. On the model of the Kleine–Levin syndrome, a unique disorder associated with spells of somnolence, hyperphagia and obesity, one might also think of the presence of some sort of hard-wired 'module' of sleep-ingestion drive that becomes pathologically activated despite the availability of food and sleep. However, food consumption is determined not only by demands on taste, smell or satiety, but is also decided by the penchant to socialize.

Food consumption is one of the easiest ways to construct the world populated by other people. The ritual is imposed on us since infancy and shapes our habits in later life. Overeating has long been observed to escalate in a group of other eaters. This contagious effect at a social event may be a part of environmental dependency syndrome. In sheep, early social experiences, social bonds (social cohesiveness) determine the choice of feeding location and the attraction for the preferred food. In groups smaller than four animals, sheep reduced their grazing time and did more aimless walking than sheep tested in larger groups. Ironically, for many humans, as in sheep, meals eating in company, either in positive or negative moods, appears to be a significant booster of meal sizes as compared to eating meals alone and in a neutral mood.[59] These phenotypes have yet to be dovetailed with molecular biology research that emphasizes other causes (e.g. inheritance, pre- and perinatal factors). It is hoped that in the future it will be possible to treat adults based on the characterization of a cluster of symptoms, their timing and severity and identification of syndrome-specific genes (e.g. those associated with mutations of the melanin-concentrating hormone, leptin feedback, orexin receptors, enterostatin, urocortin, insulin, etc.). For example, it would be interesting to explore whether a demand for immediate reward in some obese individuals may be associated with deficiencies in the central control of appetitive behaviors, such as reduced tolerance to delayed gratification. It is interesting that craving sweet foods and a shift of food preference toward sweet foods is *not* a noticeable feature in Alzheimer's and semantic dementias. However, it is overwhelmingly present in the fronto-temporal dementias. It remains to be established whether, or rather to what extent, the shift to a short term gratification in frontal patients is associated with the orbitobasal frontal lobe which is affected early in fronto-temporal dementias.

A pattern of rapid weight gain during the first four months of life in infants with low birthweight becomes a risk of overweight status at age 7 years.[60] It is conceivable that the action of N-methyl D-aspartate (NMDA) receptors, a subtype of the glutamate receptor, are crucial for inducing plastic changes that disrupt signaling mechanisms in the fetal hypothalamus or in some supra-hypothalamic sites, such as the amygdala and hippocampus thereby causing long-lasting changes in appetitive behavior. Scenarios inspired by Barker's fetal programming hypothesis (Chap. 2) portray the epidemic of obesity as adaptation of the fetus in response to influences that retard its growth. For many families, particularly those of immigrants as well as the low-income black population, a low birthweight child may suggest the need to encourage higher energy intakes. As the formerly impoverished families began their income ascent, children were encouraged to overeat, and then their energy intake was not matched by physical activity because they spent too much time watching TV shows. Some ate more ravenously and became more obese than others. One only wonders whether it is possible to identify susceptible infants before they actually develop obesity, and prevent its onset by administering the right genes to those at risk. That would certainly raise many important questions with regard to those who are 'environmentally overwhelmed.' Do those who show environmental dependency syndrome also have gene(s) for it? Are their actions predetermined? If that is the problem to fear, what can be done to help these individuals? Is the notion of environmental dependency syndrome in regard to obesity a tendency to medicalize (label as aberrant) a somewhat greater sensitivity to environmental incentives?

Some researchers are looking for inspiration in anorexia. Anorexia is no longer considered a case of resolute women over eagerly responding to cultural pressures to look trim in spite of the multitudes of environmental temptations. The fact that behavioral therapy fails more often than not to build on their 'resolution' speaks for something else. The appetite suppression effect could be thought of, rather mechanistically, as a result of a disproportionate response to appetite-suppressing stimuli. The same system of neuropeptides apparently plays a crucial role in determining 'behavioral anorexia phenotype' particularly its aspects such as hyperalertness, anxiety, enhanced locomotion, sensitivity to environmental stressors, and obsessiveness. Alternatively, an excessive sensitivity to fever-inducing cytokines or stress hormones could imaginably contribute to anorexia as well. Adipose tissue is capable of expressing and releasing a proinflammatory cytokine interleukin-6 that may be a warning sign within the feedback system controlling excessive accumulation of fat, somewhat akin to the signals from an inflamed bowel communicating to the brain to stop eating. If these signals are ignored by the hyposensitive central mechanisms in the obese, a heuristically promising way of producing a magic 'diet pill' could come via examining anorexia developing consequent to injury and/or infections.[61]

Assuming that multiple phenotypes of obesity are real and that multiple neurotransmitter disorders do exist, it is easy to understand why catecholaminergic drugs might affect only one network while serotonergic drugs modulate the other one and be irrelevant for many more. The system of appetite control conceived of in terms of monoaminergic neurotransmission, leaving outside histamine, GABA, the glutamatergic system and numerous peptides as therapeutic targets appears to be sadly inadequate. The pace of neurosciences is truly amazing. A more molecular description of what is wrong with each subset of a patient is promised by the success of the Human Genome Project. Such molecular diagnoses will be available to a practitioner along with more specific appetite-modulating agents in the not-too-distant future. Yet, even when these dream drugs are created, obese people will not be able to ingest high-energy food with impunity, hoping that new remedies would protect them from weight gain. For the majority of the obese in the industrialized West a struggle with the bulge will nonetheless require the onerous path of overcoming the self in the dining room and the gyms.

SO WHAT?

With the current epidemic of obesity there is an urgent need to identify those factors that are responsible so that appropriate interventions can be introduced.

The idea of environmental dependency as a determinant of obesity has been an essential initiative in neurosciences for more than 30 years. It has its roots in three areas: psychological, neuropsychiatric, and experimental. The neuropsychiatric experience is perhaps the most fundamental. It helps to refocus the view of obesity from 'traditional' environmental factors and lifestyle changes to those dominated by a more 'individual-centered' perspective in which different modes of causal attribution are thought to be appropriate.

This epistemological evolution was prepared by the notion of stimulus-bound behaviors, which introduced the idea of the environmental cause as secondary to the internal state of the organism.

The neuropsychology of obesity is yet to become part of today's agenda of obesity research. The neuropsychological profile is *that which determines appetitive behavior in a defined situation*. Regrettably, textbooks in psychology, physiology and neuropsychology discuss the themes of obesity, cognitive processes, and motivation (drives and drive reduction) in different places with no cross-referencing between them.

Although this section calls attention to the role of 'individual-centered' factors, it does not discount the possibility that low-income young adults might be more easily subverted by specific contextual and familial factors that are associated with an interest in foods.

In established obesity, the task of reversing metabolic machinery is intimidating. We still need to know how to target fat deposits by diet and exercise, so as to selectively mobilize specific fat depots (e.g. metabolically active visceral fat) and not to lose body protein. We also need to learn when weight reduction is a good idea for marginally overweight people in terms of health benefits.

A characterization of obesity, based on a cluster of symptoms, their timing and severity might hopefully lead to the identification of syndrome-specific molecular machinery, and allow the prediction of individual phenotypes that will respond to a particular therapy.

Our current insights do not lend themselves to personality-related treatment regimes, but as more weight-controlling genes are discovered and phenotype-genotype correlations are drawn, obesity therapy will be based on specific molecular findings. Using molecular biology to find new ways to maintain normal weight is slowly becoming a reality.

4b

Cognitive Decline:
Factors and Targets

The British have a way of honoring the elderly. Queen Elisabeth II sends congratulatory telegrams to those of her subjects who reach their one hundredth birthdays, a custom embraced by *NBC* morning shows in the US. Impressed by a dramatic rise in life expectancy in the world, Cyryl A. Clarke was curious about longevity on the British island. He asked the Queen's secretary to give him numerical details about Britain's centenarians. The reply confirmed his expectations; in 1955 the office sent 300 congratulations. In 1970 the number was 1,200 and by 1987 it reached an impressive 3,300.[1]

Life expectancy in the US also increased dramatically, from 47.2 years in 1900 to 67.2 years in 1954–1955. In 1980 it approached 73.3 years and kept rising. Internet releases of the U.S. Bureau of the Census and the National Center for Health Statistics *www.aoa.dhhs.gov/aoa/stats/profile/#older* indicate that in 1997, individuals 65 years of age and older represented 12.7% of the population, about one in every eight Americans (34.1 million). Compared to 1990, the number of old Americans increased by 2.8 million (9.1%). The ratio of women to men is 1.43 and increasing with age. The old population itself is getting older. In 1997, the 65–74 age-group (18.5 million) was eight times larger than in 1900, but the 75–84 group (11.7 million) was 16 times as large and the 85+ group (3.9 million) was 31 times as large. By 2030, people 65+ years of age are projected to represent 20% of the population. This will have numerous social implications. In their paper, 'The graying world: A challenge for the twenty-first century,' Alexander Kalache & Ingrid Keller[2] call the aging population a "silent revolution" that is likely to have a worldwide impact on all aspects of life. One of them is dementia. A decade ago, the dementias were upgraded in the fashion of the time to a silent epidemic. The number of individuals with severe cognitive impairment is likely to exceed 12 million. The number of patients with Alzheimer's disease is also projected to quadruple over the next 50 years. Assuming that life expectancy continues to climb as expected, aging and dementing disorders are feared to throw industrial nations into a severe economic and social crisis within just two decades.[3] The picture of the growth of dementias is difficult to fathom.

Neuropsychiatric Perspective on Alzheimer's Dementia

The term 'dementia' denotes a severe impairment of mental functions. It apparently originated from a slangy invective, which is still evident in the French word, *un dementi* or the Italian *mentita* for a tendency to lie or a contradiction of judgment. Unreliable behavior, the inability to plan and untrustworthiness were considered grave social stigmas in 'suave society.' For years, dementia has eluded precise definition and characterization in terms of the margins where social or cognitive deficit and functional loss signal the presence of a disorder.

The focus of this chapter is neuropsychiatric impairment associated with Alzheimer's disease. The latter is the major representative of dementing disorders. Only recently was it flippantly dismissed as a medical obscurity. In the chapter devoted to 'mythical maladies of the nervous system,' a no lesser neuropsychiatrist than Macdonald Critchley[4] lamented that there are

Critchley conceded, however, that this duo — though not quite mythological — is nonetheless "somewhat in the way of rarities." It is recognized now that Alzheimer's disease is the forth cause of death in the US, afflicting some 7–10% of individuals aged 65 years and over. When the diagnostic pointers converge on dementia, the likelihood is that in over 50% of cases it will be dementia of the Alzheimer's type (DAT).[5]

"diagnostic labels for some clinical disorders where no pathological evidence is forthcoming. Two such examples are Alzheimer's disease and Jakob–Creutzfeldt syndrome. These mellifluous labels have rather belatedly become fashionable tags to attach to puzzling cases in the clinic."

An elderly person exhibiting forgetfulness and even more so with a gradually progressing mild cognitive deficit is a suspect for DAT. Of course, this characterization is somewhat narrow. It alludes to memory "decline" along a continuum in a monitored or self-monitored process. Individuals with a mild memory loss may, indeed, feel compelled to be examined by a doctor. Amusingly, such self-referrals often have higher IQ with no evidence of a significant decline in memory when tested. After all, it is acceptable, as the famous French epigrammatist and moralist François La Rochefoucauld (1613–1680) noticed centuries ago, to complain about bad memory but never about poor judgment. It is poor judgment that matters. Ironically, as cognitive impairment creeps in and when poor insight becomes evident to everybody, an individual might become oblivious to his weakness since *anosognosia* might cut into the syndrome. It is in this narrow territory of mild cognitive impairment that neuropsychology must be very useful by refining its prognostic instruments.

Several decades ago, 'dementia' was an umbrella term indiscriminately applied to a number of overlapping syndromes of dissimilar origin. Today, it refers to a condition characterized by a *progressive* cognitive impairment (deficiency of learning and judgment, poverty of language, poor visuomotor skills, and the failure to attend to environmental cues or to divide attention). It is a gradual loss of memory that leads to and signals a complete depletion of intellectual resources, feelings, social strategies, and passions. As the ancient Greek tradition has it, Zeus, the chief philanderer of the Olympic pantheon was so taken by Mnemosyne, the goddess of memory, that he visited her quite a few times. After each encounter she had born him a daughter. Nine of her daughters, known as Muses, were believed to control all initiatives, innovations, resourcefulness, as well as abnormalities associated with imagery, creation and cognition. With them, Mnemosyne became an influential goddess who would not be scorned. Not surprisingly, this memory decline provides a convincing alibi for many aberrant aspects of social life, as well as spiritual and intellectual depletion. Thus, although memory decline is the first complaint heralding the possibility of an impending cognitive poverty, a thorough testing usually reveals that the patients may have numerous psychopathological aberrations, other than poor memory. They may not attend to a question and are often completely lost outside of dyadic contact. Their responses may thus seem incongruous and silly. The ring of the derogatory word 'absurd,' which was initially used to characterize someone who was more than just a bit hard of hearing (*ab-* + *surdus* deaf, stupid), gives away its origins. It has long since been evident that the most frequent type of paranoid psychosis is that observed in *deaf people.*

Psychopathology may emerge in the context of any neurologic condition that disrupts limbic or frontal structures. They are often encountered in patients with DAT. Among behavioral aberrations experienced by the majority of demented patients are: growing apathy, delusions, hallucinations, and depression punctuated by agitation, irritability, infrequently with physical and verbal aggression. Occasionally, dementia begins as general anxiety or disguised as panic disorder and phobias. The presence of these symptoms yields an unfavorable prognosis, particularly in terms of the quality of life of caregivers, and increase of direct and indirect costs. DAT patients are frequently disoriented. The tendency to wander and get lost in a familiar environment occurs in patients with all levels of cognitive impairment. There is a rising tide of cases in which disoriented seniors get taken into custody after they stray from their homes or caretakers. A subset of DAT patients can certainly have deficient visuospatial orientation. Posterior cortical atrophy might possibly herald slowly progressive dementia with cognitive and perceptual deficits suggestive of DAT.[6,7] Recently, Gainotti's group[8] reported that patients with DAT were impaired in performing both visuospatial memory tests and delayed recognition of Rey's Auditory Verbal Learning Test. Finally, in a subset of patients, the picture of cognitive deterioration could be complicated by an asymmetrical decline of the brain.[9] There may be a need in the future to examine visuospatial attention within the context of genetic analysis. According to some studies, even healthy middle-aged adult ApoE ε4 carriers show deficits in spatial attention, particularly shifting spatial attention following invalid location cues and adjusting the spatial scale of attention during visual search, that are qualitatively similar to those seen in clinically diagnosed DAT patients.[10] That study, however, brings to light an important question that we may confront in the future: how many genes would it take to 'pull together' and run a function, such as visuospatial attention?

The word 'disorientation' is a colloquial term for the state of bewilderment, confusion, perplexity, puzzlement, and lack of understanding. Such recurrent episodes of getting lost might well be associated with ictal events or postictal confusional states and transient epileptic amnesia,[11] inasmuch as impaired visual-perceptual deficits and spatial disorientation may be present in the absence of a parallel significant impairment of episodic memory. Outside of the intellectual/emotional connotation of the word, the term 'orientation' is defined as one's ability to choose a course in space with regard to the relevant environmental reference system as well as private reference ('internal maps'). This definition implies the loss of 'geographic orientation' (*extrapersonal space maps*) or the loss of the ability to match the environmental cues to the person's representation of the selected course, monitoring its changes and updating of the internal maps (*egocentric spatial ability*). Yet, a geographic map is relevant only when a personal and an extrapersonal *functional map* is competently spread over the surface of a regular topographical map (that of a neighborhood, town or a shopping mall). It has yet to be tested whether a failure to arrange the hierarchy of goals using the functional map or the loss of their subjective importance gradient might also cause spatial disorientation. The latter may also include time cognition, since it answers the question of "when" such goal-search is relevant.

Anybody who has closely observed geriatric patients, even if informally when they are one's parents, family members or friends, might admit that initially they are capable of disguising their helplessness by nodding and laughing when everyone else did, but soon they convey an impression as though they are deeply immersed in thoughts from which they are occasionally distracted. This may not be all that abnormal and may hint at a different source of 'disorientation.'*

Impostors of Alzheimer's Dementia

Ever since Alzheimer's discovery, the neuropathological hallmarks of dementia are recognized as extracellular neuritic plaques and intracellular neurofibrillary tangles. These 'holy grails' of dementia are beyond the resolution of *in vivo* structural imaging modalities. Consequently, the diagnosis of DAT is entertained assuming that other causes of cognitive decline (e.g. space occupying brain lesions, encephalopathy, drug addiction, chronic infection or stroke) are ruled out. That may not be a simple feat due to a group of dementing disorders that could be defined as 'DAT impostors.' For example, visuospatial impairment can be also encountered in late-onset Parkinson's disease. When combined with

---

*An anecdote, likely apocryphal, but nonetheless relevant for the present theme, was related by Keith Devlin in his book *The Math Gene*. As the story goes, Norbert Wiener, one of the great minds of the 20th century, and his family moved into a different house, and his wife reminded him in the evening to keep in mind that he has to return from the office to their new house, not the old one. To make sure that he has an extra reminder, she even handed him a slip of paper with their new address. Alas, he found himself walking to his old house and began frantically exploring his pockets for the slip of paper with his new address. There were many other slips of paper albeit with mathematical scribbles, but not a trace of the required

verbal memory decline, gait instability, and bradykinesia, the syndrome becomes difficult to tell apart from DAT, in the absence of biological markers of the disorder. Paraphrasing Slater[12] of 1943, dementias are diagnosed by making qualitative differences in intelligence and for the most part disregarding quantitative differences in psychopathology. "The time will come," he foresaw, "when attack will have to be made along both these lines." A brief sampler of the 'impostors' is given below. It can be supplemented by an excellent summary by Jeffrey L. Cummings,[13] which is still relevant regardless of its age.

Dementia with Lewy Bodies

The hallmark pathological finding of this disorder is the presence of intracytoplasmic aggregates of α-synuclein and other proteins in limbic or cortical areas, i.e. 'Lewy bodies.' Its features include early-onset, persistent, well-formed, visual hallucinations, the spectrum of motor features reminiscent of Parkinson's disease, as well as excessive morbidity and mortality. The syndrome is the second most common type of dementia.[5]

Vascular Disorders

Cerebrovascular disorders which share some risk factors (e.g. hyperhomocysteinemia is a risk factor for atherosclerotic disease; aging; menopause; and a low plasma level of vitamin cofactors, such as folate, vitamin B6, and B12) are common impersonators of DAT. Clinically, they show blunted affect, depression, emotional withdrawal, and low motivation punctuated by periods of irritability and anxiety. Actually, 'vascular dementia' itself is a disorder of variable etiology (multi-infarct dementia, lacunar dementia, Binswanger's subcortical encephalopathy, cerebral amyloid angiopathy, white matter lesions associated with dementias, single infarct dementia, dementia linked to hypoperfusion and hemorrhagic dementia). The risk of vascular dementias is correlated with the epidemiological risk of stroke (hypertension, hyperlipidemias and diabetes). Dementias may also arise consequent to hypoperfusion following cardiac dysrhythmias and pump failure.[14] The rates of vascular

---

one. Just then he noticed a child sitting on the porch of his old home. "Little girl," he asked, "Do you know where the people that used to live here have gone?" The girl looked at him and smiled. "Yes, Daddy, of course I do. Mommy said you would go to the wrong home and would lose the address, so she sent me to fetch you." This amusing case of an absent-minded mathematical genius portrays the daily exasperation of caregivers of demented patients. More about it will be mentioned in a later section on prospective memory.

dementia vary from 10 to 50% of all dementia cases. As the average age of the population increases, the prevalence of cerebrovascular disease also promises to rise. Old black people are considered to be at higher risk of vascular dementia, and manifest more severe white matter lesions, as compared with whites.[15] There is considerable public interest in vascular factors, because DAT may entail important potentially controllable pathophysiological processes that are implicated in vascular dementia (hypertension, deficient blood-brain barrier, accelerated cognitive aging, and type 2 diabetes).

Pick's Dementia

Pick's dementia, named after Arnold Pick (1851–1924) in the 20s, was often confused with DAT. The term 'Pick–Alzheimer disease,' which is no longer in use, is a reflection of this earlier confusion. It accounts for about 5% of all dementias. Pick's disorder usually begins with changes of character and social conduct, and lack of self-restraint, followed by diminished drive and apathy reminiscent of dementia of the frontal lobe type. In fact, it was described first in a 71-year-old man with advanced shrinkage of the frontal cortex on autopsy. Microscopically, the picture is dominated by the presence of 'swollen neurons' with displaced nuclei (Pick's cells). Although memory deficit in Pick's dementia may be absent at the stage of florid changes of behavior and drive, clinically the two disorders are often difficult to tell apart.

Frontotemporal Dementia

Some dementia syndromes are easily diagnosed, at least in retrospect. A good example is dementia dialytica, which was described elsewhere in the context of metabolic encephalopathies.[16] Other dementias are real imposters and their signs and symptoms can be easily found in DAT. Fronto-temporal dementia (FTD) is such a syndrome that blends seamlessly with Pick's dementia. It is an insidious disorder with early loss of insight, decline in social and interpersonal conduct, social misconduct, mood changes and emotional blunting, self-neglect, language production deficits, and a lack of insight followed by apathy and stereotypies, but relative sparing of episodic memory and visuo-spatial functions. All said, this makes FTD a syndrome of significant change from premorbid social functioning and altered personality. Also, in distinction from DAT patients, who are more likely to relinquish their religious habits if they had them, FTD patients often exhibit hyperreligiosity.

Another interesting feature of a subset of patients with FTD is their enhanced interest in food and greater appetite. DAT patients, by contrast, do not overeat. If anything, they are more anorexic than insatiable. DAT is one of the leading causes of a dysregulation of food intake (dysorexia) leading to weight loss in the elderly. Unlike DAT, fronto-temporal dementia is considered to be an asymmetrical brain disease.[17] It would be interesting to explore whether the extreme interest in food in FTD is associated with unmitigated responsiveness to environmental cues by the right hemisphere, akin to the environmental dependency syndrome discussed elsewhere (see also Chap. 4a).*

Diogenes Dementia

Diogenes syndrome is a condition characterized by extreme self-neglect, leading to abysmal living conditions, syllogomania (a tendency to hoard rubbish), lack of shame, refusal of aid, and social withdrawal.[18] In German, Spanish, and British literature, the syndrome appears under the name of 'social breakdown of the elderly.' Often it is considered a variant of FTD, even though the unity of the syndromes is uncertain. This geriatric curiosity with an estimated annual incidence of 5/10,000 of the population over 60 years of age is hardly the implementation of the teaching of Diogenes (412–323 BC), a cynic Greek philosopher, who advocated the principle of self-sufficiency and disregard of material possessions as the major principles in achieving happiness. Socrates, too, was disheveled and barefoot but his name was not associated with the syndrome. Even better still, would be to immortalize fictitious 'Uncle George,' who according to Paul Meehl, used to store uneaten pancakes in the attic. What justifies, of course, the name of Diogenes is the fact that these patients represent a population that might have had successful professional careers, higher than average intelligence and good family backgrounds. There is a possibility that Diogenes dementia is an endpoint of individuals with premorbid personality traits that include unfriendliness, secretiveness, obstinacy, eccentricity, independence and detachment.

Dementia Diabetica

Diabetes is recognized to be associated with cognitive deficits and an increased risk of dementia, particularly in the elderly. In 1997, The Expert Committee on

---

*As this volume was concluded, *Annals of Neurology* devoted its supplement to Frontotemporal Dementia and featured a Pick's Disease Conference Proceedings, which certainly are desirable updates on the problem.

the Diagnosis and Classification of Diabetes Mellitus subdivided diabetes into two major categories. The most common forms are type 1 diabetes, characterized by an immune-mediated destruction of pancreatic β-cells, leading to insulin deficiency, and type 2 diabetes, characterized by insulin resistance and relative (rather than absolute) insulin deficiency. The aging brain is possibly more sensitive to the effects of hyperinsulinemia. Gispen and Biessels[19] marshaled a number of pathogenic processes associated with diabetes and diabetic complications that are also implicated in brain aging and an increased risk of dementia, such as oxidative stress and vascular dysfunction, amyloid deposition, and an impairment of neuronal Ca^{2+} homeostasis.

Prion Dementia

Prion dementia is an outcome of some infectious and hereditary disorders. A typical representative is Creutzfeldt–Jakob Syndrome (CJS), which is associated with infection. Other than CJS syndrome this group may be expanded by other infection-related dementias, such as AIDS dementia, neurosyphilis, viral encephalitis, chronic meningitis and others.

CJS is a progressive mental deterioration similar to DAT. In its prodromal stage it may manifest sleep disturbances and dysautonomia. Some rare cases of fatal familial insomnia resemble sporadic CDJ. Unlike DAT, CJS' progress is rapid, and it invariably manifests neurological signs (visual, vestibular, cerebellar and extrapyramidal). Vertigo, diplopia, or blurred vision may be the first sign of impending danger. Yet, DAT and CJS are often impossible to tell apart based on clinical findings alone. CJS peaks between the ages of 55 and 75 years, but may debut in young people. There are three categories of CJS: familial, sporadic (the main form) and iatrogenic (e.g. in recipients of contaminated human growth hormone or blood transfusion from presymptomatic CJS patients). It was first identified in 1921 as an infrequent syndrome (1 per million). However, its prevalence varies from country to country, and there are fears that its incidence has increased among the young.

Parkinson's Dementia

At least 20–25% of DAT patients manifest extrapyramidal symptoms (slowness of movements, resting tremor, bradykinesia, rigidity, and impaired postural reflexes) along with concomitant brain lesions that complicate the diagnosis. Histopathological changes typical of DAT are present in at least a third of patients with Parkinson's disease (PD). Like other extrapyramidal disorders (Huntington's disease, Wilson's disease, progressive supranuclear palsy, idiopathic basal ganglia calcifications and others), PD may exhibit cognitive decline and even outright dementia. Its rates vary widely from 15–20% to over 70% of PD patients. Thus, dementia hardly belongs to the category of the secondary manifestations of PD. Its signs can be readily detected on formal neuropsychological testing in those with right-sided motor abnormalities (left-hemisphere Parkinsonism), rigidity and bradykinesia, rather than in those with tremor. Demented patients have difficulties forming intentions ('self-generated programs') and enlisting motor acts when such intentions are present. They manifest loss of scheme of action; reduced speed of cognitive performance; deficient self-initiated planning, and slowed initial steps of cognitive action. When the behavior of patients is triggered by external cues, their attention functions appear normal, but when they depend upon internally generated cues, they turn out to be deficient.[20] Thus, there is a considerable overlap between DAT and PD dementia.

The most common complication of PD that masquerades as dementia is depression, encountered in as many as 40–50% of patients. Depression in PD is atypical and usually does not involve ideas of worthlessness and suicidal thoughts. A denial of depression is attributable to a profound dopamine deficit of the right hemisphere,[21] as well as the disruption of prosodic competence.[22] Curiously, a significant number of PD patients who have objective evidence of swallowing problems are seldom concerned about their disturbing difficulties,[23] which can be interpreted as a sign of indifference. The histological hallmark of PD is the presence of abnormal neuronal inclusions, Lewy bodies in the substantia nigra.

Medication-Induced Dementias (Tardive Dysmentia)

Wilson and co-authors[24] have suggested that the pattern of approach behavior, coupled with edginess and excessive affect, represent a new, neuroleptic-induced syndrome which they called "tardive dysmentia." In typical cases, tardive dysmentia consists of a triad of symptoms: excessive episodic emotional reactivity, enhanced consumption of environmental stimuli, and indifference to or reduced awareness of abnormal involuntary movements.[25] Strikingly, tardive dysmentia patients may often be found trailing behind doctors or nurses with a number of somatic complaints, yet completely oblivious to their grotesque motor disturbances. Such *anosognosia* is ubiquitous in the elderly but may also be easily seen among younger, cognitively unimpaired dyskinetic patients.

Brain Imaging and DAT

A definition of dementia as a chronic progressive condition characterized by reduced mass of neuronal tissue and its neuropathological deterioration allows in-principle recognition of disease before cognitive decline results. Magnetic resonance imaging (MRI) is one of the most expensive diagnostic tests in neuropsychiatry that was hoped to add the rapidity and reliability to *in vivo* DAT diagnosis, particularly vis-à-vis cerebrovascular diseases and DAT impostures. However, even the signs of MRI white matter abnormalities (such as foci of high signal intensity on T2-weighted images) that initially were taken for granted as authentic markers of vascular lesion proved to be quite common among the asymptomatic elderly.

The literature is replete with findings of associations between cognitive decline and a varying degree of atrophy of the hippocampus and amygdala, ventricular dilation, enlarged spaces occupied by the cerebrospinal fluid, and white matter lesions described using MRI, but these markers were shared to a different extent by all dementing disorders. In individual cases, the measurements of brain structures are commonly undertaken in the context of comorbidities so that their changes may not discriminate among the causes. It was also expected that structural changes in diverse anatomical locations would permit one to relate to specific syndromes of DAT. Yet disappointingly, MRI studies share with autopsy the inability to establish whether or not individuals with early pathological changes who were symptom-free before death would have developed DAT, and if they would "convert" — when. In short, morphological brain scans are unhelpful in geriatric psychiatry outside specific "rule-out" diagnostic goals. Gratifyingly, a volumetric analysis of brain anatomy is among the best diagnostic accomplishments of MRI in that it allowed one to see significant group differences, such as the presence of somewhat greater atrophy on the left side, particularly in the temporal lobes in patients with FTD as compared to more symmetrically atrophied brains with DAT.[17] Such selectivity of anatomical impairment might be useful in differentiating corticobasal ganglionic degeneration or dementia with Lewy bodies that are often characterized by asymmetric motor and cognitive manifestations, as well as imbalanced MRI findings. However, like other DAT studies that convincingly demonstrated group differences between demented patients and age-matched controls, they were of very little help to a practicing neuroradiologist examining a single patient.

Perhaps, the rapid improvements in functional modalities of brain imaging could restrict the need for the painstaking processing of unrevealing structural brain images. Among them, particularly attractive are positron emission tomography (PET), single-photon emission tomography (SPET), and *in vivo* proton Magnetic Resonance Spectroscopy (^{1}H MRS). In the future, PET images will permit us to visualize the characteristic markers of DAT in living patients and follow up their dynamics under treatment. Images derived from PET and SPET provide useful functional information that spurred DAT research. The caveat is that activity within neuronal ensembles is not necessarily synonymous with their 'competence' or degree of dysfunction and may not prove either a decline or a greater activity of those regions in function maintenance. Resource depletion in such circuits can show up as increased signal intensity at baseline or during cognitive tasks in presumably compromised areas. In addition, the reading of data acquired with these imaging modalities is compromised by relatively low spatial resolution and variable anatomical specificity. Although the interpretation process can be enhanced considerably by co-localization techniques, this remains a costly option with a limited diagnostic yield.

MRS allows for the noninvasive study of cerebral biochemistry. It has been used to investigate cerebral metabolic changes associated with mental illness and represents one such modality that shows potential to distinguish between probable DAT and normal aging. One of its widely used markers is *N*-acetylaspartate (NAA) that is singled out as an indicator of neuro-axonal integrity and neuronal metabolism since it is present at high concentration only in living neurons and is virtually negligible in glial cells. It thus is expected to mirror the time course of grey matter atrophy. Indeed, NAA was confirmed in a number of studies to decline primarily in medial temporal lobe and parietal lobe gray matter. It is of interest that the left hippocampus showed consistently larger differences between patients with DAT and controls, and in addition showed larger changes over one year than did the right hippocampus.[26] Recently, it has become possible to measure glutamatergic markers (as glutamate + glutamine) that are particularly significant in view of the increasing attention to the role of glutamate release and oxidative stress in dementing brain disorders. Glutamate appears to be reduced in DAT,[27] meaning that a loss of neurons is paralleled by a decrease in glutamate + glutamine in gray matter cells, and that cellular death may be associated with the state of excessive activation of glutamate receptors (e.g. epileptiform activity due to deficient regulation of endogenous antagonist of NMDA receptor (Mg^{2+})?). By contrast, in the epileptogenic human hippocampus resected at surgery, the cellular glutamate content was increased to above-normal levels with no significant relationship to the degree of neuronal loss (neuron losses could reach 30–50% in epileptogenic hippocampi with normal appearance by clinical MRI criteria).[28]

Alzheimer's Disease: What is in the Name?

Although it might be possible to tell the various forms of DAT imposture apart, their clinical similarities are considerable. They include commonalties of clinical and neuropsychological profiles, as well as electrophysiology, cellular, and neuropathological phenotypes. In a number of cases a differential diagnosis of dementias on clinical criteria may be confusing. The spectrum of molecular risk factors for cognitive decline strongly suggests that there may be a variety of related or overlapping dementing disorders, which share defective genes and pathogenetic mechanisms. There are numerous indications that the day is coming when these phenotypes will have to be named after specific genetic causes or relevant pathophysiological events *before* they all converge on a final picture of devastating cognitive discoloration with blurred clinical borders.

In the meantime, like all taxonomies, that of the dementias is a linguistic quagmire. Terms are added through historical periods; new names are supplemented on the same chronological skillet when knowledge and judgments change. Some names are a part of *eponymania* of the past that gave credit to observant neuropathologists and psychiatrists (Alzheimer's, Parkinson's or Pick's dementia); others point to the presumed anatomical locus of the disorder (Frontotemporal dementia), the associated metabolic deficit (Dementia diabetica), the leading neuropathological condition (Vascular dementia), its timing with regard to medication (Tardive dysmentia), and neuropsychological profile (Semantic dementia). Still other labels emphasize etiology (Prion dementia), triggering iatrogenic procedure (Tardive dysmentia, Dementia dialytica), whimsically allude to a metaphor (Diogenes dementia) or give a precise histopathological 'address' (Lewy body dementia), which may actually be shared with various other referrals, and a recently recognized member of the group, named FXTAS (fragile X-associated tremor/ataxia syndrome), a disease associated with tremors, balance problems, short-term memory loss and anxiety.

These labels are nothing but convenient abstractions. When juxtaposed in terms of their onset, progression, and the emerging phenotype, they may not indicate whether or not, or to what extent the 'imposture' conditions, described above, share gross neuropathological and histopathological patterns, etiology, genetic liability and course. On inception, there is no reliable diagnostic test or biomarker of these disorders. The molecular profile of FTD may overlap with Parkinson's dementia owing to a mutant *tau* gene on chromosome 17 (ftdp-17). With a departure from inadequate localistic and eponymic nosology it may thus earn the name of *taupathy*. Yet, the neurofibrillary tangle composed of tau protein that becomes aggregated is also found in DAT. In fact, Trey Sunderland's[29] group at the National Institute of Mental Health provided by far the strongest weight to an emerging consensus that a 'tandem' of tau and $A\beta_{1-42}$ levels in the cerebrospinal fluid (CSF) is needed as a biological DAT marker. In their cross-sectional study (in 131 DAT patients and 72 controls) placed in the context of meta-analysis of 17 studies that provided an additional group of 3,133 DAT patients and 1,481 controls, the presence of a significant decrease in $A\beta_{1-42}$ peptide along with an increase in CSF tau levels was shown.

Interestingly, there is a subset of patients with symmetric frontal and temporal atrophy[30] who appear younger at disease onset and show greater overall atrophy. Two of the three such patients reported in the cited study appear to be ApoE $\varepsilon4$ carriers, suggesting that FTD is a heterogeneous condition overlapping with risk factors for DAT. The area is in a flux; a fact that lends support to the view that in the future when reliable biological markers are delineated, some syndromes might be either united into a single construct, or fragmented into different disorders. Recent efforts to define the nature of neurodegenerative diseases at the molecular level suggest that several syndromes might not stem from mutations within the active domain of the proteins, but rather from mutations that disrupt their three-dimensional conformation. These diseases are as diverse as DAT, Creutzfeldt–Jacob disease and diabetes and may be designated as 'amyloid diseases,' 'protein aggregate disorders,' or 'conformational diseases.'[31]

By the same token, some DAT syndromes with epilepsy might be attributed to the latent channelopathies (e.g. mutations in genes encoding ion channel proteins) (see also Chap. 3). Suggestively, the genetic locus for DAT,

Down's syndrome and the Unverricht-Lundborg type of progressive myoclonus has been mapped to the same human chromosome 21. In the broad picture of complex inheritance in DAT and given our current knowledge of its disparate phenotypes, it is important to explore the role of ion-channel genes. Thus far, ion channel mutations are a common cause of rare monogenic idiopathic epilepsies, but not of common epilepsies. For example, autosomal dominant juvenile myoclonic epilepsy was demonstrated to be a channelopathy associated with a $GABA_A$ receptor-α 1 subunit mutation.[32] It is conceivable, however, that similar ion channel defects underlie the common idiopathic generalized epilepsies with complex inheritance more frequent than currently acknowledged as well as late-onset epileptiform abnormalities due to immune, iatrogenic, and toxic mechanisms that are designated as multifactorial. The notion of a multifactorial cause implies the expectations that DAT proximity estimation based on the person's history from conception and one's genetic, neuropsychological, biochemical, physiological and endocrine profiles, along with MRI data, would result in the future in a comprehensive 'index of risk.' In reality, the emphasis on this interconnectivity obfuscates the few proximal causes of DAT and nutures impractical hopes that collecting more peripheral factors for such a synthetic pointer would provide a reliable and inexpensive magic estimate on which a physician would advise on treatment intervention and lifestyle modifications (see Chap. 7 for a discussion).*

It has long been known that structures such as entorhinal cortex continue to develop postnatally thereby suggesting that the time window for DAT 'programming' by responding to hormonal changes, viral infections, and early traumas stretches into several years of postnatal development. One might imagine that a more selective early attrition of NMDA receptors located on GABAergic interneurons would add a syndrome of psychopathology to memory decline when DAT would début as aggressive behavior or delusional syndrome. Collectively, this evidence suggests that the classification of disorders by clinical phenotypes is inadequate. Until a new taxonomy of

---

*The word 'multifactorial' is a euphemism for causes we trust very little and even less about how to rank them. Let us assume that of all factors in Fig. 4.4 only four are implicit in a response to a change in a redundantly controlled system of brain plasticity and vascular permeability. By accepting this assumption one would also agree that each factor in itself is either genetically controlled or environmentally dependent. By reducing these secondary factors to the minimal two would yield us a staggering 1,024 combinations between genetic and environmental variables (i.e. $2^2 \times 2^2 \times 2^2 \times 2^2$). Clearly, this is a mammoth amount of data to consider for a usable index of diagnostic utility.

dementias is available, all markers and paths outlined above would be treated as the equivalent indicators of impending functional decline of cognitive processes. Although clinical descriptions based on common symptoms or inclusion criteria ('group portraits') seemed satisfactory in the past for pharmacotherapy, they make no sense in a search for more specific phenotypic features of disorders caused by mutations of genes and even more so in proteomics, and 'proteotype-phenotype' correlations. Even skeptics who have a bone to pick with health psychology over its role in geriatric psychiatry would agree that psychologists would be uniquely useful in future attempts at splitting DAT into clinical subgroups.

Epileptogenicity Perspective on DAT: 'Out of the Shadows'

Alzheimer's disease is a known risk factor for seizures even though frank epileptiform syndrome in DAT is infrequent, at least not before dementia is quite advanced, when between 5 and 10% of patients seemingly have seizures.[33] However, episodes of nonconvulsive *status epilepticus* may often present as a recurrent state of confusion when repeated EEG examinations may be needed so as not to miss the episodes. By contrast, epilepsy is comorbid in Down's syndrome associated with DAT.[34,35] Of 191 adults with Down's syndrome, one study[34] recorded epilepsy with a prevalence of 9.4%. This value may possibly represent an unmasked epileptogenicity owing to improved longevity rather than a rise in the number of new cases since life expectancy in Down's syndrome patients has markedly increased in recent decades. Indeed, by the age of 50 and over, rates of epilepsy increased to 46%, and would be considered even more prevalent if diagnosed exclusively on the basis of EEG records (background slowing, bursts of generalized spike-waves or polyspike-wave discharges occasionally associated with myoclonic jerks). Epileptiform activity may also be spurred by a higher rate of vascular pathology in some groups.[36]

Epilepsy is often defined as impaired voltage sensitive Na^+, K^+, and Ca^{2+} channel functioning. Its other pathophysiological components are deficient inhibition (e.g. dysregulation of the GABA chloride ion channel or the shortage of GABA in the synaptic cleft) and excessive excitatory neurotransmission. These mechanisms are overlapping with those that set in motion a course of events leading to neuronal damage, cell death, and cognitive impairment. Not surprisingly and commensurate with cognitive decline in DAT, brain imaging studies have described the landscape of glucose *hypometabolism*, particularly in the posterior association cortex.[37–39] Another recent study,[40] reexamined hippocampal atrophy and posterior cortex hypometabolism controlling for disease severity in a sample of 11 patients with probable DAT and mild to moderate dementia. It found a significant and consistent positive correlation between the magnitude of right hippocampal atrophy and the degree of glucose hypometabolism in the ipsilateral inferior parietal and temporo-parietal association cortex. Such widespread hypometabolism is reminiscent of that recorded in the majority of patients with temporal lobe epilepsy, in its interictal periods. Although the decrease in glucose uptake in PET studies in DAT patients is often attributed to neuron death, careful studies in patients with lateralized epileptic foci tell us that hypometabolism may not necessarily be dependent on neuronal loss.[41]

Signs of *hyper*metabolism in epilepsy are seen during seizure discharges accompanied by increased local blood flow, and glucose and oxygen use. Studies in epileptic patients using ^{18}F-labeled deoxyglucose PET, demonstrated the presence of ictal *hyper*metabolism in the epileptogenic region and its projection fields[42] that may exceed six times that of an interictal state.[43] Why then were no 'hot' foci ever reported in early stages of DAT? Not a preposterous question, one might submit, especially considering that the endogenous epileptiform process assumes energy expenditure on a massive scale. Unlike ischemia and hypoglycemia, epileptic discharges could be maintained for several minutes without neocortical and hippocampal damage,[44] but in distinction from epilepsy, DAT imaging cannot be gated by EEG analysis with the same degree of accuracy. As long as oxygen tension and plasma glucose concentrations are upheld, metabolic rates increase above normal until the number of cells is drastically reduced. Then, does hypometabolism portray the 'closing stages' of DAT reminiscent of reduced energy requirements in the postictal state? This might be possible assuming that enhanced cellular glutamate concentrations in the epileptogenic human hippocampus are responsible for the hippocampal epileptic state,[28] rather than for postictal exhaustion following a period of massive self-sustained epileptic discharges.

An example of AIDS dementia might suggest such situations.[45] Of course, AIDS dementia is not identical to DAT, at least not in terms of the intensity of immunological processes. Yet, circumstantial evidence is compelling that the initiating events in the cascade of reactions leading to an influx of Ca^{2+} into cellular elements are contributed by an early infection and consequent development of glial neurotoxicity. It is worth noting that relative subcortical (thalamic and basal ganglia) foci of *hyper*metabolism have been found in early stages of AIDS-dementia, whereas disease progression was accompanied by cortical and subcortical gray matter hypometabolism. The latter thus represented a stage of the disorder when the brain is already irreparably depleted of its metabolic resources, perhaps, in a way similar to that in DAT.[46]

Excitotoxic Brain Damage

When clinical seizure manifestations are not recorded, this does not imply that subclinical epileptogenicity is absent. "A convulsion is but a symptom," declared Hughlings Jackson in 1870 of "a sudden temporary excessive discharge" of the brain. A century later, such "excessive discharges," were designated as epileptogenicity. The final common pathway of epileptogenicity, as well as of hypoglycemic or ischemic insults is represented by excitotoxic mechanisms, such as increased availability of excitatory amino acids (e.g. glutamate), and uncontrolled Ca^{2+} influx into the cells.[44] The processes associated with incessant stimulation of NMDA/AMPA receptors leading to chronic neuronal overactivity and ultimately death of postsynaptic neurons has become known as the 'excitotoxicity hypothesis.'* Olney[47] pioneered the view that a protracted presence of glutamate in the synaptic cleft in some brain structures would lead to impaired function of N-methyl-D-aspartate (NMDA) glutamate receptor system and ultimately NMDA hypofunction. The excitotoxicity hypothesis implies several scenarios of when that might happen. One (seemingly the most likely) prospect is that of glutamate release during mechanical trauma or ischemia in early ontogeny. Another is cumulative damage due to subclinical ischemic episodes. Even ingested glutamate, like endogenous glutamate, might conceivably bind to cellular membrane receptors and contribute to neuronal attrition, particularly with advancing years. It was suggested,[48] though never proven, that glutamate commercially added to many foods could be a source of excitotoxicity and neuronal

---

*At resting membrane potentials, the NMDA receptor ion channel is physically blocked by a Mg^{2+} ion so that no current flow occurs when glutamate binds to the receptor until the membrane is depolarized by AMPA-related activation to at least −50mV. In such a state, the Mg^{2+} block is reduced so that excitotoxic cascades can be initiated even by inputs that are normally subthreshold. By providing inflow of Ca^{2+} into the cell, chronic neuronal glutamate hyperactivity becomes an engine of the primary insult which is delivered to the same circuits that normally mediate plastic changes in the brain responsible for learning and memory formation.

damage, particularly in the elderly with deficient blood-brain barrier. Finally, endogenous detoxicants that normally remove glutamate from the extracellular fluid might be deficient. Such a deficit could be caused by the cytokines that are always present in inflammatory processes, and their quenching is a recognized therapy option in DAT.

The neutotoxic theory of DAT received a significant boost in a line of research on the generation of 5-hydroxytryptamine (serotonin), and the formation of kynurenine along the kynurenine-anthranilate pathway. The pathway is important not only for tryptophan degradation, but also for the generation of niacin as well as three other products which have marked effects on the brain.* L-kynurenine in this pathway is a substrate for the synthesis of *neurotoxic* 3-OH-kynurenine as well as *neuroprotective* kynurenic acid. As such, it has become a parent for several groups of compounds that are now being developed as agents for the treatment of epilepsy and stroke. The last relevant kynurenine, 3-hydroxykynurenine, is involved in the generation of free radicals and is also neurotoxic.[49] A little over a decade ago, quinolinic acid attracted a considerable interest after it was implicated in neurodegenerative disorders, especially in the AIDS-dementia complex. Since the discovery of the specific neurobiological activity of components of the kynurenine pathway in 1981 and 1982 by Trevor W. Stone, kynurenins have evolved during the last two decades from relative obscurity to some of the major players in the pathogenesis of depression, anxiety, decrease of libido, muscular abnormalities, deficit of pain control, and psychopathology.[49]

How Many Factors Does it Take to Cause Alzheimer's Dementia?

When reviewing the list of DAT risk factors, the first question that arises is: How one can judge the plausibility of each of the mechanisms? What are the cracks that open the doors to the pathophysiological cascade which leads to dementing disorders? Which of these factors are modifiable and might thus be prevented, and which are not? As there is no cure for DAT thus far, another question of traditional interest for health psychologists is: what preventive measures are there, if any? In order to introduce some order in the chain of molecular targets, all major risk factors are commonly organized around the

---

*During immune response, interferon-γ stimulates indoleamine 2,3-dioxygenase (IDO) converting tryptophan to N-formylkynurenine followed by kynurenine in an ensuing step.

widely debated 'amyloid cascade' hypothesis. The 'amyloid cascade' has the advantage of telling the story in its 'womb-to-tomb' sequence, even though many dots cannot be connected without speculative exertions. This is not a 'monistic' hypothesis and several independent pathophysiological tiers are to be call upon to portray an outcome.

Genetic Liability

Mutations to three separate genes are associated with early-onset DAT (35–65 years of age). These are the amyloid precursor protein (APP) gene on chromosome 21, the presenilin-1 gene on chromosome 14, and the presenilin-2 gene on chromosome 1. All three genes are expressed in neurons. Their mutations cause an enhanced production of the long form of β-amyloid (Aβ) that is at the core of neuritic plaques. The process leading to DAT is portrayed as initiated with the proteolytic actions of β-secretase that clips from the APP the fragments of 40 to 43 amino acids (particularly $A\beta_{1-42}$). However, a smaller fragment of Aβ ($A\beta_{24-35}$) possesses much of the biological activity of the full-length peptide.

There is another apparently significant susceptibility factor associated with the apolipoprotein E (ApoE) gene, located on chromosome 19, which to an extent predicts an outcome of aging. ApoE is highly polymorphic. Among its three most common allelic products are ε2, ε3, and ε4. Pairings of the alleles give six possible genotypes, of which ε2/ε3 is found in about 60% of the US population. Only ApoE ε4 allele appears to be associated with the development of DAT (about 2% of the U.S. population), albeit for unknown reasons, mostly in white people. About 30% of the population has at least one ε4 allele. It accelerates dementia at an intermediate age by about a decade as compared with individuals having ε2, ε3 copies (the latter may not develop sporadic DAT before the age of 90). The majority of DAT patients in the US (64%) have at least one ε4 allele (a frequency twice that in the general population). Even then, all of the above molecular markers explain no more than 50% of all cases of early-onset DAT. Despite its low specificity, the advantage of early ApoE genotyping is in an accuracy up to a robust 97%, if ε4 allele is recognized. The latter allele guarantees that DAT would develop in *all* individuals who have the dubious fortune of reaching an age of 120–140 years. The stark fact that everybody is at risk of developing DAT justifies an exhibition of the long laundry list of other risk factors to distinguish those who will get there sooner.

Gender

DAT is likely to occur 1.5–3 times more often in women than men. This is often emphasized since contrary to dementia with Lewy bodies, males are preponderant with a ratio of about the same order in the opposite direction. The susceptibility of postmenopausal women to DAT is attributed to the loss of estrogen, a steroidal hormone produced in the ovaries. Estrogen has numerous other effects, such as promotion of the breakdown of the amyloid precursor protein, and increasing glucose utilization and cerebral blood flow, as well as causing less atherogenic serum lipid profiles. More importantly, in the context of this perspective, is the fact that estrogen has neuroprotective functions at various cellular levels. In the kainic acid model of epilepsy, estrogen delays the onset of seizures, and reduces seizure-related mortality.[50]

The view that estrogen enhances memory is widely shared. Part of this conviction is based on the findings that estrogen promotes the growth of dendritic spines and new synapses in various brain regions (including the hippocampus). However, reports that women on estrogen replacement therapy are superior to those who do not use the hormonal supplements in a variety of cognitive tasks, are balanced by reports suggesting that the value of estrogen treatment is rather limited.[51]

Trace Elements

Under physiological conditions, Aβ is a soluble cellular metabolite that is produced by a variety of cells and is found in the cerebrospinal fluid and plasma. Why a soluble, nontoxic Aβ is converted to a bundled and neurotoxic Aβ is unknown. A number of studies are beginning to converge on the potential role of trace elements, such as zinc (Zn^{2+}) in the aggregation of β-amyloid. Zinc is found in high concentrations in mature amyloid plaques in human tissue, thereby suggesting its contribution to a potentially neurotoxic process.[52] It is a cofactor for many enzymes in all tissues and is present in particularly large concentrations in the zinc-containing neurons that originate in numerous brain areas of the limbic system that carry the brunt of injury in DAT.[53,54] Small portions of the total Zn^{2+} in the brain (not more than 10%) are sequestered in the presynaptic vesicles. It is co-released with glutamate at excitatory synapses and functions very much like the Ca^{2+} neural signal. Under pathological conditions (e.g. following an episode of ischemia, or seizure activity in the hippocampus), extracellular concentrations of Zn^{2+} can easily reach neurotoxic levels. In this form, known as 'radicalized,' it becomes an oxygen radical generator responsible for producing dysfunctional cells.[55] Therefore, Fig. 4.4 grants a special place to the zinc-containing pathways that co-release Zn^{2+} together with glutamate into the synaptic space upon presynaptic activation. As with Ca^{2+}, the generation of reactive oxygen species might be crucial to both rapid and cumulative effects of Zn^{2+} neurotoxicity. One of its effects is mitochondrial damage followed by increased membrane lipid peroxidation and Aβ aggregation. Extracellular Zn is now thought of as a contributor to a suppression of GABA-induced currents, gradual failure of inhibition in regions such as the hippocampus and amygdala and ultimately in epileptogenicity that is reflected in background EEG slowing, generalized 'spike-and-dome' or polyspike-wave discharges which are occasionally associated with myoclonic jerks. Other trace elements, such as iron (F^{2+}) might also enhance the propensity of β-amyloid protein for aggregation which is important in view of the gradual increase of iron levels with advancing years. The role of ferrous iron is of interest in view of its capacity to promote oxidative stress via oxygen free-radical formation. The pro-oxidant iron which is normally bound to proteins may be available for free radical reactions in the presence of a deficient blood-brain barrier, particularly in the areas with high density of calcium (Ca^{2+}) channels. Excessive F^{2+} accumulation in the brain is a potential risk factor for neuronal damage, particularly by increasing the cytotoxicity of neuromelanin and dopamine.[56]

Free Radicals

Chemical species (atoms, ions, molecules) that possess an unpaired electron (e.g. ionized water molecules and the highly reactive OH^- (hydroxide), are endowed with excessive oxidizing potency. Such 'electron hungry' species are produced during normal physiological processes (e.g. catecholamine metabolism, immune reactions, or excessive calorie content in diet), thereby contributing to *oxidative stress*. The term implies a state of imbalance between the production of reactive oxygen species, such as superoxide anion ($\cdot O_2{}^-$) and hydroxyl radical ($\cdot OH$) (termed 'free radicals') and antioxidant protective mechanisms. A common example of the process whereby free radicals are produced is a conversion of H_2O_2 in the process of the Fenton reaction in which an essential trace element, iron acts as a catalytic agent:

$$H_2O_2 + F^2 \rightarrow \cdot OH + OH^- + Fe^3$$

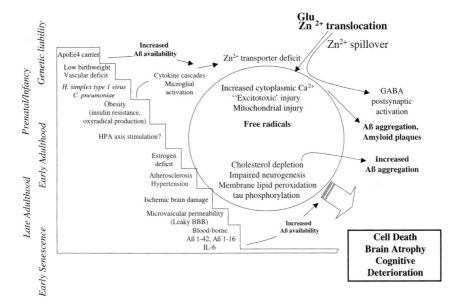

Fig. 4.4   Hypothetical gradient of DAT pathophysiology, and sources of perturbations in neuronal functions. The pathophysiology of DAT is portrayed as a relentless descent along the steps from perinatal insult to cognitive decline and death. The implicit idea behind this schematic of injury mechanisms is that although the effects of each pathway (and its marker) may be quasi-independent of each other, the simultaneous activation of several pathways is associated with greater decline in function and ultimately, substantially greater cognitive impairment. The 'equipotentiality logic' implicit in the portrayal of each step is not proven and has a good chance of being misleading.

ApoE4 is the first step in the descent and the major inauspicious marker. It seems to predispose people to cardiovascular disease, worsen outcomes after traumatic brain injury, amplify hypercholesterolemia, lower bone mineral density, and fuel inflammatory responses to infections. Excitotoxic injury is portrayed as the central part of the scenario. In it, Zn transported into presynaptic vesicles of glutamate-containing neurons by the vesicular transporter and co-released with glutamate (Glu) into the synaptic space upon presynaptic activation is the central trigger of the cascade. Cytokines damage the Zn transporter that helps to maintain low cytosolic Zn levels. An extrasynaptic 'spillover' of Zn makes it available for Aβ aggregation. Rapid Zn entry through Ca-A/K-receptor channels can cause mitochondrial dysfunction and reactive oxygen species generation, which result in neuronal injury. In order to reduce the complexity of the schematic, some pathways had to be omitted. One of them is related to the aggregation of tau proteins, which leads to neurofibrillary tangles. The coupling between amyloid production and tangle formation is poorly understood. It has yet to be elucidated how all these pathways dovetail or when intrinsic or acquired vulnerabilities determine individual propensity to early-onset familial DAT or late-onset disorder.

Mitochondria are the chief providers of energy for the cells, and in the process of energy production, free radicals become an unavoidable nuisance of metabolism that is capable, if uncontrolled, of causing rapid peroxidation of lipid membranes. Each mammalian cell suffers about 70 million spontaneous DNA-damaging events/year that are contributed by free radicals.*

With the accumulation of genetic damage caused by free radicals, various mutations of the amyloid precursor protein gene, presenilin genes 1 and 2 and others, become unavoidable. Those with the ε4 allele are at a particular weakness by being susceptible to peroxidation. In order to curb the onslaught of free radicals, a number of defense antioxidant and detoxifying mechanisms evolved. They restrain oxygen species offering protection or repairing various types of oxygen-inflicted injuries to cellular membranes, mitochondrial DNA and functional proteins. Yet, the neurons are relatively deficient on radical-eliminating enzymes, which are localized mostly in glial cells. This fact raises the possibility that glial-neuronal interactions are an integral component of the microenvironment in which the mending of neurons is achieved. The weakening of this 'patch-up machinery' is a cumulative process. It takes years to reach the level of incompetence when the antioxidative defenses succumb and disease begins. Aging is the major reason why the mending processes are ultimately overwhelmed. With its high lipid content, the brain presumably becomes the prime target of free radical-mediated damage, leading to age-related neurodegenerative disorders.

Neuroimmune Mechanisms

Another tier of DAT pathogenesis centers on the role of infection and immune processes. Senile plaques are highly insoluble, a fact which contributes to an enhanced inflammatory response thereby triggering harmful reactive oxygen species as well as other events leading ultimately to cellular destruction. Evidence is compelling that infections, such as caused by *Herpesvirus hominis, H. pylori,* or *C. pneumoniae* contribute to DAT. Some steps pictured in Fig. 4.4 allude to environmental factors, such as the

---

*By comparison, ionizing radiation at a dose of 2.2 mSv/year contributes no more than 5 DNA-damaging events/year. To give an idea of this effect, consider that the average individual dose accumulated from the fallout of a nuclear test conducted between 1961 and 1964, was about 0.35 mSv.[57]

likelihood of being infected by pathogens very early in life, so that the damage often remains subclinical for several decades. Herpes simplex type 1 virus (*HSV1*) is particularly likely candidate because of its predilection for limbic regions that are critical for normal memory processing and recall. Viruses can move into the brain by neuronal routes, as typically occurs with HSV, which can exist in a latent state within the CNS. The former is the most common mode of access prenatally or neonatally. HSV1 has been detected in the brains of many elderly people. When the virus resides in the central nervous system of ApoE ε4 allele carriers, the carrier might be at risk of DAT.[58] The spread of infection via blood circulation may also occur if the blood-brain barrier is impaired.

Activated astrocytes are invariant components of Aβ plaques and IL-1 overexpression is seen in conditions that confer risk for DAT (e.g. head trauma, Down's syndrome), or in conditions that accelerate DAT-like neuropathologic manifestations (chronic epilepsy). DAT patients show a heightened, spontaneous and IL-2-induced release of IFN-γ and TNF-α from NK cells as compared with healthy individuals.[59] It is important to add that astrocytes can be effectively activated by 'sterile' compounds from the extracellular milieu since, besides having homeostatic and immune functions, they possess signal transduction elements including voltage- and receptor-operated ion channels, as well as receptor-operated second messenger systems. Although astrocytes are devoid of synapses they can release neurotransmitters thereby providing an addition feedforward process of depolarization to stimulate latent epileptogenicity.[60]

Inflammatory factors acquired the status of a signal of the impending cognitive decline *ex-juvantibus*, so to speak, after it appeared that the long-term use of nonsteroidal anti-inflammatory drugs may decrease the risk of DAT.[61] The presence of coronary heart disease and/or obesity may further add to the inflammatory and immune responses by generating pro-inflammatory cytokines. Chronic overexpression of IL-6 in transgenic mice can lead to significant neuroanatomical and neurophysiological changes in the CNS, similar to what is commonly observed in various neurological diseases.[62] The sites at which cytokines act within the brain have yet to be identified, but act they do, particularly insofar as sickness behavior and cognitive functions are concerned. Microglia cells might disrupt the bidirectional traffic of the Zn^{2+} across the plasma membrane by damaging the capacity of its transporter to maintain low cytosolic Zn levels.

Obesity

The role obesity plays, particularly visceral adiposity, is occasionally mentioned due to its association with increased rate of cardiovascular morbidity, increased production of cytokines, oxidative stress, along with microvascular flow deficit due to impaired endothelial regulation of nitric oxide formation.

Brain Trauma

Brain trauma is a difficult variable since many individuals with mild head injuries may not recall a specific one. For example, children or adults playing soccer may sustain head injuries during heading. A modern football has a weight of about one pound and can reach a speed of 130 km/h. Recreational players, doing at least six headers in a regular game might collect a considerable number of tough impacts that could lead to neuropsychological impairments of 'uncertain origin' within a few years. One study, concluded recently, showed that the ApoE ε4 allele is a marker for a poor clinical outcome of brain injury.[63]

Blood-Brain Barrier Deficit

Excitotoxic brain damage has a predilection to regions facing the ventricular and subarachnoidal spaces, suggesting that part of ventricular atrophy might be mediated by a fluid-borne toxin, most likely glutamate and aspartate. A likely blood-brain barrier dysfunction might be contributed to by excitotoxins with the NMDA-receptor affinity. Such a possibility was modeled in rats infused with quinolinic acid (250 nmol/0.25 microl/ventricle) into both lateral ventricles. It appeared that quinolinic acid significantly increased the extracellular tissue concentration of albumin in the hippocampus proper (but not in the subiculum, entorhinal cortex and dentate gyrus) and in the striatum. These regional differences in brain microvascular permeability may depend on the density of NMDA receptors in the capillary barrier, thereby suggesting that a dysfunction of the blood-brain barrier is a complicating rather than a primary DAT causal factor.[64] By the same token, they reveal that the enhanced permeability of microvessels may operate in some cases of dementia, but not in others that show the earliest evidence of neurofibrillary tangles.

Not only is pre-morbid vascular disease a significant risk factor for DAT but over half of patients manifest underlying vascular pathology. Aging is likely to make brain arteries less compliant to blood pressure transmitting it to the capillaries. Vascular changes, such as decreased capillary density, complicated by thickening of the capillary membrane are part of the patho-physiology of experimentally induced and clinical diabetes (for a review, see Ref. 19). Aβ is apparently capable of inducing the release of the vascular endothelial growth factor, which is a possible culprit of vascular dysregulation causing endothelial damage and angiogenesis. New vessels are devoid of the blood-brain barrier so that the brain would be flooded with the blood-borne substances that are normally excluded by the barrier (e.g. protein molecules, protein-bound metals, β-amyloid protein, $A\beta_{1-42}$ or $A\beta_{1-16}$). In addition, $A\beta_{1-42}$ acting as a vasoconstrictor would increase vascular resistance, decrease brain blood flow and facilitate thrombotic and ischemic events.

Cholesterol Paradox

The role of cholesterol in DAT pathogenesis is possibly dualistic: the height-ened levels of cellular cholesterol contribute to DAT development by elevat-ing Aβ secretion; however, the increased amount of oligomerized Aβ reduces cellular cholesterol levels, and is a potentially dangerous outcome since cholesterol is an indispensable material in regeneration and synaptic plastic-ity.[65] In addition, cholesterol depletion in cells is implicated in the parallel scenario that accounts for the shift of tau to a hyperphosphorylation state leading to neurofibrillary tangles.

ApoE is a regulator of lipid metabolism. It is involved in cholesterol 'house-keeping' by extracting its surplus from the cells. This duty is carried out by ApoE ε2, whereas ApoE ε4 is unhelpful in this regard. In ApoE ε4 car-riers, cholesterol thus disrupts the capacity of cells to internalize Aβ, which instead undergoes gradual aggregation. Thus, drugs that boost intracellular cholesterol removal in ApoE ε4 carriers are seemingly an interesting adjunct to DAT therapy of pathophysiological significance. Be that as it may, a higher allele frequency for ApoE ε4 is not necessarily associated with increased risk for DAT in some ethnic groups (e.g. African Americans), whereas its low frequency may be nonetheless associated with higher DAT rates (e.g. in Israeli Arabs).[66] Part of the problem could be of technical character, i.e. an extensive clinical and pathological overlap between DAT and Dementia with Lewy bodies, where the role of ApoE ε4 is less prominent.

There is still another thrilling "but" in stock. A recent case-control study by Bogousslavsky's group in Switzerland[67] has reported that patients with early poststroke seizures appear to have *lower* mean serum cholesterol values. The authors raise an interesting possibility that cholesterol exhibits "antiepileptic" as well as "neuroprotective" properties with regard to cerebral ischemia and seizures. This explanation makes sense. The effect was compared with that of a high-fat ketogenic diet, an old therapy, still used with some amendments in children with intractable seizures.

Adrenal Axis Functions

Intuitively, a perturbation of the adrenal axis would further complicate DAT by interfering with a biochemical endpoint such as catecholamine levels, as they are particularly susceptible to alterations in adrenal axis functions. However, the role of psychological stressors in DAT remains problematic. It has long been observed that enhanced sympatho-adrenal response with high levels of catecholamines ameliorates the ischemic damage.[44] Another mechanism whereby stress or depression would lead to hippocampal damage is through a glucocorticoid cascade.[68] Excitatory corticofugal pathways are known to contain glutamate and aspartate. Consequently, stress-induced increased impulse flow can, under certain conditions, damage neurons with deficient self-repair machinery. However, the evidence available so far is not sufficiently strong to implicate emotional stress in DAT. No dynamic stressors or their combinations can predict the age of onset, speed of progression, and unique manifestations of DAT, which are quite variable. Given that the role that stress plays in DAT has yet to be established, all events which detail its contribution to the disease are left out of Fig. 4.4, so as not to complicate the already knotty scenario. That leads to the next section.

Therapeutic Outlook

In total, the process of Aβ deposition seems sluggish. It takes numerous participants and then years, even decades to lead to clinical manifestations. By the time patients become symptomatic, extensive — and potentially irreparable — damage to neuronal circuits will be made. That poses numerous questions: What needs to be prevented? What has to be repaired? What endogenous excitotoxicity hypothesis is suggested in terms of slowing down the juggernaut of dementia? And what should be done first?

The story of DAT is being told in many voices and themes. Each shows that the progress toward an understanding of dementing disorders has been frustratingly slow. As it looks now, each story is not DAT pathophysiology;

at least none seem to exhaust it. Ultimately, the veracity of each theme will be validated by unequivocal practical achievements, such as a set of reliable dementia pointers or "risk profiles" that would enable the application of the specific medical efforts.

Realistically, an ideal drug against DAT is hoped, at the minimum, to delay the progression of cognitive deterioration, or to stabilize cognitive functions on the level consistent with self-help, at least for some time; it should improve patients' mood and some behavioral aberrations, if any (e.g. agitation, vocal and physical aggression, apathy, hallucinations, and wandering) that are so burdensome to caregivers. Finally, given the potential of significant underlying morbidity, an ideal drug should not aggravate patients' somatic condition or add the burden of untoward side effects when combined with ongoing medication for other non-DAT conditions. There numerous trials at a variety of levels (e.g. offsetting a cholinergic presynaptic deficits; controlling an excessive opening of the GABA chloride channel; making GABA available in postsynaptic sites; inhibiting of β- or γ-secretases; immunizing against $A\beta$, acting at hormonal, plasma lipid, trace metals, immune levels and others). Thus far, no drug has been really helpful, even though none were ever anticipated to approach the power of the Fountain of Youth.

It is not sensible to hope to reverse the whole gamut of somatic and vascular changes, potential infections, obesity, and brain deleterious evolution, which may overlap in time. It is even less certain whether the tweaking of the repair processes would help since their targets have to be better defined qualitatively and quantitatively at the clinical, pharmacological, instrumental, and molecular levels, as well as the level of clinical phenotypes. Therefore, it now seems a gamble of the past to hope to bypass that overwhelming problem by a quick 'cognition first' approach by augmenting cholinergic neurotransmission via precursor loading and acetylcholinesterase inhibitors, and hitting with the same remedy $A\beta$ production via increased expression of amyloid precursor protein. Precursor loading strategies have been, for the most part, disappointing. The effects of acetylcholinesterase inhibitors tacrine and donepezil have been somewhat more promising (see Ref. 69 for a review). But then one might be wary that the outcome looks attractive due to the inclusion in the sample, patients with dementia with Lewy bodies who are particularly responsive to cholinesterase inhibitors. The other problem is that the increasing popularity of acetylcholinesterase inhibitors in DAT requires awareness that donepezil, less toxic and better tolerated than tacrine, and even galantamine,[70] might potentiate existing circuits of enhanced epileptogenicity. Occasional benefits of the latter family of drugs, mostly of palliative nature, have been offset by the emergence of troubling untoward effects. Common side effects of tacrine are gastrointestinal discomfort, vomiting, nausea, and abdominal pain. Although seldom categorized as epileptiform reactions, they might as well be contributed by epileptiform discharges in the limbic systems.[71,72]

Glossing over all subtleties, one might see that the central event depicted in Fig. 4.4 is the creation of free radicals even though it remains uncertain whether and to what extent oxidative stress acts as the major catalyst of the progressive downhill course of DAT. Free radicals are implicated in aging, dementias, cancer, and cardio-vascular disorders. One property of free-radical reactions is that of self-propagation, which continues until quenched by endogenous or exogenous free-radical scavengers. The body contains an elaborate antioxidant defense system that works well when all is well. It is supported by dietary intake of some water-soluble agents (glutathione, vitamin C), lipid-soluble vitamins (α-tocopherol, β-carotene) and the endogenous production of agents such as glutathione. Thus, prevention of oxidative stress is a recommended health promotion strategy. However, an 'antioxidants first' strategy has been difficult to support by their efficacy.

To date, the pharmacological therapies approved for the treatment of DAT are given to alleviate symptoms of cognitive decline at the stage when a widespread neurodegeneration in corticolimbic areas make such intervention palliative. The epilepsy-DAT linkage might provide an alternative logic, at least therapeutically, as well as a paradigm for a search for other useful agents. Currently, the center stage of trials of drugs is occupied by memantine, a noncompetitive NMDA antagonist.[73] Memantine is not a novel drug (e.g. it was used to suppress acquired pendular nystagmus in patients with multiple sclerosis), nor were the anticonvulsant effects of this low-affinity channel blocker pronounced when the drug was given alone. It did, however, reduce kindled seizures in rats when co-administered with the AMPA (α-amino-3-hydroxy-5-methyl-4-isoxazolepropionic acid) receptor antagonist.[74] Based on its better therapeutic window, memantine was launched in Germany by Merz in 1989 as a neuroprotective agent for the treatment of dementia. It is now seen as a more rational treatment for DAT as compared to cognitive enhancers. Although introduced as a neuroprotective agent, it is actually dissimilar to other drugs of this category (e.g. amantadine or selegiline), whose neuroprotective effects in PD were thus far rather disappointing. If the science holds true in humans as in rats — and there is a good chance that it will — then memantine and similar glutamate/NMDA receptor antagonists might, before long, be able to change prescribing practices in the US. So far, memantine remains a harbinger of optimism in controlling the previously hopeless condition through the search for an efficacious and well tolerated drug with a long half-life. It may lead to a revision of treatment strategies in geriatric psychiatry. Perhaps, it would be safe to add, for some time.

In science, as in life, there is always something "on the other side." The role of the NMDA receptor antagonists as solo drugs or as adjunctive neuroprotective compounds is limited because of concerns over their ability to cause neurodegenerative changes in corticolimbic regions in rodents and produce psychotic reactions in adult humans.[47] The hypofunction of NMDA receptors is thus certainly undesirable. Their effect may be illustrated by the NMDA-antagonist ketamine, a short-acting anesthetic that causes dissociative thought disorder, depersonalization and catatonic states. Ketamine was forsaken in veterinary practice as a drug of addiction and a psychotogenic agent regardless of the fact that it seemed an efficacious anticonvulsant.[75] Even in a single dose, let alone in the course of repeated administrations, ketamine appears to cause neuronal injury in the limbic cortex. Under such conditions, persistent suppression of NMDA receptor function with untoward psychopathological effects would be imminent. One recent electrophysiological study conducted on prefrontal rat brain slices made use of two distinct activity modes of pyramidal neurons. The authors report that the regular spiking of pyramidal neurons turned to repetitive bursting when glutamate or NMDA were focally applied to the apical dendrites. Such repetitive bursting has long been recognized as a sign of epileptogenicity, but it is not all that bad as it has a greater chance of engaging GABA interneurons. The two different firing modes were further used to study the effect of NMDA antagonists. As Fig. 4.5 demonstrates, ketamine effectively decreased the number of intrinsic bursts as well as inhibitory postsynaptic potentials.[76] This result provides strong evidence that ketamine leads to a weakening of the potential to connect to GABA inhibition. It follows that a better choice for antagonizing this kind of neurotoxicity might be to add some anticonvulsant agents that activate the GABA$_A$ receptor.[77]

The GABA$_A$ receptor is a complex system of transmembrane proteins arranged around a central chloride channel. Although its effects are multifaceted, dodging the complexity, it is possible to say that GABA works to counterbalance the excitatory action of glutamate in the CNS. The most compelling evidence for

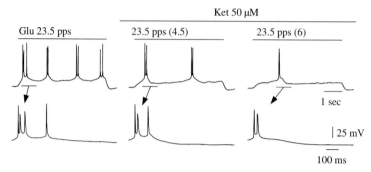

Fig. 4.5 Effects of ketamine (Ket) on bursting induced by dendritic glutamate (dGlu). Representative recordings from a prefrontal cortex pyramidal cell showing that ketamine decreased the number of bursts induced by dGlu and changed the temporal characteristics of the bursts. In this cell, glutamate was applied via pressure ejection. After Fig. 8B of Shi & Zhang,[76] with permission.

the epileptogenicity hypothesis of DAT is the fact that patients with progressive memory impairment initially attributed to DAT showed improvement when they switched to antiepileptic medication on the basis of epileptiform EEG findings.[78] Likewise, the amnestic wandering of presumably DAT patients was reported[11] to decrease after treatment with antiepileptic drugs. Apparently, any new late-onset epilepsy in the elderly with a diagnosis of cerebrovascular disease, small vessel ischemia or DAT can be successfully controlled with anticonvulsant monotherapy.[79] Therefore, the rule of thumb in DAT is to medicate first-onset seizures as opposed to the policy of waiting for a repetition in younger patients. However, glutamate receptors, like that for GABA, form a family of currently eight subtypes subdivided into three groups with different specific functions in regard to neuroprotection.

In summary, the psychopharmacological treatment of DAT has thus far been directed by a search for ways of improving the cognitive state of patients and delaying their deterioration. NMDA and GABA receptors are emerging as leading targets for medicating DAT. Novel anticonvulsant medications (e.g. Lamotrigine, Remacemide, Rilutek, or Harkoseride) are beginning to be entertained as potentially effective in the treatment of DAT. This new generation of drugs might promise to provide the framework within which early pharmacological intervention directed at controlling NMDA receptor-ionophore complex or enhancing GABAergic activity would prevent deterioration and modify the course of the disorder thereby leading to a more favorable long-term outcome. There is some teleological wisdom in the need to preserve the role of the excitatory synapses that play such a fundamental role in cognitive functions. Their hyperactivity might be a hint of some feed-back processes directed at recovery of the lost synaptic network that, ironi-cally, leading to neuronal self-destruction. This represents a classical example of malfunctioning homeostatic preservation in older persons suggesting that regardless of whatever else is considered necessary to keep the neurons from dying, we must also take into account the need to maintain the activity of the NMDA and AMPA receptors albeit by balancing their hyperactivity with GABAergic drugs. Memantine is the first step in this direction.* Not all cases of dementia would respond to this therapy, which might only prove the view that it is time to represent DAT as an etiologically diverse syndrome. Its ther-apeutic targets are complex. Activation of subtypes of group-II or group-III of metabotropic glutamate receptors seems to be neuroprotective *in vitro* and *in vivo*. By contrast, group-I receptors need to be antagonized in order to evoke protection.[80] The recognition of the fact that the latent (subclinical) excitotoxic epileptiform process might be a significant player in DAT pathophysiology and even predate other major events described above suggest that in the patho-physiology in DAT, epileptogenicity is getting "out of the shadows."[†]

Options for Health Psychology

Neuropsychiatric Perspectives on DAT Continued

The chief executive officer at Dallas County Hospital in Perry, Iowa, forgot to take her 7-month-old daughter to the baby sitter, leaving her in a van for nine hours. A NASA engineer who intended to drop his 9-month-old son off at a day-care center forgot him in the car for eight hours. In each case, the child died. According to research conducted by General Motors, dozens of deaths occur because infants are forgotten by reasonably young parents in hot, unventilated, cars (*www.vindi.net/editorials/275986281500270.shtml*). *The Washington Post* of February 22, 2003 placed on its first page an article

---

International Journal of Geriatric Psychiatry published *Memantine Workshop* of 2001 held in Barcelona (Spain) in its supplement of 2003.

†The notion of 'shadows' had a different connotation when the Pan-American Health Organization (PAHO) announced its *Global Campaign* for the control of epilepsy "Out of the Shadows." But it is the source of my borrowing.

reporting that a Manassas man inadvertently left his youngest daughter strapped in her car seat in the family's van on a hot day. Although convicted by the jury of involuntary manslaughter and child endangerment (which could put him behind bars for up to 15 years), he was spared all but symbolic jail time by a judge who ordered him to do volunteer work (two hours each week). Court testimony during the Manassas trial showed that the man was having difficulty taking care of the family's 13 children while his wife was out of the country, ultimately causing him to *lose track* of time and his youngest daughter with it. Essentially, that charitable verdict implies that he was exonerated because of the multitasking operations his central nervous system was unable to cope with. More colloquially, such cases are branded as forgetfulness or described as "goal-neglect."

In neuropsychology or cognitive psychology, such memory failures projected into the future are known as deficits of *prospective memory* (PM).[81] PM must be a recent evolutionary device.* Being effortlessly deployed for any routine activity of contemporary mortals, PM essentially keeps our lives organized by the 'thinking-off-line style,' such as planning to shop, arranging a meal, keeping appointments, ordering prescribed drugs, meeting a partner at the tennis court, paying the bills or coming on time to a party. Quite naturally it is expected to decline with advancing years and most certainly to fail with a general cognitive deterioration in DAT. Surprisingly, in some studies, the elderly were surprisingly competent when tested with 'ecological' tasks, such as sending postcards or making telephone calls on request some time in the future.[82,83] Even patients with DAT showed no inferior performance in simple tasks, such as selecting a colored coupon from an array of lures and offering it to the experimenter after a week's delay. When following one-week retention of the initial task, a different coupon became the new training target, and all participants were able to shift to the new task requirement.[84] Moscovitch[82] and later other workers[83,85] attributed the paradox of 'immortal' PM to the fact that the participants were keenly aware of their forgetfulness and tried to compensate for it with greater efforts to remember, particularly when they had access to external memory aids.[83]

The course of PM is understood to consist of a host of concurrent and interactive processes, such as encoding of intention and response selection;

---

*In Greek mythology, only the Titans like Prometheus (*pro-metheus* — one with foresight) were initially endowed with the power of planning and prediction.

mapping of the potential retrieval cues on time vectors when the retrieval options must be worked out from a variety of task materials; potential foreground operations; the length of time the goals must stay in the background; emotional states of a person. This indicates that PM is a basic feature of the high-level system that provides 'Gestalts' for maintaining the systematic flow of goal-directed behaviors[86] in the presence of foreground cues and cognitively generated orienting arousal that captures attention automatically and without awareness.[87] The possibility that such cognitive orienting responses ('insights') disrupt the orderly progression to planned actions is not at all speculative. It thus becomes imperative to clarify why even demented individuals retain certain control over their delayed goals.

A distinction has been made between event-related (or cue-related) and time-based tasks, which may account for the paradox of ageless PM.[88,89] Remembering 'what' (a cue) may be easier as compared to remembering 'when' because remembering the former is *automatic*, stimulus-driven, and thus exclusively dependent on the strength of environmental prompts (recognition) whereas remembering 'when' rests on self-generated impulse.[90] Characteristics of time-cued goals and the existence of concurrent competing tasks strain working memory thereby making their completion more vulnerable to distracting, or task-irrelevant intrusions in elderly individuals with limited attentional resources.[91,92] In one such experiment, participants were required to perform an action every 10 minutes (a time-based task). In a parallel experiment, they were asked to remember to act whenever a certain word was presented (an event-based task presumed to be low in self-initiated retrieval). Age differences were found in the former but not in the latter task.[93] The pattern of age differences was replicated in other studies.[83,94] These observations might suggest that not only does DAT manifest spatial orientation deficit, but that inferior time-perception might be its obligatory feature.*

---

*Unlike the accuracy of biological self-sustaining oscillators which is close to physical time, prospective time assessment is the most vulnerable module. The John Gibbon's Scalar Expectancy Theory,[95,96] requires three major components for time monitoring: clock, memory, and evaluation producer. The clock is essentially an accumulator of the pulses from the pacemaker; the cumulative number of pulses is viewed as 'time' or 'absolute time.' This is a multipurpose device onto which semantic information must be mapped. It is run continuously like the molecular circadian timer, but can be reset at any arbitrary time by prospective motivations. The latter turns a 'switch' on, so that the time passed by can be approximately computed ('perceived time') against the one known to the accumulator as the number of pulses multiplied by the unit (i.e. a period of the pacemaker).

Time is monitored within two dissimilar reference systems: "shared" and "subjective personal."[97] The first is set by recognized or institutionalized time-keepers and measured in terms of specific precise components (minutes, hours) that are referred to as a clock. Less precise 'shared' units of time are fragments of the day (afternoon, lunch-time, martini-time), or even less specific time segments (skiing period, summer, or the next semester). People may or may not act in accordance with 'shared' time, or have different compliance with institutionalized behaviors (because they skip lunch or do not drink martini), nonetheless they are instantly aware of the scale, and it remains highly relevant. Within both shared and personal reference systems, PM may be pronounced deficient when a person acts on intentions much earlier then projected, or too late for an act to be pertinent. The former happens due to underestimated time or impulsiveness whereas the latter may be associated with a time overestimate or a deficient system of prompts, such as can be exemplified in *dynamic akinesia*. All may be illustrated by brain pathology when such a deficit is easily observable.

Prospective memory implies a variety of dissimilar incentives requiring various levels of attentional demand to enhance control over time,[97,98] as well as different hedonic values of the tasks themselves (e.g. pleasant, neutral, aversive, relevant, or unrelated to life events).[99] It requires a significant degree of reliability of various neurotransmitter systems, including the dopaminergic neurons that are believed to process the time and are activated by reward-predictive stimuli.[100] I thus declare myself to be among those[101] who believe that this area of brain research would yield a place in neuropsychiatry as visible as that occupied today by retrospective memory. At the very least, it could probe an isle of spared mental health that involves decision making for voluntary behavior in cue-related prospective actions, on which some rehabilitation strategies might be built.

Increasing 'Brain Reserve'

Your mother might have admonished you, "If you don't pass your spelling test, you'll never get a good job." In fact, given the availability of contemporary computerized spellcheckers, you may. But this admonition is a metaphor for the role of education in cognitive longevity. The risk of DAT has been shown to decrease by approximately 17% for each year of education.[102] According to Mortimer,[103] a fraction of the population with high educational levels, or those who presumably were able to 'get a good job,' had either a greater number of neurons, or their interconnection density in youth, designated as 'brain reserve.' Mortimer believed that intellectual stimulation in early life, as well as nutrition and prevention of cerebrovascular disease in early life, contribute to the expansion of 'brain reserve,' as revealed by the practical ability to solve problems and do well in neuropsychological tests. One study supporting the notion of brain reserve examined the association between linguistic ability and dementia in a group of 74 nuns, primarily from convents in Milwaukee, who provided their handwritten autobiographies completed some time between the ages of 19 and 37. The participants died on average about 62 years after writing the autobiographies, when they were between 78 and 97 years old. Tellingly, the density of wording of ideas (propositions), which is a standard measure of the content of ideas in text samples, had strong inverse correlations with the severity of DAT pathology in the neocortex. Correlations between idea density scores and neurofibrillary tangle counts were -0.59 for the frontal lobe, -0.48 for the temporal lobe, and -0.49 for the parietal lobe (all highly significant). By contrast, the severity of atherosclerosis of the major arteries at the base of the brain and the presence of lacunar and large brain infarcts were unrelated to idea density scores.[104] Unlike semantic and pragmatic aspects of language, syntax appears to be buffered from the effects of advancing years and dementia. In an earlier study on the same group, both idea density and grammatical complexity were assessed in 93 participants. It was found that a 'low density of ideas' in early life had stronger and more consistent associations with poor cognitive function than did low grammatical complexity.[105]

Scholastic 'calisthenics' notwithstanding, cognitive longevity, intelligence and the risk of neurological disorders are determined to a significant extent by heritable factors as well as pre- and perinatal events. Even mild brain impairment may foil the child from reaching full maturation and cognitive capability (as reflected in poor learning ability and scholastic achievements). There are intriguing observations that small brain size, as assessed by head circumference, is a marker of reduced brain reserve. After adjusting for age, sex and education, head circumference appears to correlate with the Cognitive Abilities Screening Instrument score, but not with diagnosis of probable DAT. When the data are stratified by diagnosis, no association is obtained among controls, whereas a strong effect appears for DAT patients.[106] These findings, as well as those discussed in Chap. 2, indicate that the deterrence of prematurity is the primary measure in establishing brain reserve.

Other investments into brain growth and development of children may be as modest as adding a safe and cheap nutrient, such as essential fatty acids. The effects of the long-chain polyunsaturated fatty acids on membranes of excitable cells of the central nervous system, and thus on perceptual and cognitive function may not be limited to infancy but may also be seen during school age and adulthood. Preterm infants fed for a month, within the first 48 hours after birth, with a nutrient-enriched preterm formula have been said to show a higher verbal IQ than those who were given standard infant formula when tested at about 8 years, when cognitive scores are highly predictive of adult ones. This indicates that when adequate nutrition is not available during the critical period of intrauterine brain growth, or if human breast milk (rich in long-chain polyunsaturated fatty acids) is not offered and the fatty acid composition is not maintained in infant formulas during 2-year postpartum, infants become deficient, in particular in language-based skills. This also promises memory decline in a more remote future.[107] Scientists have yet to understand fully what happens prenatally and why cognitive disabilities originate as the fetus adapts to survive starvation in the womb.

From the standpoint of potential therapeutic intervention there are a number of questions to clarify. What are the cellular (molecular) analogues of the learning burden that identify superior learners that are relevant to humans? What neuronal machinery offers maximal payoff? Whether or not markers such as superior linguistic skills are genetically endowed or education affected? Does learning remedy genetic or prenatally compromised cognitive longevity? Are there variants of complex semantic structures decided by cultural evolution that are relevant for the prediction of the rate of cognitive decline? There are too many potentially relevant endogenous molecules to sort through in different regions acting concurrently or simultaneously.

One molecular candidate for promoting cognitive longevity is the brain-derived neurotrophic factor (BDNF), a recently discovered protein that has been mentioned above. It has been proposed to play a critical role as an intercellular synaptic messenger in the long-term potentiation in the hippocampus. It promotes the function and survival of the major neuronal types afflicted in DAT, including hippocampal, cortical and basal forebrain cholinergic neurons. BDNF is also considered to act as an endogenous therapeutic agent whose deficit retards the recovery of traumatic, chemical and ischemic lesions in the brain. We have yet to establish the contribution of activity-dependent synaptic release of BDNF, its role in the regulation of synaptic transmission and synaptogenesis in the brain in early ontogeny, a role for functional BDNF gene polymorphisms on learning and memory and its relevance to 'brain reserve.'[108] BDNF mRNA expression is reduced in DAT, which among other effects might have contributed to a declined food intake in DAT, known generally as "anorexia of aging." It is of interest though that BDNF modulation of synaptic plasticity and spatial learning may require a 'compliance' of cyclooxygenase, which was mentioned in Chap. 2 as playing a crucial role in inflammation and muscular activity. The above-mentioned discovery that non-steroidal anti-inflammatory drugs significantly lower the risk of DAT is hoped to provide a lead in developing agents for treating or precluding cognitive deterioration. And yet, the need not to be casual about anti-inflammatory drugs cannot be overstated. Shaw and colleagues[109] report that the broad-spectrum cyclooxygenase inhibitor, ibuprofen, hinders the induction of long-term potentiation, the major marker of synaptic plasticity in animal models. The fact that it may also affect memory performance is confirmed by the fact that the same rats were impaired in spatial learning performance in a water-maze. It is of further interest that a 4-day activity in a running wheel *prior* to ibuprofen appears to reverse endogenous BDNF levels and reinstate long-term potentiation. In terms of 'scholastic calisthenics,' this experience might mean that mental stimulation, particularly focussed cognitive activity in later life, is capable of reactivating cellular energy needed for the preservation of adequate synaptic transmission. Thus, well-defined cognitive and motor challenges might have a crucial role in the restoration of learning and memory in the context of pharmacotherapy.

SO WHAT?

Lord McCall[110] recalled a pediatrician who at a conference shared a chestnut that the first minutes of life are the most dangerous. An old heckler in the audience shouted out, 'the last few minutes are pretty dangerous too.' There are many suggestions of what might fuel DAT processes and what actually happens to the brain with advancing years so as to lead to dementia. There are a few 'proximal' (specific) causes of senescent cognitive decline as well as numerous 'distant' or 'modulating' variables.

DAT is a neurodegenerative disorder characterized pathologically by highly insoluble senile plaques, neurofibrillary tangles, and synapse loss. The etiology of DAT and its molecular triggers remain elusive. It is accepted that genetic factors play an important role, but numerous other factors have been suggested. They include infections, hormonal and neuroimmune dysregulation, brain trauma, reactive oxygen species, endogenous neurotoxins, trace elements, vascular and blood-brain barrier impairments, and others.

With the recognition of the fact that impaired function of the NMDA glutamate receptor system plays an important role in the pathophysiology of DAT, the center stage of trials of neuroprotective drugs is currently occupied by NMDA receptor antagonists. This concept poses a general question of whether early pharmacological intervention directed at controlling NMDA deterioration and channelopathies will result in a more favorable long-term outcome.

The allusion to a cumulative multifactorial injury enmeshed in contingencies and uncertainties will only inundate the argument with irrelevant details due to delayed 'maturation' of DAT. Thus far, such complexity of factors seems to have diverted intellectual resources from efforts to elucidate the minimal number of proximal genetic determinants of dementia.

It is hoped that DAT will become an area of molecular neuropsychiatry that promises to split 'dementia epidemic' into several disorders of genetically distinct types, each with its own pathophysiological scenarios and medication armory.

The major domain of practical relevance for health psychology in this competitive area will remain in:

(i)   collaborating with molecular geriatric psychiatry in splitting DAT into clinical subgroups;
(ii) examining prospective memory;
(iii) exploring the role of brain reserve as potential tools for improving the quality of life of the elderly, as well as participating in the management of DAT.

4c

Self-destructive Behavior:
The Cultural Perspective

More than 150 Shakespearian characters either contemplate or actually commit suicide. Death by suicide was even dubbed an 'English malady' (*'mal anglais'*) a label that sounds like a thinly veiled insult since in the past, self-destruction was condemned and criminalized. Suicidal individuals were considered unrepentant sinners because they usurped the God-given command over life. Their banishment continued even after the 17th century when medicine replaced the church as the custodian of the mentally ill, and it was gradually recognized that people who took their own life are not so much evil or sinful as unfortunate 'misfits.' Shakespearian testimony notwithstanding, the rate of suicide in Protestant Britain was actually lower than the European average. Yet until the 'Suicide Act of 1961,' death by suicide was a criminal offence on the island and its rates could well be underestimated. As early as in 1542, Luther lamented that in Germany suicide had reached epidemic proportions. He could not have foretold that several centuries later, suicide would again be labeled as epidemic, although the American Foundation for Suicide Prevention recommend using a more benign word — "rise" — in connection with suicide rates.

In 1999, the Surgeon General[1] called attention to an alarming increase in the rates of contemplated or committed suicide among children and adolescents in the US, where it ranks as the third cause of death among young people between 15 and 25 years of age for 2001[2] (*www.nimh.nih.gov/Suicide Prevention/suifact.cfm*).*

The clusters of suicides among the young who often 'copy' the particular methods of self-destruction suggest the existence of 'contagious' effects of self-inflicted death and so creates in the public eye a mood of a mini-epidemic.[3] The urgency of dealing with suicide is that each such avoidable death is estimated to intimately affect at least 6 other people. Nonetheless, mortality by suicide, though tragic, is hardly a novel epidemic, even among the young. The Suicide Data Page released in 2003 (*USA Suicide: 2001 Official Final Data*) indicates that in children 5–14 years old, rates of suicide fluctuate between 0.8 and 0.7, for 1990 and 2001, respectively. For the age group 15–24, the rates vary between 13.2 in 1990 to 9.0 per 100,000 in 2001. Likewise, overall, the rates of suicide seem to be steady or falling. In 1970, suicide was ranked the eleventh cause of death; it moved up to the eighth place in 1990, then the seventh in 1992. Subsequently, it retreated to the ninth cause of death in 1996 and dropped to the eleventh cause of death in 2001. A dependable source on the history of suicide[4] has indicated that in 1850, the suicide rate in Italy was 3.1 per 100,000, whereas in Denmark it reached an impressive 25.9 per 100,000. Over a century later, the rate of suicide in Italy tripled whereas in Denmark, the rate remained about the same (24.1 per 100,000 took their own lives). The peaks of suicidal death in the US were recorded in the first decade of 20th century and again in the 30s (*www.afsp.org/statistics/USA.htm*) and dropped considerably after that. A plot of suicide rates by gender released by the WHO in 2002 for the US (Fig. 4.6) does not show any rate increment during recent decades. It provides a useful opportunity to review the rhetoric about the suicide epidemic. Suicide has been sufficiently visible through out the centuries so as to warrant a more modest 'endemic' rather than an 'epidemic' label. Only in a few European countries have suicide rates appeared in excess of 20 per 100,000. These countries are Belarus, Finland, Estonia, Poland, Russia, and Hungary. It is difficult to find a common explanation for all of these nations, but some

---

*The National Institute of Mental Health (NIMH), the Centers for Disease Control and Prevention (CDC), and the Substance Abuse and Mental Health Services Administration (SAMHSA) sponsored a workshop on October 22–23, 2003, entitled *The Science of Public Messages* for *Suicide Prevention* (*www.nimh.nih.gov/ SuicideResearch/suicprevmsgwkshop2p3-26.pdf*). The meeting provided a meeting ground for experts in suicide, suicide contagion, public health decision-making, hoping to promote health literacy, public messaging campaigns and discuss the complex issues underlying effective suicide prevention.

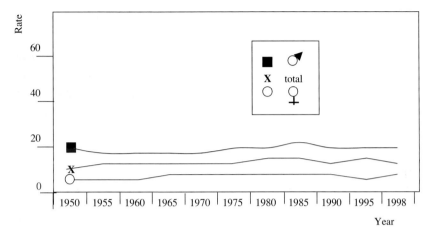

Fig. 4.6. Suicide rates (per 100,000), by gender (USA 1950–1998). Source: WHO, Geneva, 2002.

of them are among world leaders in per capita consumption of hard liquor. Social problems are also a potential trigger of suicide. Yet, for many other countries, including those with deplorable human rights records, crime and poverty, suicide rates are surprisingly low.

Risk Factors of 'Garden Variety' Self-destructive Behavior

Risk factors lend themselves to grouping in several dissimilar ways, socio-cultural, psychological, neurochemical or psychoneurological. Suicidal deaths are frequently explained by early exposure to violence, indoctrination, and cultivation of religious and national hatred, child abuse and neglect, as well as poverty. Some of these themes are not unfamiliar in the US, where the public passionately blames violent movies, graphic TV shows, bloody computer games and excessive broadcasting of suicidal accounts for the rise in aggressive behavior and violent suicidal acts in schools. AOL Time Warner, Palm Pictures, and 11 video game makers were being held responsible by the families of victims of the Columbine massacre in the US in 1999 for allegedly influencing Dylan Klebold and Eric Harris. Perhaps, more important, as many claim in retrospect, is that bullying was the primary cause of their suicidal murder. Bullying is commonly defined as a persistent teasing or verbal and physical assault in order to execute control over a person perceived as subdominant. However, in hurting the weak, the cumulative effect of their resentment may also harm the offenders. Initially, the antipathy of the weak may be limited to just an ideation of the offender's suffering or death, but it may be a dry run for real revenge. Audrey Hepburn as Eliza Doolittle looks overwhelmingly charming when protesting Professor Higgins's bullying in My Fair Lady. But her daydream of his execution by firing squad was deadly serious. Not only have Harris and Klebold fantasized openly about committing acts of violence, they made a video in which they executed their nemesis on school grounds. Undeniably the power of contemporary mass communication, especially invasive and graphic journalism, may fuel discontent and provide examples to copy; it may perhaps provoke those who are uncertain of the value of their lives. Also, social indoctrination could offer an explanation for hostility and brutality, but hardly suicidal violence. At least 45% of first graders in Washington, DC have witnessed assault or murder with a deadly weapon.[6] However, it is commonly recognized that the possession of firearms by a psychologically impaired individual is what matters, and sometimes decisively so.

The rates of suicide in US schools do not co-vary with the rate of unemployment, whereas those barred from schools and snubbed by their peers, only infrequently turn their guns on themselves, let alone kill a dozen of their schoolmates in revenge for alleged injustice done to them. It is more likely that some misfits collectively create environments of their own, since, using Morris Kline's[7] line, their "mind contains furniture into which their guests must fit." What is this "furniture"?

All factors of suicide summarized in Table 4.1 converge on those that lead to or are associated with helplessness, despair and ultimately, clinical depression (all of them are shown italicized). Normally, therefore, neuropsychiatrists would be right to look for signs of depression in anybody who wishes to die. The question is how *not* to misjudge its presence. Another major suspect is that of genetic liability. Given that some genes have a role in forming more than one characteristic and most characteristics are formed by more than one gene, the question to ask is, what is being inherited? Is it a predisposition to depression, self-directed aggression, or some central deficits causing a downward social drift due to the inability to establish interpersonal relations, poor problem solving, certain metabolic or neurochemical deficits causing self-image problems or impulsivity? Some answers to these questions call for a great deal of resourceful animal modeling. But suicide is a difficult problem because it does not call for reproducing an ambivalent psychopathological state, potentially leading to a deadly outcome, but an unmistakable outcome itself. Therefore,

Table 4.1   Rick factors for suicide.

Demographic
   Gender (men/women ratio is about 4:1)
   Marital status (*being single, having disrupted marital relations, particularly for men*)
Personality and life events
   Low self-esteem
   Loneliness
   Fatalism
   Pessimism
   Withdrawal from others
   Little interest in activities
   Poor concentration
   Poor peer relations
   Shame, humiliation
   Entrapment
Psychopathology
   'Subsyndromic' mood disorders
   Prior suicidal behavior
   Sleep disorders
   Depression, anguish, pain
   Drug abuse
   Alexithymia
Upbringing
   Sexual and physical abuse
   Emotional neglect
   Law family cohesion
   Lack of pride in one's family
   Imitation behavior
   History of bullying or being bullied
Biological
   Family history of suicide
   Genetic liability
   Low plasma cholesterol
   Impulsivity
Medical
   Chronic illness, malignancy
   Recalcitrant, medically unexplained symptoms

---

animals replicating some 'pathologically submissive displays' or learned help-lessness postures in captive animals are unlikely to demystify the nature of sui-cidal acts, particularly when disguised as arson, murder, or associated with disinhibitory personality traits and others kinds of reckless behaviors. They do not tell us whether a 'humiliated' animal 'wishes' to die or responds with ideation of death when its family or sexual bonds are cut off, whereas for human beings, thinking about death is a fundamental feature of our character. As Kurt Goldstein[8] has taught us, suicide more than any other disease is a disease of humanity; it is "a voluntary act, and, with that, a phenomenon belonging to abstract behavior and thus characteristic to human nature alone." That does not imply that suicide is completely resistant to modeling, except that modeling would be deemed successful only when some inventive simplifications are found. Deploying simple models, such as Harte's[9] teasing invitation to *Consider a Spherical Cow* nudges medicine toward looking and performing more like physics. Yet, even emulating suicide with a 'spherical cow' in the laboratory setting might only be relevant for some of its basic components.

Recently, the serotonergic system has been implicated in impulsivity, depression and suicidality. Depressed patients and victims of suicidal attempts showed reduced serotonergic transmission as reflected in decreased numbers of brain and platelet serotonin transporter binding sites, which is paralleled, as an adaptive upregulation, by the increased density of brain serotonin (5-HT) receptors. Genes that code for proteins involved in regulating serotonergic neurotransmission (such as the tryptophan hydroxylase, 5-HT transporter, and $5-HT_2A$ receptor genes) have therefore been major candidates for association studies of suicide and suicidal behavior. Among the genes implicated in suicidal ideation is the 102C allele in the $5-HT_2A$ receptor gene.[10,11] Low output or low stability of the serotonin-containing neurons may be a marker of genetic predisposition for suicide, independent of, or additive to, a psychiatric disorder.[12–14] Still another lead has been offered by a study by Avshalom Caspi[15] and associates, who studied the promoter activity of the serotonin gene. The latter exists in two structural variants (alleles), i.e. the short ("s") allele and the long ("l") one. It appeared that only individuals with the short allele of the gene have impaired serotonin transmission and this predicted depression symptoms, an increase in symptoms, depression diagnoses, new-onset diagnoses, and suicidality in relation to stressful life events, such as bereavements, job crises, or romantic disasters — as compared to individuals homozygous for the long allele. Although neither causal nor diagnostic in and of themselves, their findings lend further credence to the notion that significant life events may feed on psychological vulnerabilities. The question is what kind of life event is capable of triggering the depths of despair leading to a fatal outcome.

Thus far, most credible factors have been proposed by G.W. Brown,[16,17] whose studies are essential reading for health psychologists interested in suicidology. They emphasize that feelings of humiliation and/or being trapped following severely threatening events predict depressive episodes in individuals with the background of psychosocial vulnerability, to a more significant degree than other traumatic life events. In a very thorough recent study, Brown[16] admits, nonetheless, that background vulnerability factors such as low self-esteem ('internal' factors) are capable of propagating an environment of their own. And so, such 'envirotype' or core relationships ('external' factors) might be quite highly correlated with 'internal factors.' He thus posits:

Psychological vulnerability might also appear as memory left by humiliation and gloom. One might guess that selective long memories of previous offences might thus become insulated from mitigating circumstances or cognitive therapies unless a special psychologically acceptable rewarding situation is created to facilitate the 'forgetting.'

One more mechanism of psychological vulnerability may appear as impulsivity since neither depression nor suicidal ideation is an act of death unless an urge of sufficient force is generated. Seymour Kety[18] proposed that a defective gene might reduce the ability to control untoward and self-destructive impulses in situations of adversity leading to depression. Parenthetically, it is conceivable that the impulsivity trait may have some evolutional advantage and thus that suicidal individuals were not discarded by evolution. History can furnish us with quite a few examples when the knack to trust one's instincts and act on a whim, or even recklessly, on deficient information, has led to the significant achievements, or financial, military or scientific gains. Such success is a momentous pheromone that might have been acting to restock the suicidal gene for the next generations.

The severity of impulsive behaviors might be related to frontal lobe abnormalities. Raine[19] conducted a rare brain imaging comparison of

> "... the two perspectives are complementary — and just what emphasis is given is likely to depend on the point at issue. In considering life events and depression in those with a diagnosis of non-fearful personality disorder, one would obviously be particularly concerned with an individual-level perspective, but one would also want to keep in mind the possibility that the propensity of such patients to create their own depressogenic events will interact with the level of social integration in their culture when viewed as a whole" (p. 369).

metabolic brain landscapes that underlie affective, impulsive brutality with those that underlie planned, predatory violence. The volunteers for brain glucose metabolism studies with positron emission tomography were 15 predatory murderers, and nine affective murderers. The assessment of their left and right hemisphere (medial and lateral) and subcortical structures (amygdala, midbrain, hippocampus, and thalamus) regions showed that predatory murderers have sufficiently robust prefrontal functioning, presumably capable of regulating aggressive whims. By contrast, affective murderers showed reduced left and right prefrontal functioning, thereby suggesting that they lack prefrontal control over the regulation of emotion.

A small frontal lobe region, the supplementary motor area, seems to be particularly essential for higher-order motor planning and temporal organization of movements that demand retrieval of motor memory, especially in sequential performance of multiple movements. Its anterior part sets in motion circuits triggered by cognitive demands. Lesions restricted to this area (bilaterally or on the subdominant side) contribute to a syndrome characterized by impaired initiation of volitional movements and a severe deficit in the self-initiation of language production (akin to dynamic akinesia), as well as motor neglect. The supplementary motor area is implicated in Parkinson's disease, and in keeping with expectations, Parkinson's patients manifest quite consistent hypoactivation of this region in positron emission tomographic images.[20,21] The fact that Parkinson's patients are disabled in executing complex cued actions and in producing cognitively generated movements might possibly explain the paradox of their low rate of suicide. They are inferior in motor ideation (i.e. the willed conceptualization of motor action), and self-initiated actions. This state of dynamic akinesia is possibly reflected in more specific *suicide apraxia*, i.e. the incapacity to see through the plan of action and generate an impulse leading to death.[22] One might wonder whether decreasing the vigor of the supplementary motor machinery in the potential candidates for suicide (e.g. by turning it 'off' for a short period of time, say by transcranial magnetic stimulation) would provide the required waiting period to delay or foil death in some depressed patients when they show a dangerous level of suicidal ideation. However, impulsivity is a typical feature of other pathological states recognized by the American Psychiatric Association's *Diagnostic and Statistical Manual* (DSM)-IV (312.31), where pathological gamblers reside under the same roof as sufferers of intermittent explosive disorder, kleptomania, trichotillomania, and pyromania. The result of gambling may be suicidal, but gambling itself is hardly driven by a desire of death. Thus, impulsiveness is mostly an executive arm of suicide, not its cause.

Human Bombs

With September 9/11 in fresh memory, one clearly sees the need to take a closer look at a new kind of brazen suicide that is carried out in order to kill others. This eruption of suicidal aggression has established a strong foothold in countries where suicide was virtually unknown. It has shifted a perspective from a 'personal impulse' of someone who no longer wishes to live to that of a group lined up for death. Ironically, for the first time in history (that is, since the glory of Andalusian and Sicilian Islamic civilization from the 11th to 15th centuries) what happens inside the Muslim community has a direct bearing on the world at large.* What are we dealing with: criminal homicide (parasuicide) caused by injured honor and pride, ideologically goaded low-intensity warfare that is getting increasingly bolder, or a result of frank depression prompted by social triggers in a few that have become exploited by ideologues? These questions are not just *a propos* suicide; they are about the sickening effort to kill others at the same time. After all, many patriotic Russians did the same to the Nazis during WWII. So, are suicide bombers instruments of hatred swelled out of control under the impact of group loyalty, as some believe?[23] Be that as it may, the Middle East has become the major breeding ground, an almost world-size laboratory to examine the nature of suicidal violence. It is not just another item on the agenda of health care for it promises to grow into an item of concern for the entire planet.

In the following, let us consider in more detail the Middle Eastern epidemic of suicidal terrorism or rather omnicide, inasmuch as one of the major authorities on the topic, Ariel Merari[23] made it somewhat easier by recently

---

*Suicidal death as an instrument of war is not monopolized by any culture. Although considered to be a product of the punitive and domineering authority of Wahhabi Islam, murder by suicide was known in Europe. Among fathers of terrorism are the Russian-born political philosopher and anarchist, Michael A. Bakunin (1814–1876), who advocated small-scale group actions for "propaganda by the deed," or Germans, Karl Peter Heinzen (1809–1880) and later Johann Most (1846–1906), who contributed the idea that murder-suicide is a form of revolutionary struggle. Many websites now contain useful and balanced information on the topic (e.g. *http://faculty.ncwc.edu/toconnor/429/429lect02.htm*).

proposing, among other factors, the following challenging itemized declaration of what it is *not*:

- Terrorist suicides do *not* fit the characteristics of ordinary suicides;
- Religion is neither a pre-requisite nor a major factor in the etiology of suicide terrorism;
- There is no evidence that the wish to take revenge for *personal suffering* plays a major role in an individual's readiness to carry out a suicide attack;
- Suicide terrorism is the product of manipulative group influences, rather than the result of individual characteristics.

In order to understand suicidal acts of this kind, we require explanations on at least four levels. First, we should gain some inkling of the experience that lies behind those who were unable to die and can thus be interviewed, or their relatives who volunteer to comment on the motives of the deceased and thus permit a glimpse into the mind of the suicidal terrorist through their eyes. Second, we must understand whether the realization of death arises from a model of escape from the burden of living with pain or as a purchase of a better life. Third, at the neuropsychiatric level, we need to consider how and when the state may be rephrased in terms of underlying brain dysfunction(s). Finally, we must have some insight into what is behind 'manipulative group influences.'

Suicidal Terrorism: Is it Parasuicide?

The outbreak of aggressive death by suicide in Islam is often attributed to unmitigated hatred of infidels. Reuters of Thursday, January 23, 2003, quoted Muslim cleric, Sheikh Abdullah el-Faisal as urging women followers to raise their sons to be part of the holy cause by murdering nonbelievers: "Your male children must have the Jihad mentality ... At 15 your Muslim boys must become soldiers. Jihad training must be compulsory."* Joseph Lelyveld cited in his essay *All Suicide Bombers Are Not Alike*, published in *The New York Times Magazine* (October 28, 2001), a scandalous confession

---

*Mr El-Faisal, 39, of Stratford, is a Jamaican-born convert to Islam, who denied the charges arising from taped addresses (*www.guardian.co.uk/religion/Story/0,2763,888706,00.html*). A search for 'Jihad' via Google on the Web gives 135,000 hits with many historical and regional differences in the way the term is used. Although commonly conceived of as 'striving,' 'struggle,' or a (non-violent) 'holy war,' it also has a subjective meaning as the internal war for self-improvement, and yet crueler connotations.

by a columnist from *Al Arabi's*, a weekly that speaks for the remnants of the old Arab nationalists: "I cannot restrain my joy," its author confessed. "For the first time in my life, I witness with my own eyes the defeat of American arrogance, tyranny, conceit and evil." (See also, *www.gamla.org.il/english/article/2001/sept/memri2.htm.*) It is unfathomable that someone whose religion demands justice and compassion as major virtues should spout such bloodthirsty rhetoric and be overjoyed by the deaths of innocent people. Granted, it is within the scope of Islam to be able to inflict death. The question is, why by suicide?

As always, sociopolitical nuances obscure the role of neuropsychiatric factors in suicide. Unmitigated atrocities are seldom considered as a mental health issue when they are sanctified by a struggle for freedom or dominance. The underlying motives are mainly treated as a human, political, social, and legal or religious issue, or their combinations. Not surprisingly, those suicidal bombers are often regarded as cultural idols of their nation. We might ask though, with Kurt Goldstein[8] and Ernest Becker,[24] how empirically valid the cultural hero system that sustains and drives those who die by omnicide is? If we are to peel away the heroic camouflage, we would arrive at Becker's view that much of what motivates this kind of heroic death is fear and 'the struggle for self-esteem at its least disguised.' Thus, what is labeled by Islam as martyrdom, and by law as crime, psychiatry may suspect as a cynical usage of sickness for achieving political goals. After all, personal frustrations in the context of social upheaval, including attributions of injustice to religious intolerance are potent catalysts of atrocities by confrontational groups.

The inclusion of individuals in different categories of violent death alters statistical analysis and ultimately interferes with the search for definite causes of suicide. One needs to be aware of circumstances when a relentless murder is staged with a full appreciation of the personal peril that nonetheless has an option not to be fatal. Such acts are often designated as *parasuicide*. These villains are by and large *not* completely sane. In some cases they suffer from episodic dyscontrol syndrome and their family members describe personality traits that are indicative of minimal brain dysfunction or pseudoepilepsy. In fact, organic cerebral disorders have been recorded in as many as 94% of individuals suffering from this syndrome.[25] Its complicating factors are being a woman, with mental disorder, given to substance abuse, and comorbid somatic illness. Previous parasuicide was found in 60% of young men and 80% of young women.[26] Annual rates of parasuicide in recent decades range from 2.6 to 1,100 per 100,000, and lifetime prevalence rates range from 720 to 5,930 per 100,000.[27] Parasuicide is understood to be a reliable predictor of suicide, and whose risk persists without decline for a long time, years or decades.[28] Other potentially lethal performers belong to the pool of sufferers of borderline personality disorders (antisocial and histrionic), who easily manifest destructive aggressive tendencies, particularly when they hope to obtain immediate postmortem stage-center and glory. We might guess, without being able to prove it, that the misfits' inventory of possible outcomes may be quite long and variable, but suicide or suicidal ideation will be a salient landmark on their cognitive map.

Suicide as a Search for Award

Some explanations of the readiness of Arab terrorists to die through mass slaughter are plainly anchored in the way sexual behavior and the achievements of carnal satisfaction are regulated in their societies. These adolescents and young men are convinced that, as 'martyrs', they will be alive in Heaven and in addition fittingly rewarded with a heterosexual party. One would-be bomber resident of Taibe who turned himself over to security forces was an exception. He explicitly said during his interrogation that he wanted to be reunited in Paradise with another suicidal murderer, Tsadek Elhafaz of Kalkilya, who blew himself up in Karnei Shomron, killing two and wounding 30. He certainly believed that God authorized this wicked reunion. With such an inspiration, terrorism does not promise to end any time soon. It obeys the "law of the corset": if you tighten it in one place, the bulge will be elsewhere. It can only be contained within Islam, not outside of it.

During the preparation for the mission, the instructors of the would-be killer from Taibe assured him that:

1. He would feel no pain (that is an honest assessment for a quick death). Clearly, any form of death is painful and final only for non-Moslems kuffar (infidels), whereas martyrdom for Muslims is mercy from Allah. Therefore, a suicidal terrorist feels holy, 'protected' and eternally alive, whereas nonbelievers are damned and dead. "You should feel complete tranquility," Mohamed Atta, one of the 9/11 suiciders who rammed an airliner into the World Trade Center Tower, is said to have assured his accomplices, "because the time between you and your marriage in heaven is very short."

2. His body will not rot in a grave (also a plausible promise since in most cases there will be no body to speak of to assemble in a grave).
3. He will travel to paradise to meet other martyrs and virgins.

The death of a martyr is routinely announced in the Palestinian press not as an obituary but as a wedding "to the Black-Eyed." The same Muslim cleric in London, Sheikh Abdullah el-Faisa, mentioned above, explicitly guaranteed that the boys would be rewarded for their martyrdom in paradise with 72 virgins: "Religious martyrs are not dead." The *Jerusalem Post* of November 14, 2002 also tells us that the future terrorist was assured that even if he didn't succeed in causing fatalities he would still go to paradise. The question is who would be ready to deprive these men of having a unique chance to exercise their right to have fun with 72 beauties when they wish to? Do we have a duty to compel them to abandon that hope?

Humans are the only creatures aware of and intimidated by their irreversible finality. They dread:

> "The undiscovered country, from whose bourn
> No traveler returns, puzzles the will,
> And makes us rather bear those ills we have,
> Than fly to others that we know not of."
>
> *(Hamlet, Act III, Scene 1, William Shakespeare)*

The awe of death was acquired in the cultural evolution with the formation of a symbolic self and the appreciation of the risks of its abrupt termination. The realization that a life is not ours, that the body is death-bound, that it might become at any time a food for worms when the self will no longer *stand out* (i.e. exist) individually, must have been a devastating discovery, leading to anxiety or panic[24] (see also Chap. 5). The consciousness of a living thing, of its being just a fleeting creature, is apparently more shocking in cultures whose members are also ambivalent of religious faith and the notion of life after death. It may be less awful to those who have a chance of an eternal gift, such as a harem full of innocent maidens who would not be distracted from their connubial responsibilities even by the menstrual cycle. Amazingly, in a ritual unknown to the high-risk suicide wishers of any other faith, the martyr-grooms are instructed to have clean underwear for the heavenly reception following their successful self-destruction. Recall an old line attributed to the immortal wisdom of the Jewish mother: "Make sure you wear clean underwear, in case you're in an accident." An example of the unmitigated happiness of impending death was exhibited recently on the other side of the world by Amrozi bin Nurhasyim, the self-confessed perpetrator of the night-club bombings in Bali (Indonesia) last October, which killed 202 people, many of them Australians tourists. He was dubbed the "laughing bomber" by the Indonesian press for the often happy expression on his face during the trial. As the judges pronounced him guilty and sentenced him to death for organizing the bombing, Amrozi shouted in giggling delight, "Allahu Akbar" (God is Greatest), much to the revulsion of his victims' families.

But of course, this postmortem license is mostly for males. Only for them does suicide provide a channel for an escape into personal manhood. Given that most bombers die in confidence that God will deliver on his promises or rather on the promises of his clerics, one has to find a way to dissuade the brainwashed. Should not Amrozi be taught to be more skeptical and to ask as Prophet Abraham (*Ibrahim*) did: "My Lord, show me how you raise the dead." The Lord said, "Have you no faith?" "Yes," said *Ibrahim*, "But I wish to reassure my heart. ...."

Parenthetically, until very recently, Muslim clerics did not approve of women enrolling in the army of suicide bombers regardless of the fact that they would be a better choice for a suicide mission. They are less conspicuous, have a better chance of disguising a bomb on their body; they are less likely to be searched, let alone stripped to show their skin, which would create an outcry in the Middle East media. By contrast, about 30% of the suicide operations in Sri Lanka have been conducted by women. Rajiv Gandhi, the Prime Minister of India from 1984 to 1989 is the best known victim of a woman suicide-bomber.

Suicidal Aggression and Depression

Ideally, to make a diagnosis of depression with suicidal plans, one needs to examine those who intend to commit suicide. The second best is to talk to those who fail in suicide attempts. In some cases, an empathetic interview yields an honest answer. The would-be suicide bomber, Thauriya Hamareh, certainly leaves an impression of a miserable woman with low self-esteem, insecure, hopeless and helpless. This 'TV diagnosis' is admittedly confounded for it is not made in the privacy of a doctor's office and is not based on observations of adequate length. To what extent is the verbal presentation of suicidal thoughts valid in determining the risk of suicide? Can we rely on the answers that potential terrorists give when they are questioned by police? Well, no. Quite incredibly, however, her rational for contemplating to murder others with her suicidal death — "to create a just and equal, non-corrupt and non-criminal society by the spread and unification of Islam"[29] (pp. 1, 13) — seems sincere to this listener. The question is whether she is depressed or cognitively impaired? Some psychological impairments might be conceived of as 'reaction forms' when the focus of biological psychiatry research shifts from the alleged mental "disorders" to disordered psychological domains.[30] Or rather would her suicide be a 'reaction' of a lonely, submissive and unhappy woman who otherwise would not be heard in Muslim society? We may never know. The notion of feminine modesty in Saudi Arabia implies that a woman cannot make intimate disclosures to a psychiatrist. The same could be true elsewhere in the Arab world.

Alas, one does not see suicidal failures that often. Most people who commit suicide might have communicated such ideation in a more or less disguised manner to friends and family members often months before the act. Such ideation is well worth exploring in the encounter with potential terrorists since very little is known about the intersection between mental health and Islamic practices. Therefore, a less orthodox way to learn about a suicidal mind is to consult veteran prisoners acting as observers. Having spent 18 years in an Israeli prison, Walid Dakah spoke with many security prisoners and interviewed every youngster he could among those whose plans were thwarted. It is not easy to trust the stories about such events when the narrator himself was not only their spectator, or a victim, but a willing perpetrator convicted for life. On the other hand, beggars cannot be choosers, inasmuch as Dakah was skeptical about the authority of the study conducted by the antiterrorism unit of the National Security Council (about which he learned from a report in *Haaretz* of December 29, 2002). His mistrust was based on the conviction that the prisoners under study were unlikely to 'behave naturally' with authorities. With this disclaimer in mind, I went through the portion of transcripts of three such interviews, reported by Amira Hass of *Haaretz* Friday Magazine (03/04/03). All of them confirmed an impression that the expectation to "meet the master of the universe and to live a better life" in paradise was "the main thing." One terrorist was essentially illiterate, a rather unusual case for a Palestinian Arab, who also confessed with a line almost lifted from Sartre: "Life is a headache [sic] ... The things we see on television are nauseating and make us lose our taste for life." Another was "involved with a group of *worthless people*, until [he] met someone who scolded me and ... started to give me lessons in prayer." Two of them offered their bodies in the name of Islamic Jihad, the third on behalf of Fatah. They prefer an explosives belt over a rifle since the former requires no cognitive effort, "you need to train to use a rifle." There were also obligatory words of hatred and nationalistic rhetoric since all youngsters grew up in the hotbed of repressed fury and revenge. Reading the excerpts selected from his interviews it was difficult to escape the impression that these would-be suicide bombers (all three from the West Bank and aged 18 to 20) are utter misfits regardless of the efforts to edit their account. Walid Dakah was quite qualified to edit his own story. "As a young man," he intimated, "I acted on emotional impulses, not for rational ideological motives. The ideology came later." In his diary, too, he might have appended some ideology later as he wrote it.

It would be fair to surmise that some indications of personal suffering, inadequacy, addiction or sexual aberrations communicated in the process of such interviews sheds a little light, however distorted, on the pool of suicide candidates. Drug addicts (often branded "*worthless people*"), gay youth and those afflicted with AIDS as well as women suspected of romantic affairs may be compelled to offer their deaths as a dignified liberation from the inevitable honor killing and thus purchase a one-way ticket to martyrdom and immortality. According to a report by the Al Jazeera TV station (though unconfirmed by other sources), the 16-year-old who blew himself up as border policemen approached him near Kibbutz Bahan, north of Tulkarm, in the morning of June 18, 2002 was a carrier of the AIDS virus. An association of suicide attempts with HIV positive status has been registered in suicidology, and suggests the need to investigate other 'shameful disease' associations. The same holds for sexual misbehavior. When one survey examined sexual abuse in a randomly sampled group of 652 Palestinian undergraduate students, their rate appeared to fall within the range of other societies and had a similarly strong psychological impact on victims. Sexually abused participants (both female and male students) expressed significantly higher levels of psychoticism, hostility, anxiety, somatization, phobic anxiety, paranoid ideation, depression, obsessive-compulsiveness, and psychological distress compared with their nonabused counterparts.[31] It is doubtful that the families of those who are indoctrinated into a heroic homicidal mode would share any compromising details of sickness, particularly psychopathology or sexual problems of their children, or indeed know about it more than is permissible in their culture. Informants queried in the West Bank do grant some material, if they provide it at all, for socially cognizant interviewers. They speak of 'occupation,' 'control,' 'hegemony,' 'religious conflict,' 'depravity' and 'economic hardships.' Only seldom do they indicate that suicide bombers are socially isolated, 'retarded,' sick, or might feel threatened by their families. The choice of being a martyr aligns some deep personal weakness with motives suggested by religion, and makes such altruistic death not only acceptable, but desirable and rewarding.

Religious affect (fear and guilt), particularly when spurred by thoughts of having committed an unforgivable sin, is sufficient to trigger numinous experiences changing all future life events. It would not be outlandish to imagine that the teens are coaxed to die with honor and to become martyrs rather than to slowly perish disgraced and ostracized by their own people. In their sick logic they fight for acceptance by killing others so as to heighten their "social integration," in Emile Durkheim[32] parlance. Statistics on this controversial subject are scarce, and most of the evidence about honor threats, banishment of those alienated from God, tormented by anxiety disorder after admitting to their consciousness some unlawful ideas, exhibiting unorthodox behaviors, or seduced by strangers or family members, is impressionistic and anecdotal.

Psychiatric Cultures

In societies where psychopathology is stigmatized, suicide is not a part of disease; rather, it becomes a righteous act when it is also accomplished by killing non-Muslims in order to fulfill one's social, political and religious obligations. Admittedly, much of what has been learned until now may has been distorted due to the censored disclosure of information owing to socio-cultural norms or deferential recording by health professionals. A conventional way of learning about victims of suicide is by conducting clinical interviews with proxy informants structured on *The Diagnostic and Statistical Manual of Mental Disorders* (DSM-IV) adjusted for use in the Middle East. Surprisingly, I found very few studies in the countries with endemic political suicide that have described changes of mood over time. The analysis of psychopathology in the context of professional psychiatry of the Mediterranean basin is also limited. An authoritative volume on *Culture and Psychopathology* edited by Ihsan Al-Issa in 1982 contains multiple references to the ancient Greeks but not a single reference to Arabs in its Index. A single passing allusion to Muslims is related to cardiovascular disorder (!) in India. One might find some allusion to contemporary depression and anxiety sandwiched in a historical examination of psychiatry in the Pharaonic era through the Islamic Renaissance. To be sure, such studies must be terribly difficult to conduct due to cultural variations that may not necessarily fit into the Western concept of mental disorders, depression, in particular. Also, standardized diagnostic criteria for depression must be applied consistently over time so as to understand when and why the incidence of attacks are changing; how it is influenced by economic incentives, social status and age. One has to be prepared that some or many of the informants would not accept the notion of depression as a factor motivating suicide.

Consistent with the DSM, depression may be defined broadly as emotional suffering that arises from a biological, behavioral, or psychological dysfunction within the individual. This characterization follows the trend of considering mental aberrations as true diseases, which are discrete entities with their own causation, course, and outcome. However, anxiety as a core component of the depressive syndrome may be consequent to culturally sanctioned responses to noxious events (i.e. stimuli an individual is unable to assimilate), such as bereavement reactions to death of a loved one. Its symptomatology may thus have significant variability between people and cultures in terms of its severity and rapidity of development. The problem of diagnosing mental illness and anxiety in particular is that it is often a *polythetic* category, meaning that it rests on a number of classifying features that can be found in other individuals who are considered healthy by their peers and health professionals. According to the *International Statistical Classification of Diseases and Related Health Problems* (ICD-10), the core symptoms of depressed mood (depressive thoughts, ideas of self-harm, sadness), loss of interests, loss of pleasure and reduced energy levels, are sufficient requirements for establishing the presence of a depressive episode. However, there are others that might be relevant, such as a diurnal variation of mood, somatic distress, headaches and pains, as well as psychomotor retardation and *inability to feel any emotions*. Ironically, the latter symptoms in suicide candidates or failing terrorists are dubbed 'calmness' and 'equanimity' to prove that they are actually not depressed. Raine's[19] findings mentioned above are consistent with the fact that individuals with 'proactive aggression' are calmer than those who display 'hot,' angry aggression, and plan ahead their destructive and self-destructive acts. All recent cases of desperate violence have a mark of premeditated behavior. Curiously, the protagonist of Jean-Paul Sartre's *Erostratus* explains in a letter written prior to his carefully planned intention of indiscriminate massacre of innocent people:

It did not escape Sartre that 'calmness' might characterize an individual ready for suicide.

One study coming from the Department of Psychiatry of United Arab Emirates University (a more tolerant place of such

"You understand then that I am not 'furious.' I am, on the contrary, quite *calm* and I pray you to accept, Monsieur, the assurance of my distinguished sentiments" (p. 49, italics added).

studies than elsewhere in the Arab world), showed marked cross-cultural differences in rating depression using Hamilton's Depression Rating Scale, mostly in terms of higher scores on 'retardation' and 'somatization' among participants.[33] Ironically, the retarded 'somatizer' might be a determined assassin who may insist on somatic treatment when depressive symptoms appear to be subthreshold or do not meet criteria for depressive disorder, and who may not accept psychotherapy as a medical solution. Consequently, the conclusion of this study is that the scale's internal consistency would be violated thereby causing a reduced recognition of depression. Until the frequencies and modes of expression of depressive symptoms in different age groups in Arab countries are examined consistently using the instruments widely used in Western countries, we run the risk of missing some signs of depression. Even in Western patients, depression can easily be overlooked if they are not systematically and compassionately interviewed in order to understand the person's tendency to "externalize" dysphoria.

In the Muslim community, the risks of suicidal ideation, attempted suicide, and death by completed suicide is provided with influential socio-cultural attributions that must contribute to a pervasive underdiagnosis of depression. In general, although presentation with physical symptoms is expected to be a regular form of psychiatric presentation in the Western community, the studies mentioned above suggest that it must be infinitely more prevalent in the Muslim countries where self-depreciation, guilt and worthlessness belong to the prayer rather than primary care physicians. While harboring evil sentiments and planning revenge, such individuals might present numerous gastrointestinal and autonomic symptoms, anorexia, weight loss, insomnia or hypersomnia, and decreased energy.[34] At a certain point many healthy individuals might think of death by suicide, but in no way act on the idea, unless it comes as a pathological insight to a sociopath (e.g. as in Sartre: "One night I got the idea of shooting people.") Suicidal terrorists who sincerely believe that they procure the eternity of happiness for their sacrifice have an easier transition to the last stage. Given that they are making a therapeutic 'trip,' so to speak, even if disguised as an altruistic act, their distress signals or plea for help are not communicated on the wavelength codified by Western psychiatry.

Another profound difficulty in understanding suicide behavior is associated with the need to make out idioms of distress, and interpret conceptions and formulation that determine the quality of mental health care in Third World countries. Brown[16] ranked humiliation as a sense of being devalued (with three subcategories: separation, other's delinquency, and put down). In his sample based on women, typical examples were learning of a husband's infidelity, a boyfriend saying he wanted to end a year-long relationship, and a woman who found out that her 12-year-old daughter had been stealing from her and playing truant from school. None of these events are applicable in our case. Brown clearly saw the need to supplement the spectrum of depressogenic events by taking account of the cultures that create dissimilar events, states or their series, say, by sending girls away to be 'married' before menarche for religious reasons, or on a similar model, by dating someone outside of the permitted selection, being shamefully sick, or collaborating with perceived enemies, and many others.

As ethnopsychiatrists observe, Western psychiatry may seem inadequate for the Middle Eastern psychiatry culture that is based on a Mediterranean family- and/or tribe-centered attitude and the *androcentric* ethos. That psychiatry service is run by men, for whom diagnoses are artificially constructed; they are fictitious items with no roots in their cultural genesis. The depth of the cultural divide was unexpectedly brought to light in the 70s when scores of foreign physicians, many of them from Arab countries, were relegated to state residencies regardless of their former training, status and abilities. Pearl Katz,[35] writing for a volume on ethnopsychiatry, portrays a scandalous picture of the work ethics of psychiatrists in Ken Oak hospital in Maryland, most of them from Middle Eastern countries, who objected to being evaluated on the basis of their performance. All responded with the "rhetoric of complaint" that the rules of practice are irrelevant and hateful. Their roles in the past were determined by the external locus of control when the yardsticks of success were based on kinship, family ties, fate, age, and professional relationships. In short, it is not at all surprising that only now are we beginning to understand the acquisition of the concepts of psychological morbidity, death and homicide by adolescents and the way they are shaped in Muslim culture. The level of training must have improved since the time when Ken Oak physicians were assessed because the majority of Arab psychiatrists are now trained in the US or Europe. However, given that ultimately the outcome is conceived of as decided by the Higher Authority (whatever God wills, happens, or *in'shallah*), the quality of diagnoses and care will not depend only upon professional qualifications. Psychiatry in the Middle East has yet to acquire the culture-making power it has in the U.S., Europe or other Western societies.

Herostratus Syndrome

Some people who do not appear to be clinically mentally ill might still manifest an inability to handle their relationships and end up perpetually dejected, demoralized and frustrated. Their weakness is expressed in low self-esteem, lack of self-control, suicidal ideation and inadequate social and work functioning. Socially, shame, humiliation and a sense of not belonging builds upon preexistent susceptibility. By dramatizing personal doom such individuals may tend to blame others unjustly for their failure. The Islamic jihad is to a considerable extent a resentment struggle of unhappy people. Religion provides a binding glue to all those who feel kinship in the fight against infidels. A potential 'martyr' accomplishes his goal twice since on a personal level, each is assured the rise from the paltry anonymity of his past to the glory of posters on the walls of his town. This leads to the point that the tendency to commit suicide as an act of retribution for personal deficiency is so abhorrent that it is given the name of *"Herostratus syndrome."*

Herostratus is a villain of 356 B.C. whose claim to immortality is in burning down the great Temple of Artemis at Ephesus, one of the seven wonders of the ancient world. DSM-IV acknowledges the relevance of pyromania, albeit as a form of impulse control disorder rather than due to an intellectual and affective disorder of humiliated individuals akin to (regrettably discarded) monomania of Esquirol (1772–1840). The Russian poet S. Nadson (1862–1887), the 'bard' of hopelessness, humiliation, misery and death was more on target in trying to explain Herostratus' unfathomable crime by his acute sense of being a loser, a pariah who was "mistreated by chance and pushed aside as drifters are ..." looking for a way to get even with the more successful others. His was a horrific crime meant to deprive those who were ahead of him of the reasons for their aspirations, pride and enjoyment. An important nuance of Nadson's thesis is that Hersotratus must have lived with the painful realization of being { *Червяк, раздавленный судьбой, Среди толпы многомилльонной!* } a 'maggot squashed by destiny, in the midst of the countless hordes' in the author's English translation. Nadson did not try to diminish the scope and magnitude of the crime by an effort to understand it in Esquirol's terms. Nor does this chapter diminish Herostratus' repugnance by medicalizing it. Personal and shared despair as well as unmitigated loneliness are familiar motives for retribution directed at specified 'them,' but we often lack methods to deal with such motives adequately when their triggers are centuries away from our grasp, let alone the capacity to understand crimes of such magnitude. Also, depression is considered 'real' when caused by an internal psychological dysfunction and not if symptoms are a reaction to a standard (common) 'negative environment.'

Strangely, anxious and timid vulnerable people might be "driven to establish a minimal level of acceptance from closeness to others, presumably because those of our forebears who behaved in such a manner were more likely to survive in our difficult ancestral past" (Ref. 36, p. 32). That is why anxious and depressed people tend to monitor their peers' attitudes. Miller[36] makes it clear that those who are easily hurt are particularly concerned with the normative appropriateness of behavior, and are more motivated to avoid rejection by others. Nations, like people, can be depressed. They tend to think that other nations persistently measure their decline and pay more attention to their actions than they actually do. One might add that depressed nations, like depressed individuals, are excessively sensitive to the attitudes of others, quite unlike those with power, influence and self-respect, who may show a degree of disregard of their surroundings. That is particularly true of the groups and communities that adhere to the code of behavior which demands monitoring and protecting their 'honor.' Individuals who fail to establish a reputation as tough fighters and cannot protect themselves from potential insult are unlikely to deter potential thieves of their property. As a result, violating honor, perceived or real, is unbearable without settling of scores sometimes delayed for years and generations. Nisbett and Cohen,[37] who designated such populations "cultures of honor," show that they develop in environments where there is little law enforcement (such as frontier communities) and/or where wealth is easy to lose (e.g. herding economies). The presence of the culture of honor in the U.S. South as opposed to the North is an example of the validity of this psycho-anthropological conceptualization. Submitted to laboratory staged affronts, Southerners display more anger, manifest more physiological changes characteristic of stress, and behave more aggressively than Northern subjects. Nisbett and Cohen's book is not about terrorism, but about the world-views of people bound to clash in interacting with one another. It is abundantly clear that the culture of honor does not overlap precisely with the geographic map. Such suicidal murderers as Dylan Klebold and Eric Harris, mentioned above, were driven by perceived offences committed against them by their peers and fantasized about regaining their honor. But of course, some parts of Africa and the circum-Mediterranean that evolved from 'herding economies' in Nisbett and Cohen's parlance still retain in their code of behavior violence and homicide in the form of honor-related killings as protective devices against threat, displays of disrespect, or insults. We must not forget that Middle Eastern culture is not inferior, but different with dissimilar ethics, relationships with oneself, others and with God. The culture creates a psychological process of preparation in advance of perceived humiliation thereby determining the process termed, by Ariel Merari,[23] a mission with no return. Disconsolate, embittered, and depressed Arabs with their overblown sense of historical role, and guided by corrupt, tyrannical regimes that offer nothing to their insecure population following several bitterly fought and humiliatingly lost wars, speak of suicidal terrorists as the strategic answer to the dominance of the West and an offset of its military supremacy.

So what are the components of Herostratus syndrome? Let us consider the following six items:

- Signs of deep humiliation due to public revelation (actual or imagined) of either personal inadequacies (assumed or genuine) or those presumably shared via the membership in groups;
- Attribution of unhappiness and resentment to individuals who belong to salient factions or institutions;
- Relative prosperity of adversaries that is considered unfair;
- Feeling of being trapped in a punitive situation with no way of recovery from the current bleak state unless the enemy suffers recognizable injury or pain;
- A culture of redemption and recovery through retribution;
- Unquenchable craving for recognition and immortality.

These are not unusual requirements. "Is it not remarkable," Eric Gans[38] pondered in 1997, "that no one in history has equaled, let alone improved on, Herostratus' example?" Those who crashed the airplanes into the World Trade Towers or who self-explode in the marketplaces, hotels or restaurants of Israel, Bali or Kenya answered his question. Herostratus was certainly unearthed in the image of Osama Bin Laden. But the same applies to his less spectacular followers, even some comic creatures who were caught before they delivered the bomb. One might recall that in Jean-Paul Sartre's story, the protagonist was labeled *Erostratus*, even though he did not commit his intended crime, a wanton act of indiscriminate shooting on a busy street. He had only six bullets in his revolver and was ambivalent whether to leave six holes in the belly of the prostitute he wanted to see undressed, or to kill passersby. He never quite got the moods and messages of the world that passed by him and lives with a burning desire to kill, *seeing* 'revenge' in his mind's eye. He was thrilled in a Dostoevskian way by visualizing the panic-stricken victims "knocked off like clay pipes." In the court of law, the penalty for this pathetic, obsessive-compulsive and sexually incompetent thug might have been meager, assuming that his single victim remained alive. Moreover, in the end he had no nerve to commit suicide as imagined in this melodramatic scenario. Why then, use the ultimate name for a scoundrel? The beauty of Sartre's insight is in trivializing wickedness. 'Herostratism,' it seems, is not a unique mutation, but a common phenomenon, a symbol of vain, bizarre and blind vindictiveness that can easily possess many histrionic personalities. One of the readers of this chapter, Prof. N. Milgram, fittingly observed that even if the 'Final Solution' never happened, Hitler would have remained a member of the Herostratus club just because he ordered that Paris be burnt to the ground. One might wonder who are those who would be overjoyed had such a monstrous act happened.

Perverse Social Capital and Suicide

Herostratism might be rephrased in terms of a theory of comparison developed in the early 1950's by Leon Festinger (1919–1989), one of the dominant figures in social psychology in the US. The theory derives from the principle that people (and groups) have a need to socially compare themselves with others who are similar in some relevant aspects, particularly when they are uncertain about their abilities or find themselves participating in presumably inequitable relationships. Such 'information-seeking' is exhibited when the standards for comparisons on the issue in question are pretty fuzzy. In a contemporary society, a person may be unpopular or downright rejected for a number of reasons, not necessarily justified. In keeping with Festinger's theory, people tend to protect themselves against unfavorable social comparisons in the realm of possessions, marital relations, sports achievements, and economic and scholastic success since the view could be a potent source of mood changes. The same is true for group comparisons.

Illness can be described in terms of psychology, behavior and culture. Cultures of honor may well pose the question of "why we are not as successful as they are" in social comparison. This question is answered in a variety of ways since the channeling of frustration into political dialogue and political action in oppressive societies is limited. Unable to live by a code of honor, their chieftains moralize on the benefits of honorary death. It is intriguing that suicidal acts are common among humiliated people, particularly among adolescents with a sense of severe anxiety due to peer-group pressures or rejection regardless of their social circumstances.

This gives access through the back door to the notion of 'social integration,' interpersonal trust and norms of reciprocity. Admittedly, people living in societies with a high degree of social cohesion characterized by strong social networks and high levels of interpersonal trust may not be healthier than those living in socially disorganized societies, but they are less exposed to destabilizing stressors. As an equivalent of protection given by material capital, this sense of control, mutual ties and trust is known as '*social capital*.' There is a strong association between indicators of social capital (mistrust in government, crime, quality of work relations, civic engagement in politics) and life expectancy, as well as mortality rates.[39] Criminal behavior, also creates the sense of belonging (e.g. to a gang, mafia or terrorist group), not unlike that which is contributed by the membership in clandestine organizations, ethnic and religious groups and that often frees people from family ties and acts as their surrogates. The latter relations provide what was defined as '*perverse' social capital*.[40] Little is known as to how social capital might affect suicidal ideation and suicidal attempts. If I understand his view correctly, Merari appears to be partial to the role of 'perverse' social capital as the major determinant of the loyalties to the mission of terrorist's groups. It seems though that such militant groups simply map directly into the personal problem of potential victims, by shrewdly working on blowing up their misery to claim their allegiance. The allegiance

becomes bilateral since 'perverse' social capital presumably acts as a polariz-
ing factor by enhancing the sense of offence in those who feel exposed due to
failures in relationships, shameful infections, loss of jobs, collective (cultural)
insults and injured respect in honor cultures, i.e. adding to the list of demoral-
izing events and further fueling existing (subclinical) reactive depression. If we
assume that the potency of environmental triggers would be particularly convincing for those with deficient serotonin transporter genes then such indoctri-
nations might conceivably recruit the willingness to die. Here one might see
why Aaron Beck's[41] influential notion that depression is not a primary disorder
of mood, but the consequence of how the patient thinks about himself, his
world and the future seems so fitting to describe the state of health and mind of
suicide candidates.

The classical treatise of Emile Durkheim, *Suicide*, emphasized the role
of society, particularly the loosened bond among its members and the value
of communication. Promotion of such bonds was believed to mitigate
impulses of self-destruction. Durkheim's[32] notion that a desire to destroy
oneself is inversely related to the "degree of integration" in society still has
some currency with psychologists, sociologists and anthropologists. Perhaps,
such a communication deficit alluded to by Iyad Sarraj, a Palestinian human
rights activist and psychiatrist, may be akin to *alexithymia*. The latter term
was coined by Sifneos[42] to denote emotional malfunctioning and poverty of
fantasy life, inability to verbally describe one's emotions, as well as externalize one's thoughts. This is not entirely consistent with Arab culture, where
fantasy life is hardly impoverished, but might be consistent with deficiencies
in the ability to externalize as 'social capital.' Many ideas of Emil Durkheim
were continued into the cognitive domain by noticing that distress cannot be
effectively 'fragmented' and cushioned within the social network when one's
linguistic palette is inadequate to communicate sorrow, gloom and anguish.

Dr. Sarraj, who was interviewed by Bob Simon together with Dr. Merari
in the same show of *60 Minutes*, mused about the 'double-layer' wall of consciousness, so to speak, one for external and another for internal consumption:
"In this tribal society," admitted Sarraj, "we have two sets of language —
one for the public, which is a language of steadfastness ... a language of
being macho ... a language of being proud ... even of dying. Underneath of
course we're human beings and we suffer."(CNN.com; August 9, 2001.) He
believes that the suicide bombers do *not* have a violent trait: "[Suicide
bombers] usually were very timid people, introverted; their problem was

always *communication* ... ." He further acknowledges that many of them have had a problem with power in their childhood, and most of them have had personal experience with serious traumatic events in their lives, and particularly, witnessing the helplessness humiliation of their fathers. Ariel Merari (personal communication, February 23, 2003) indicated that the failed suicide bombers do not have a history of acting out, criminal records, or running away from home, and that the psychological profiles of some of them is consistent with Sarraj's description. These *calm* individuals would be quite likely to translate indoctrination into a determined suicidal assault. Given that Merari[23] has a unique experience, including that of conducting psychological autopsies on the majority of suicide Palestinian terrorists in the period of 1993–1998 (that has yet to be published), this admission carries significant weight. It remains to be seen whether Sarraj had alexithymia in mind, and if he did whether his comment was based on rigorous studies. His observation suggests, however, that the fact that the vast majority of terrorists do not appear to be suicidal in any clinical sense does not mean they do not have the common 'seeds' of vulnerability. The overall rate of mental disorders among the perpetrators of completed suicides based on psychological autopsy studies in different cultures may be as high as 90%.[43–45]

Coda

Let us sum up then. What has been affirmed is that suicidal *homo religio* belongs to the garden variety of suicide in that actions can be understood as contributed by (but not limited to) anxiety and depression. Scientists will continue debating whether there is a common denominator for all cases of suicidal death, including that of political terrorists, or, like cancer, it has numerous causes and dissimilar processes in different ages and places. Although sociological explanations of suicide are still popular in some quarters, the viewpoint presented here sides with a stance that the days of searching for the explanation of suicide in the inadequacies of the social order are numbered, and an awkward truce in neuropsychiatry is over. Recall George Minois's[4] warning:

"In spite of the innumerable sociological treatises that have appeared, we cannot say that the question [of the nature of suicide] has made any real progress on the plane of understanding since the day of the philosophers" (p. 328).

The agenda of contemporary psychiatry is hardly dominated by the question whether individual, "psychological" grounds for suicide are just a façade of the psychoneurological (read, molecular biological) causes, but rather by the question of what those are. This suggestion does not deny the fact emphasized by Merari,[23] that suicide bombers thrive in the backwater of hatred and indoctrination that facilitates the process of recruiting and training the bombers for their mission and loyalty to the group's goals. One might only add that such programming shapes up those deeply unhappy, frustrated, more vulnerable, lonely, and humiliated individuals into a determined and calm assassins. Suicidal behavior is known to be associated with greater manifestations of anger,[46] and aggression may well be associated with clinical depression.[30,47] Depressed patients score significantly higher on the Buss–Durkee Hostility Inventory, particularly on items of 'total aggression' (irritability, negativism, resentment, suspicion and guilt) and on 'inhibited aggression' and 'covert hostility.'[48]

Of course, not all examples of wickedness are psychopathology. The trick is in telling which is which. Bereavement-provoked hatred and the experience of wrath demanding retribution can complicate a lingering personal unhappiness and provide it with meaning. Yet, we would be somewhat out of touch pretending that there is nothing wrong with the psyche of terrorists trying to cremate people alive. In Eric Gans's view,[38] Herostratus is inflamed by an acute recognition of personal inadequacy combined with failure of 'marketability': "The more he realizes how justly the 'rational' social order evaluates him, the greater his resentment against humanity …." Sartre's insights demonstrate that Herostratus's state cannot be mitigated. Either he is mad for being recognized for what he really is or he exaggerates others' disdain and attention to his persona. In either case fighting contemporary Herostratism is a treacherous business because its religious fervor further rekindles a self-righteous rage.

Electing the problem and proposing its 'understanding' begs the question of what is its solution, its therapy. The term 'therapy' derives from the Greek word '*therapeia*,' which meant 'to serve' in an elevated sense of the word, 'to honor,' 'to show respect,' to furnish or supply with something desired, to answer the needs of a troubled human — but has evolved to become a term for medical or psychological intervention. Mass resentment and unhappiness can hardly be treated by medical means. Besides, the villains expect restoration of their sanity in revenge, and their grateful society applauds the effort. That does not mean that change is impossible. But the change calls, at a minimum, for a revaluation of some sources of personal humiliation. That is likely to happen. Queen Victoria was reluctant to let her physician examine her even with a stethoscope. Sir James Reid, her trusted physician for 20 years did not even know about her umbilical hernia and a prolapsed uterus until after her death. At this time, no presidential candidate can hope to be elected without submitting himself or herself to what once was considered a humiliating physical. It is more difficult when humiliation is nurtured in culture and we are polarized along religious and cultural lines. The question is, Can we hope to reduce the marketing of omnicide, say by sending the surviving villains to the state forensic facility? Highly esteemed psychoneurologist, Kurt Goldstein's[8] answered in his limpid prose:

"... voluntary suicide is sometimes the last way out in the attempt to preserve the personality. One has to be very careful in the evaluation of self-sacrifice, because it is often nothing more than an escape from the difficulties of normal self-actualization. If society has to ask for general self-sacrifice on the part of its members, then there is something wrong with the organization of that society" (p. 236).

It is doubtful that suicidal terrorists exhibiting manifestations attributable to humiliation/entrapment depressogenic stimuli[16,17] could be forcibly treated under current civil commitment law, unless we acquire a certified biological marker to medicalize criminals. The findings of molecular markers of depression inspire some hope that in the future, people at higher risk might be offered certain preventive procedures that would pre-empt the progression of depression to the stage when nothing is left to live for. Yet, given that over half of the Caucasian population has the short allele of the promoter region of the serotonin transporter gene[15] we have yet to learn when depression, aggression/irritability becomes directed against the self as opposed to its being directed against others (externalizing symptoms) or, more generally, when humiliation and hardships breed an unquenchable desire to overcome personal failing, rather than forcing innocent people into a personal hell. Besides, suicide bombers do not acknowledge their mental incompetence or express a need for treatment. In the culturally endorsed concept of depression, these individuals are considered fully capable of acting in the interests of *their* society as well as *their own* best interests. Thus, this question must await more research and its final 'therapeutic' solution should be provided *within* the insular and incendiary Islamic culture. It eludes me how exactly that has to be done. But eventually, everyone will be forced to look for an answer and health psychologists have to be proactive. I thus put the question before the prospective student of health psychology adding to it some thoughts in the following 'so what?'

SO WHAT?

When discussing suicide, investigators start dotting their papers with the term 'epidemic.' Epidemic metaphors can grow irksome. There are epidemics of depression, exploding obesity and diabetes, a juggernaut of aging baby-boomers, the cardiovascular scourge, crime, social plagues (e.g. ethnic cleansing in Rwanda and Sudan), the blight of AIDS and SARS, and now we live in the midst of epidemics of allergy. The word speaks to a deep and historically imprinted fear of being invaded by invisible agents, which in the past reduced the population of Europe by a quarter. Compared to all other epidemics, suicide is a distant rumble. We are *not* in the grip of an epidemic of suicide. And yet, of all afflictions discussed in this chapter, suicide associated with political terrorism has evolved into a complex international emergency that undermines the social and economic fabric of nations.

It is branded here as 'Herostratus syndrome,' a disorder of hostility, suspicion, blame of others, hatred and resentment along with insatiable longing for recognition. Nothing is known regarding the heuristics employed in selecting suitable candidates for suicidal missions. Despite the extensive literature on the nature of suicide from clinical studies, there is relatively little cross-cultural clinical evidence to make obvious predictions of suicidal scenarios. More experimental work in the natural cultural environment is needed.

The mass media is a powerful manipulator of public opinion. It thus becomes the major target of terrorists and their constituents. The citizens of Ephesus were so appalled at Herostratus's act they issued a decree to put his name out circulation. They did *not* succeed. In *Erostratus* by Sartre, the protagonist was easily exposed by a simple co-worker who correctly guessed his fantasies and his tendency to act out so as to compare his character with that of an ancient arsonist. The following exchange follows:

"And what was the name of the man who built the temple?"

"I do not remember," he confessed. "I don't believe anybody knows his name."

"Really? But you remember the name of Erostratus? You see, he didn't figure things out too badly."

With this revelation of the accessibility of postmortem fame, the evolution of the next villain was preordained.

This dialogue has another implication. Words count. They may inflame contemporary Herostraus on being immortalized by the media before he sees the glory of paradise. They can sway a member of an insular Islamic culture perhaps more effectively than they could the deranged Frenchman. Even a 'regular' suicider would find it more satisfying to die when assured of sympathy and respect of others. Incidentally, in Hungary, which has one of the highest rates of suicide, the media portrays it in romantic light.[49] Therefore, by avoiding the dramatic or quixotic representation of suicidal behavior in television reports, large sensational headlines in newspapers and lengthy depictions of morbid suicide in literature and movies are likely to deter some uncertain candidates. It would be helpful if reporting on suicide followed recommendations for the media by the American Foundation for Suicide Prevention (*www.afsp.org*).

As long as contemporary Herostratus becomes immortalized through the media spotlight before his passage into the next world, not to mention the ideological sanction, even glorification, of suicide bombing by their communities, this scourge is not likely to desist. It obeys the "law of corset": if you tighten it in one place, the bulge will appear elsewhere. It can only be contained within Islam, not outside of it.

5

---•---

Collective Exaggerated Emotions

This title is a recognizable euphemism for countless episodes of a collective psychogenic illness, such as menacing ecstatic possessions, bloody Maenadian rituals or the dancing mania of St. John the Baptist which began in 1374 on the Franco-German border and gradually spread epidemically to the neighboring Netherlands, Belgium, France and Italy. They are part of our remote history, even though a few pockets of contagious mass anxiety exist and may be easily produced *de novo*. Among them, excitement about the miraculous healing experiences within Catholic Pentecostal groups, speaking in tongues (glossolalia), sporadic episodes of prophetic frenzy, such as the 'Jerusalem syndrome,' or religious rituals like the one that occurred on May 17, 1984 when Madonna dell'Arco was said to begin to shed tears of blood. With the progressive transitions from one epoch to another, beliefs and worries from the old often transmute into the new. Their content evolves with technology and culture, which vary from one generation to another. Some individuals are in a state of perpetual readiness to react to their conscious or subconscious fears. In the Elizabethan age, people fell sick after being 'fascinated' or 'bewitched' by an evil eye. Nowadays, the public is more concerned about the mysterious effects of cosmic waves, chemicals with complex names that enter the body with food, foods which were genetically altered or exposed to high-energy photons, the malignant effects of electromagnetic radiation, the appearance of acute childhood leukemia that is associated with cumulative exposure to magnetic fields (such as those caused by police radar and cell phones) and shoplifting detectors' harm to pacemakers, as well as other concerns that revolve around hot topics such as global warming, ozone holes, pesticides, car exhaust emissions and road rage, AIDS and SARS, multiplication of unknown or mutated viruses, mercury poisoning while eating fish, genetic crop alteration, mad cow disease, or new topics covered by a popular poetic cliché, "waiting for the sky to fall," such as terrorists getting material for radioactive 'dirty bombs,' globalization, and many others. Although these frightening portents are not about to result in a devastating stampede or a mass exodus from cities, as some epidemics did in the past, they can have enormous economic repercussions. At the very least, some of these items provoke vigorous debate, animosity, and public demonstrations. In this chapter, the intention is to show that this arena of cultural psychiatry is of significant interest to health psychologists because it tells us much about the world in which we live.

Everyday Phobias

Madness, as Nietzsche pronounced facetiously, "is rare in individuals, but common in parties, groups and organizations." However, definition may be one of the most confusing parts of what signifies mass madness. That is why some authorities[1] view the notion of 'mass' or 'epidemic hysteria' to be an invention of Western psychiatry that should be replaced with the term *collective exaggerated emotions*, which emphasizes the presence of emotional excess in a bevy of vulnerable individuals, but does *not* include the obligatory components of irrationality, conversion symptoms and motor frenzy, as do such terms as 'group madness' or hysteria. Some are actually everyday events, which may not be perceived for what they are.

MMR Vaccine Scare

Consider the fever phobia that must have been experienced by parents of all socioeconomic classes when the temperature of their children approached 101 F. Poorly informed young parents are likely to panic because they believe that their child is at a significant risk for cognitive impairment. Another example of collective parental phobias is the relatively recent and continuing 'MMR vaccine scare.' It is named after the triple, measles-mumps-rubella (MMR) vaccine implicated in autism. The scare was unwittingly triggered by a consultant gastroenterologist of the Royal Free Hospital in London, Andrew Wakefield, who reported that 8 out of 12 children immunized with MMR had been diagnosed as autistic. The damage from Wakefield's publication was so great that the mounting evidence against a causal association between MMR vaccination and the risk of autism was hardly noticed.[2]

Autism is a tragic affliction. Parents see a doctor when their child shows no social reciprocity, does not try to attract attention of others when happy, or when he or she cannot coordinate vocalizations with intentions, and uses peripheral vision to look at objects. Some children with autism may recite the alphabet and recognize numbers, but may not orient to the sound of their names or follow a pointing gesture. They have deficient social communication, poor linguistic skills, and motor stereotypies. Autism may have a dissimilar course, and well over half of these children are mentally retarded. Only infrequently do adult individuals with autism gain successful employment. They almost never marry and only rarely do they form normal reciprocal friendships.[3] The overall incidence of autism might appear to have increased due to greater than before sensitivity of psychiatrists to the disorder following its introduction into the *Diagnostic and Statistical Manual of Mental Disorders* (DSM) as a pervasive developmental disorder. The incidence of newly diagnosed cases of autism increased sevenfold, from 0.3 per 10,000 persons in 1988 to 2.1 per 10,000 persons in 1999, whereas the prevalence of MMR vaccination was over 95% and virtually constant. It is not improbable that the increased awareness of autism followed the Dustin Hoffman Hollywood film '*Rain Man.*' Regardless of the reason, the pediatric 'vaccinophobia' and fear of autism acquired quite an instructive ring in the recent climate of bioterrorism as well as the controversy over the Gulf War syndrome.*

Anxiety about Mobile Phones

Electricity and mobile phone radiation from around us has created another cause for alarm. "Should you sleep on an electric blanket?" asked Allen D. Elster somewhat mischievously, in his book on magnetic resonance imaging. The question was motivated by some publications and rumors implicating electromagnetic fields in leukemia, brain tumors, Alzheimer's disease, asthma and allergies, and more recently, in itching, heat sensation, pain and

---

*The hunch that autism was caused by a pathogen, however speculative, was an acceptable hypothesis, inasmuch as it has a respectable nosological 'kin.' Since 1990, psychopathology was enriched by a new syndrome, that of *pediatric autoimmune neuropsychiatric disorders* (PANDAS).

skin eruptions (i.e. 'screen dermatitis') in people exposed to video display terminals. The current disquiet is associated with a few inconclusive publications suggesting that the low energy level emitted from cell phones, electric power lines and personal computers might also play a role in the etiology of psychological aberrations, sleep disorders and cancer. One may be able detect some neuronal responses in the future using more sensitive technology. The issue is how long it would take to achieve a harmful dose, if at all. Since such exposure is virtually unavoidable, the scare has become a well-publicized journalistic topic with allegations in the media and in the courts suggesting that cell phones and other types of hand-held transceivers cause malignancies, cognitive abnormalities, and even suicidal ideation. In spite of all the explanations and assertions that a risk from the cell phone-related radiation is physically implausible,[4,5] people feel uncomfortable.

Even Elster concludes his book with a recommendation of 'prudent avoidance,' meaning that the probable risks of electromagnetic exposure should be translated into 'decision-making processes, such as one's choice of home or job.' The understanding that the effects of chemical substances range from beneficial to harmful, depending on dosage, was voiced as early as at the time of Paracelsus (1493–1541). Clearly, the effects of bacterial agents and electromagnetic fields obey the same law. One cannot doubt Eslter's scholarship. Therefore, the incongruity between his beliefs in electromagnetic field safety and the recommendation to avoid them suggests that the dilemma of whether or not one opt for an electric blanket should be settled outside of the scientific domain.

Mysterious Gas Poisoning

In March–April, 1983, the odor of hydrogen sulfide (H_2S) escaping from a faulty latrine in the schoolyard caused a massive two-week epidemic of complaints of poisoning in three districts of the (formerly Jordan) West Bank region. The accusations in the mass media spurred public health authorities to identify and isolate the toxin. It turned out to be the emotional climate in Jenin Hospital that contributed to the generation and propagation of fears of "mysterious gas poisoning." One might think that this is a lacunar fear, only supported by the grotesque claims that Israelis intimidated by the fertility of the Arabs use chemical weapons and tear gas to increase abortions in Palestinian women, or that depleted uranium shells were used to inflict a lasting genetic damage on the Palestinian population, and so on. Yet, a similar episode was recorded in McMinnville, Tennessee in November 1998 when a teacher at the high school noticed a "gasoline-like" smell in her classroom that made her dizzy, nauseous, drowsy, and short of breath. Several students who were with her at the time and presumably watched her symptoms closely soon developed similar manifestations. As the word spread and the afflicted individuals were rushed to hospital, the fire alarm was sounded and the school was evacuated. A few days later, the school was reopened but then again, a few more students became symptomatic and were rushed to the emergency room. Overall, about 10% of people there reported symptoms seemingly associated with exposure even though 3,000 hours spent by examiners revealed nothing hazardous and helped little to allay the fears. Likewise, none of the putatively exposed persons actually became ill.[6] The symptoms were not accompanied by positive physical signs or by laboratory findings.

The commentators of Jones' paper[6] argued that volatile toxins such as hydrogen sulfide due to sewer gases causing odor/fumes could potentially cause autonomic reactions in a fraction of people. Studies carried out around hazardous waste sites in California, through which the main route of exposure was low-level parts per billion concentrations of either gaseous emissions or airborne dust particles, show that more profuse symptoms are found primarily in those who commonly complain of odors or who are worried about environmental chemicals. Interestingly, of the 94 affected individuals in the 'Jenin epidemic,' 77% were adolescent females. The olfactory system in women is far more sensitive than in men. Some researchers on sex differences in olfaction have even suggested that this female trait be added to other secondary sex characteristics (*'un charactére sexuel secondaire féminine'*).[7] Donald F. Klein's influential model of 1993 attributes spontaneous panic accompanied by the 'hyperventilation syndrome,' palpitations, tremors, faintness and a *false suffocation alarm* to carbon dioxide hypersensitivity. This theory is still a widely discussed metaphor for a complex defensive response of the respiratory/homeostatic brainstem malfunction developing in response to threat. In the present context, the issue of the veracity of his model is less relevant than the question of why this presumably phylogenetically old response of a few can be so contagious to so many. The change of emphasis of inquiry is to look at the disorder not so much from the viewpoint of individual vulnerabilities, but from the perspective of its power to propagate between individuals of a social group. What is the nature of this social contagion? Does it need to be based on fear? Recall a comic episode in

Rob Reiner's 1989 film *When Harry Met Sally* when Sally (played by Meg Ryan) fakes an orgasm while lunching in a deli. A woman seated at the neighboring table immediately orders her meal: "I'll have what she's having." Such an automatic tendency to capture emotions and bodily states of others and be swayed by them is at the core of many crowd reactions and mass hysteria that may include both corporeal and frank hallucinatory components (*http://jom-emit.cfpm.org/1998/vol2/marsden_p.html*).

Radiophobia

In these uneasy times, the public is also concerned about being potentially exposed to ionizing radiation. The fear is associated with recognized harm to pregnancy, including that of teratogenicity, accelerated aging, morbidity and mortality from cancer and all other causes in populations exposed to diagnostic or environmental radiation. Radiophobia is also costly as it requires billions of dollars annually for the protection against hypothetical risks of low-level radiation exposure. Professionals are not immune to the fear and today, more than ever before, the public media may present a regular finding to sound as an alarm. Recently, the *JAMA* (*http://jama.ama-assn.org*) published a standard epidemiological paper indicating that women who have a dental X-ray during pregnancy are three times more likely to give birth to a low birthweight baby than those who do not. The *New Scientist* (*www.newscientist.com/news*) found it of interest to inform its readers about the result. Within a little over a week after this publication, this finding was known to all. The Google search engine generated almost 50,000 hits for the terms 'dental X-rays' and 'low birthweight,' which piggybacked on this information. These findings were certainly alarming inasmuch as they challenged the current view that during pregnancy only direct exposure of reproductive organs is of grave concern. But they were intended primarily to alert radiologists.

What could be so sensitive in the head-and-neck region as to be responsible for the observed relationship at dose level of under 0.4 mGy? According to ambivalent authors of the study, the thyroid is likely to be implicated. It has yet to be established and examined why the thyroid was not protected in these patients. Every student knows that an association is not a cause. There are indications that orally induced bacteremia is intimately related to systemic health, including that of pregnant women. Periodontal disease, in itself may be associated with preterm and low birthweight babies. Those who were exposed to diagnostic X-rays were likely to have in addition some other health confounders not accounted for in that study, and perhaps, unrelated to ionizing radiation. Why then was this paper singled out as a news item? The answer is simple. Uncomplicated risk statements associated with health care delivery are the most important determinant of whether a regular professional publication will be noticed by the public media and the public.

These supposed risks are fueled by a debate among experts regarding radon hazards at low doses and dose rates, particularly due to uncertainties as to whether residential radon exposure causes lung cancer. The need for *absolute* public safety is partly driven by the linear, no-threshold model, predicting a gradual increase of the cancer risk with the dose of radiation. In accordance with the precautionary attitude, residents are encouraged to find alternative housing or engineer amendments of their habitat at a substantial cost. Despite the fact that in many scientific investigations no evidence for the danger of residential exposure has been shown, people are still not feeling secure. Many sense, in light of negative findings or contradictory evidence, that scientists missed something. In reality, a great deal of experimental and epidemiologic evidence indicates that low-dose radiation damage to DNA is negligible and the DNA damage-control biosystem is actually stimulated by low-dose radiation (i.e. exhibits a 'hormetic effect'). The gist of this protective outcome is that it presumably induces an efficient chromosome-break repair mechanism that, if present at the time of the challenge with high doses of radiation, would result in less damage after the exposure. Much of the arguments have been detailed elsewhere[8] to illustrate the point that good medicine and solid research is not enough to sway the deadly industry of litigation. The gist of it is that the fear of danger outweighs the numerous findings about the potential benefits of low level exposure.*

Concerns over the safety of irradiation of raw meat and other products that are marked with a "radura" symbol in grocery meat cases is another example of public anxiety. Efforts to sterilize foodstuffs with X-rays date from the beginning of the 20th century. Doses from 0.5 to 1.5 kGy are required to inactivate some common food-borne pathogens. A maximal dose is set by FDA at 7 kGy (for frozen beef). No damage is caused by this treatment to the nutrients, flavor, or health of its potential consumers. Only expert

---

*A useful source of information on radiophobia and hormesis can be found in URLs referring to studies by J.R. Cameron and S.M. Javad Mortazavi (e.g. *www.angelfire.com/mo/radioadaptive*).

cooking can guarantee a comparable level of safety. Cindy Skrzycki of the Washington Post of April 29, 2003 wrote in her article *Fallout over Irradiated Food in School Lunches* that fear was reactivated with an introduction of irradiated food into the school lunch program in the 2002 farm bill. Some parents were passionate about not allowing even the option of irradiated beef. "Why would you want to prohibit it," asked James H. Hodges, president of the American Meat Institute Foundation, which does research on food safety, "if there are no safety and health questions." Clearly aware of the style of debates on risk factors, he answered his own doubt with the realization that people are concerned with hair-raising 'what-ifs': "What if the sky falls?"

'Malignant Epidemic Trenditis' of Globalization

Fashion is a benign epidemic that waxes and wanes through seasons, times and cultures. It can be attributed to peer pressure or what Taylor,[9] a master observer with a quick wit, called *sheep's disease, crowd madness, the silly syndrome* and the "*lie down and be counted*" syndrome. There are some more malignant forms of sheep's disease or '*epidemic trenditis*,'[9] such as tattooing and body piercing. Body piercing and scarification is traditionally practiced by contemporary tribal societies especially in Africa, Asia, and South America, but were relatively uncommon in the Western world. Some beautiful images of African women portrayed by Amedeo Modigliani convey his fascination with their scarified necks and faces. Displayed for all to scrutinize, these young women parade an instantly recognizable record of their new roles in the tribe that were caused by puberty; they speak of what should be expected of their bodies, or tell about their pain endurance, a feature essential for childbirth. The skin mutilations are thus plainly communicative of one's personal status much like the records made in our resumés (CVs). They cannot be altered on demand nor could one evade the traditional body mutilation without escaping the tribe. By contrast, in Western civilization, being 'labeled,' was always synonymous with being 'tainted,' branded as an animal and certainly unthinkable for an honest man, particularly a man of self-control, authority and position ('*honestus*'). It was unquestionably prohibitive for women's identity since nothing is concealed under God's omniscient eyes.

   Tattoos were apparently imported by sailors, who marked themselves and their slaves, and then the practice was taken on by the underclass, such as prostitutes and criminals operating around major ports. It is said to have been some sort of language among French criminals and a sign of a positive

Wassermann reaction overall. Even in medical circles, where bare bodies were commonly seen, this fashion was improper. "Who are they," asked McDonald Critchley,[10] "those who elect to be marked — if not marred — in perpetuity?" In his essays, he showed a picture of a man who turned his entire body into a canvas. His patient's bowed back and sagging skin grotesquely contrasted with the bravado of the art, which probably looked more relevant in his younger years and communicated his social standing.

Critchley assumed that doctors could make an interesting contribution to this topic if not for the fact that "the tattooist is becoming more and more a rarity." He was mistaken. That association of criminality with body mutilation has irrevocably changed, much as the rules about hiding one's nudity. By the 1970s, skin artists were increasingly in demand since body mutilations became common practice among members of the punk movement looking for a means to shock, provoke and challenge mainstream tastes. On similar motivations, body piercing became popular with teenagers who were rejected by their family and friends due to their unorthodox behaviors or homosexual practices. It was a marker for a rebellious expression of independence from the family unit even though there is no firm data to prove that claim. Tattooing communicated a sense of social acceptance within the narrow group of misfits, their mutual social bonding, and thus by sharing a problem the label rescued its owners from their insularity and anxieties.

The tides of immigrants from Africa and Asia must have returned to body mutilations their original 'normative' marker status. One might wonder whether the identification with the poor, misunderstood, exotic, naive and often helpless in our boundary-free culture is now carved on the skin as the ID for empathy by some individuals who are more capable than others of exhibiting shared positive or negative emotions. Unwittingly, in this new interdependence of the world's markets and businesses that have dramatically broken speed limits in the last two decades as technological advances have made it easier for people to travel, communicate, and do business internationally, tattooing and piercing have become a sort of modern gobbledygook for that connectivity. Although globalization (the G-word) has become an ugly word for some, almost a term of abuse in liberal circles, it also made most of the world more tolerant of the newcomers from Africa and India, in particular when their customs were lovingly exhibited by movie idols and popularized by the media. Is this a reason why tattooing was so readily accepted? An example in point is tattooing henna (an extract of the plant

Lawsonia intermis) designs on the body, a popular oriental cultural tradition in Marocco or India, where it is called *mehndi*. It would have hardly been noticed and might have remained culturally endemic if not for the fact that Madonna had her hands decorated mehndi-style for one of her pop videos. Suddenly, henna body mehndi art has become a mass obsession and a global business, as a popular alternative to the traditional, permanent tattoo. Since the late 1990's, however, dermatologists began to report allergic contact dermatitis, attributed to a chemical agent (paraphenylenediamine) that is added to produce a faster effect with so-called "black henna" (*http://dermatology. cdlib.org/91/original/henna/wolf.html*).

With the invention of the electric needle, and the adoption of better hygienic standards, the art of tattooing and body piercing has become big business. Buzz McClain reports in *The Washington Post* (February 11, 2003) that his wife of 10 years and vice president of public relations for a large food service company, acquired a stainless steel ring and a pewter-colored glass bead where her bare navel used to be. Today, as rules and manners have relaxed, something that previously was considered 'intimate' (i.e. below the neck) is now a legitimate, if not widely shared, public rite. According to a Chicago cosmetic surgeon McClain interviewed, in the last two years there has been a tenfold increase in bellybutton piercing among customers above the age of 35. Such an ornament may not be seen by many, much as a similar jewelry placed in the nipples or genitals,[11] but there are several visible piercing locations such as the high-ear rim, nose, lips, labret (the area right above the chin), eyelids, neck, and the tongue that are widely used by a new brand of consumers. 'Love parades,' particularly the annual parade in Berlin, provides an adequate display of the art. If these tattoos and mutilations do not shock us today, it is because they have become as habitual a phenomenon as the unwearable outfits of contemporary supermodels.

The readiness of some in assimilating sanctions for personal behaviors and body changes in cues given off by others, as well as scaling personal conduct to those seen or publicized was considered in the past as suggestive of hysteria. The latter was alleged to be "the pathological intensification of a flair (*Anlage*) which exists in each person."[12] If everyone, as Paul Julius Möbius claimed, "is ... a little hysterical," hysteria may be easily invigorated by intense media attention, such as the coverage of the *Time* magazine of April 29, 2002 that ran a story on tattooing as "something not entirely negative." The media provides cognitive or emotional cues that elicit resonance in many people who otherwise would not have recognized them if left to their own perceptual devices. These cues may also be sanctioned on the fringe of our 'cultural avant-garde,' as an alluring pastime with mild symptoms of legitimate insanity.

The *Lancet* recently printed an engaging paper[11] that described and lavishly illustrated many untoward effects associated with body piercing. When presenting psychological data, its author shifted gears to plead for a sympathetic and accepting attitude, so as to "diminish any prejudices held by health professionals against people with piercings." Since body modification has become social reality, she suggests, piercing and tattooing should be "understood" and considered normal. The definition of 'normal' carries with it the risk of overlooking pathologic features in tattooing. By the same logic we should make suicide, overeating, allergy, and diabetes the norm. A climate of non-judgmental attitudes does not rule out other options, including remedial practices since the fact that individuals now tend to mark some 'special moments in their lives' on their bodies rather than on the pages of diaries or a calendar cannot be branded culturally sound. In health psychology, as in engineering or system management, one needs to establish whether the source of malfunction is external or internal before making recommendations. Without such analysis the Lancet's paper[11] becomes an example of what has been designated[13] "infotainment." By disseminating premature normative statements the infotainers are capable of misleading the therapists, particularly when there is a receptive environmental, legal, religious or sociopolitical milieu that holds together once independent individuals aggregated into a single homogenous swarm. That magic glue helps like pheromones to recognize beliefs by others as valid in the individual's subculture. It has been dubbed the "power of context."[14]

Mimesis and Mass Anxiety

What does it mean to share anxiety in a world populated by fretful people? This implies — one is tempted to say — the capacity to read other people's emotions, identify with them, be driven by them and ultimately *reproduce* them. The Greek notion of *mimesis* assumes sensual and intellectual affinity that are crucial for imitation and subsequently learning and cultural sharing. It has come to symbolize the understanding of interindividual relations and reading intentions, wishes and fears transmitted from one individual to another and the capacity to magnify them.

'Resonance' is a term, borrowed from physics, used in psychology to describe the augmenting of personal responses based on implicit input from others. It is based on an assumption that we are capable of predicting relevant intentions and behaviors of others and of taking account of their actions as though they communicate reliably what is happening in the world around us. This is not a safe assumption. Sir Kenneth C. Calman[16] reminded us of the Kantian hunch that "we see things not as they are, but as we are." An individual response to stress begins with one's interpretation of the stimulus that is carried out by an 'information processor' which takes into account one's developmental stage, education, individual and societal history, as well as one's gender and 'modes of consciousness.'[15] Essentially, this capacity builds on orienting mechanisms that identify objects and events, and establish a 'space of communicative behaviors' by providing meaning to forms and symbols, and then binding them with the trajectories of locomotion and posture. The nature of intersubjectivity is a mysterious operation of our sensory and associative networks that require an integrated functioning of the cerebral hemispheres, where according to William James (1842–1910), control of 'mental action' and consciousness reside. Recently, a more precise address for the intersubjective resonance has been proposed. That 'address' was also consonant with the sentiments of Albert Szent-Gyorgi (1893–1986): "The brain is not an organ of thinking but an organ of survival, like claws and fangs. It is made in such a way as to make us accept as truth that which is only advantage. It is an exceptional, almost pathological constitution one has, if one follows thoughts logically through, regardless of consequences. Such people make martyrs, apostles, or scientists, and mostly end on the stake, or in a chair, electric or academic."

Mirror Neurons

An Italian neurophysiologist, Giacomo Rizzolatti[17] and his colleagues at the University of Parma identified a subset of neurons in the ventral premotor area of the frontal lobes of a macaque's brain that discharge when the monkey watched someone else perform a task (e.g. the experimenter's hand picking up an object). The puzzling thing about these cells was that they neither reacted to the object nor registered the movement itself. Rather they fired when the monkey would do a similar thing to the object in its mind's eye. These nerve cells were called 'mirror' neurons, because they seemed to be endowed with an observation-execution matching capacity as though 'acknowledging' that the experimenter's activity was agreeable. The novelty of this finding was evident in light of the accepted conviction that the motor cortex is confined to the subservient, passive job of controlling movements of the opposite side of the body. The coexistence within the same neuronal system of motor and sensory properties dispelled this view. It showed that the motor neurons not only trigger actions, but also internally represent them as 'motor ideas.'

These motor ideas aid in the understanding actions made by others and might also be indispensable for the semantic categorization of objects.[18] Likewise, in the realm of feeling, sensory cells or cells in the limbic system might conceivably respond to guessed sensation or emotion as well as to real emotional stimuli. The area where mirror neurons were initially located is known as area F5, which is presumably homologous to the human Broca's region, which receives input from the inferior parietal lobule. Therefore, these findings excited a number of neuroscientists working in such diverse areas as language, consciousness, and the theory of mind. For some, mirror neurons are part of a network of *grasping* (insight through 'mimicking') what is going on in the minds of others.[19] The fact that such ideational emulation is not followed by an overt locomotion in a waking primate suggests the presence of ideational rehearsal of copying or imitation behavior with aborted output that, according to Rizzolatti, represents a larval mechanism for recognizing actions made by others. Based on the proposed homology between area F5 in the monkey's brain and human's Broca's region, they speculate that these neurons represent a prerequisite for the development of phonetic gestures and ultimately, speech. These neurons presumably bridge the notions of 'doing' and 'communicating' by turning doing into communicating. A slight benefit in survival terms afforded by this new mechanism of 'acting in the world' on learned information must have produced genetic changes for generating signals representing objects.[20] Non-human primates, like people it turns out, spend a great deal of time watching and, presumably, interpreting the actions of others. This could, indeed, be the source of language comprehension, but — no less likely — it might be the foundation of compassion and the reason for emotions being *contagious*.

Some inspired theorists have suggested an array of possibilities for mirror neurons. On the heels of this discovery, Ramachandran[21] of the University of California at San Diego proposed that mirror neurons have evolved in order to fulfill another purpose before they were utilized for language. He studied patients who developed a complete paralysis of the left side of their body following right hemisphere stroke, but were not aware of their deficit, being otherwise lucid and intelligent. Such patients are said to have anosognosia. Surprisingly, some of them not only denied their own paralysis, which was previously well-known, but also rejected the presence of paralysis of another patient whose inability to move his arm was clearly visible to them and to others. Said differently, by losing control over one's body image, one cannot *grasp* the difference of one's action from those performed by someone else. It seemed as though the right hemisphere is involved in the monitoring of visuo-motor patterns required for interactions with others. In a study conducted by Seger and colleagues,[22] functional MRI was used to monitor brain activation when the participant generated the first verb that came to mind in response to the presentation of novel and repeated nouns (priming test) and then generated either an unusual verb or the first verb to come to mind to novel nouns (unusual test). Under the former conditions, there was increased activity in the *left* inferior prefrontal cortex, whereas under the latter conditions, there was increased activity in the *right* middle and superior frontal gyri, the left middle frontal gyrus, and the two sides of the cerebellum. Thus, Ramachandran's notion seems to be consistent with the findings that the right hemisphere may have an advantage over the left hemisphere in processing distant semantic associations, which are desirable for metaphoric comprehension or resolving lexical ambiguities.[22] The other possibility is that the right superior frontal cortex aids in these tasks by securing the presence of reflection.[23]

Ramachandran attributed this bizarre 'double denial' of patients with hemineglect to the deficit of mirror neurons. This interpretation is in keeping with Trevarthen's insight mentioned above that 'intersubjectivity' is an evolutionary extension of 'intentional subjectivity.' For a human being, the ability to recognize one's own sensations and to build on them a picture of one's collective relations is the primary mission of consciousness and social intelligence. An inability to recognize the self and extend it for establishing the milieu of common signals means social demise. Thus, mirror neurons must have evolved to solve personal problems in the social domain and only much later were they utilized for tasks outside collective needs. They may be related to language in a restrictive sense of appreciating and communicating intentions of others, and particularly some scenarios of danger that might be of relevance to group activities. They helped making sensible decisions rapidly and on limited information when 'cause-effect' contingencies were uncertain. For example, emotionally charged information could have been transmitted by protolanguage with a fixed number of calls. Such emotional calls, like prosody, may be localized in the right hemisphere, probably together with the engine of orienting responses. Ramachandran further suggests that autism might be associated with a loss of mirror neurons since the afflicted child cannot understand or empathize with others emotionally or gesturally, and consequently withdraws from family members and caregivers. He muses: "It's as if anytime you want to make a judgment about someone else's movements, you have to run a VR (virtual reality) simulation of the corresponding movements in your own brain and without mirror neurons you cannot do this." Of course, 'emulating an action' is not mind reading, nor is it relevant for chatting about the intentions of others. But it seems tempting to speculate that by processing the movements of others, mirror neurons have become an instrument for *Homo* to discover himself. They might have taught the developing brain to learn by imitation and discern emotions and intentions from what the bodies of others involuntarily broadcast. Yet mirror neurons can make their owner autistic or mentally incompetent if their firing is fixed at a stage of development that imposes the view that other people's acts and thoughts merely parallel those of the observer.

Excited by the discovery of 'mirror neurons,' Ramachandran loaded on them more tasks than they could possibly carry, such as facilitation of imitative learning, tool use, and ultimately, mastery of art and mathematics. One may wonder, though, why these neurons have so hopelessly failed in evolving the monkeys' brain to a higher level of consciousness and or self-awareness. After all, monkeys are experts at reading each other's emotional expressions and behavior.[24] The answer may be that these cells might have had a more modest yet a crucial role in securing the survival of the species. They must have helped to derive from the signs of fear in others the presence of danger for the self. These neurons might have organized a network that coached the brain to represent situations that either do not faithfully represent any specific predator or the proximity of others in a limited ethological repertory of the species.[20]

A more interesting property of mirror neurons might be in extending *extrinsic exploration* exhibited by any animal to that of *intrinsic exploration*, which, as Berlyne defined it,[25] is the kind of discovery "that introduces stimuli that can be said to be rewarding in themselves, regardless of any instrumental activity that they evoke" (p. 289). In addition, mirror neurons allowed for the processing of objects and stimuli that an individual is familiar with, but which are perceptually not available in the immediate environment.[26] One may guess that hominids who had such neural machinery were proficient in acquiring a new social function, thereby obtaining a high place in the hierarchy of other hominids, previously established by sheer aggressiveness and brutal force. With this new brain engine, humans have attained the ability to 'react' off-line when reacting meant 'reflecting.' This pun is intended to remind one of the gift of generating what Irving Maltzman calls the cognitive orienting response that enables "level 2 abstractions," that is, thinking of something that does not exist in the current environment, but resembles the patterns created by past sensory input. This ability is clearly not unique to humans.

Alessandra M. Umiltà and colleagues[26] demonstrated that a subset of mirror neurons becomes active not only during action display, but also when the final part of that action, and the one that is crucial for triggering the response in full vision, is *hidden and can therefore only be inferred.* These neurons respond to the experimenter's performance (grasping an object) very much as if the latter were in full view. When the action only emulated the grasp without seizing the object (imitation control), a neuron failed to respond, although what the monkey saw differed only in his 'knowledge' of either the presence or absence of the object. Thus, these neurons illustrate, contrary to the old chestnut, as the authors posit that "out of sight" is not necessarily "out of mind." This implies that the motor representation of an action performed by others can be internally generated in the observer's premotor cortex *off-line* when a visual description of the action is lacking, thereby providing the basis for guessing an action of interest. In full compliance with the notion of Darwinian evolution, those who maintained such rudiment capabilities of inferring others' intentions ('others' minds'), and have consequently developed suspicions to cues that had previously been ignored by others, became 'evolutionary agents' (in Stephan Jay Gould's words), and the reason why mirror neurons have remained in place.

In his essay, *The Social Function of Intellect*, Nicolas Humphrey proposed that society must have been the driving force behind primate intelligence. A group functions like one big organism, almost purposefully, supporting, nurturing and punishing for mutual survival. Although predators must have posed an occasional danger, a more relevant menace came from the aggressive members of the primitive herd who jealously watched feeding and sexual privileges. Young monkeys are particularly vulnerable to threats, and juveniles were observed to be more likely to respond with alarm calls.[24] The situation of confrontation between 'strong and aggressive' and 'hungry and timid' was always asymmetrical; the winner was capable of appropriating the entire resources. Some 'clever' timid primates must have *stood out* in their capacity to monitor the dangerous impulses and moods of others. With this capacity they must have discovered their individuality, or their individual existence independent of the collective one. The word to 'exist' originates from the Latin verb *existere*, meaning to stand out, to come into being. These individuals stood out in their ability to devise an alternative strategy when outranked. A weak rhesus macaque would not fight back. Instead, he might have chosen to confront the bullies by yelling to a high-ranking mother to come to the rescue. In linguistic terms these screams were less than 'expressive' and recruiting a 'big brother' was often a bogus call, but it helped.

Trickery and shrewdness clearly indicates foresight and the ability to 'read others' intentions and to forecast their responses. This kind of smartness of the weak in a power struggle was branded 'Machiavellian intelligence.'[27] Perhaps, by providing sensitivity and ability to deploy specific alarm responses to implicit threats, mirror neurons were an obvious selection advantage, particularly for the physically weak but ambitious members of the colony. Some timid, subordinate vervet monkeys are known to occasionally emulate leopard cries that, which all other members of the colony into the trees, thus enabling them to enjoy in solitude a palatable food item.[24]

Although useful in maximizing social success, this stratagem had its limitations. In the end, in the quest to secure his genes every individual was ultimately on his own. Excessive agitation and displays of apprehension must have become a reproductive drawback whenever the repertoire of emulation posturing, threatening vocalizations, facial expressions, and gestures signaling danger to others caused false alarms ('excessive noise') in an increasingly complex social environment. One way to mitigate the effects of false alarms is via the process of habituation when the primitive herd would ignore the cheat. However, habituation is a very unreliable shield that might bring about dehabituation, and thus an even more vigorous response. The other problem is that an obsessive 'reading' of others' thoughts and motives, particularly of those directed against the observer, might lead to a dead end and ultimately be of a delusional nature. Among humans, it is typical of the schizotypic personality[28] and bona fide schizophrenic patients.[29]

People are expert at analyzing events in terms of social dangers, perhaps because the primitive herd has selected to function as a social group. As millennia went by and the manufacture of tools was perfected, the value of individual initiative became more advantageous than the collective reactivity of the protohominid herd. Therefore, it might have been preferable for the species to curtail the fright signals of their sensitive brethren, so as to thwart uncontrolled collective panic responses. The mirror neurons must have been too costly triggers of emotional group behaviors, and consequently some evolutionary 'shackles' must have gradually evolved. There is obviously an evolutionary paradox in the need to place a novel, highly sensitive mechanism of communal behavior under tight control. Natural selection might have worked to inhibit emotional responsiveness via higher-order intentionality, for example, by attributing to such panicky members either deceptive intentions (e.g. attempts to hide food) or an inability to correctly assess predators' proximity. A variation in the condition of the genetic group with an emphasis on *individual* rather than crowding, assembling, flocking and collective fight or flight responses should have facilitated a compliance with this requirement. Humans have not lost a predisposition to react to treacherous stimuli, nor have they stopped updating knowledge of their own and strangers' social relationships by deploying Machiavellian intelligence. Rather, we have acquired a wide range of personal strategies for coping with dangers by negotiating with one another, inhibiting an impulse to run, looking for the Almighty's blessing, or just nailing a horseshoe at the entrance of our dwellings. One is tempted to conjecture that by harnessing the mirror neurons, the human brain has become capable of seeing beyond the emergency of the orienting response, plotting a path for further actions, engaging in long-term planning and prediction, and contemplating the future. This course of action was probably completely new, since the panicky primitive had not been able to accomplish it before. That does not mean that with it, socially shared emotions ceased to exist. They underwent some socially acceptable face-lifting. That leads us to the next point.

Prometheus versus Epimetheus

Remote history suggests that among other causes, mass sickness and death are the most likely sources of socially shared anxiety. That makes acts of anticipated bioterrorism so dreadful. The mistake is to suppose that terrorists would use a weapon that goes off with a dramatic bang, or produce a visible cloud of germs. As an oft-quoted line from a 1925 T.S. Eliot's poem bleakly predicted, "This is the way the world ends/ Not with a bang, but with a whimper." That may be something packaged in "handfuls of ashes from a furnace." The most popular explanation of the biblical 'plague' is that of anthrax. It is interpreted as the first example of God-inspired weaponized bacteria that causes black necrotic central skin eruptions leading to the deaths of people and domestic animals on such a scale as to be recorded in the collective memory of the Hebrews. On November 21, 2001, anthrax spores were found in US Senate offices, and were spread by mail-sorting machines by postal facilities in New Jersey and Washington. The spores became airborne mostly by roughly handling or opening the envelopes. Predictably, though, the outbreak of an epidemic was contained.

"So the LORD said to Moses and Aaron, 'Take for yourselves handfuls of ashes from a furnace, and let Moses scatter it toward the heavens in the sight of Pharaoh. And it will become fine dust in all the land of Egypt, and it will cause boils that break out in sores on man and beast throughout all the land of Egypt.'"
EXODUS 9:8–9

Anthrax, in all of its forms, is certainly a dangerous illness, but it hardly tops the list of most contagious infections. There are a dozen others that we dread. Therefore, when we speak of biological warfare in general, barring the inoculation of all healthcare workers and the vulnerable population against all possible deadly infections, the systematic threat of a sophisticated terrorist system makes the cost of defense so unbearable that civilized society could hardly find an answer to any conceivable bacteriological scenario. Intruding into civil liberties and spending money to achieve doubtful public bio-safety do not seem prudent options. In a world with thousands of bacteriological labs that are potentially able to produce or modify lethal pathogens, the national budget of the Department of Homeland Security for biological countermeasure programs would never be adequate. Not surprisingly, defenses in the form of offensive warfare have become a more pertinent strategy for confronting terrorism, particularly that of radical Islam.

The question on our mind these days is what if more than a handful of fine dust is sprayed over our cities? After September 11, 2001, the poignant 'what if' is no longer a relevant question, but rather 'when' more wicked attacks will happen. An informed choice about potential options requires information that allows weighing up the benefits and drawbacks of action as opposed to continuing normal life. Yet, understanding such information requires specialized knowledge, and yet more information, and then still more. So, how much information do we really need when we feel in danger, given that anyway in most cases, people's decision-making is not strictly rational?[30,31] One cannot say. The rule of thumb is that the more information the public *desires*, the more acutely its deficit will be perceived (most of us know very little about pathogens that may be used by potential terrorists) given an urgent need for survival and safety. Much of what we fear is the novelty of menace. We would not panic if the news media were to inform us that the sanitary conditions in our restaurants are poor and that we are often served substandard foods. After all, that would just be a drop in the ocean, compared with the 76 million cases of food-borne disorders that cause 5,000 deaths annually, or the 300 annual deaths caused by 60,000 chemical leaks and explosions in the US.[32] Another eloquent example is that Americans face a more real threat in the form of cancer. On balance, 1,550 Americans die each day of malignancies. "Imagine," wrote Coffey[33] in 1997, "five fully loaded jumbo jets crashing with no survivors on the same day."

When searching for tactical options as to what to do we have been guided since the dawn of civilization by subconscious or conscious monitoring of other people's unease. One might wonder why our 'mirror neurons' do not trigger a contagious scare more often than they commonly do? As speculated above, a possible reason might be that mirror neurons cannot easily find output to our motor system for flight because evolution managed to place them under tighter neuronal control. That must have caused dissociation between an individual's and the crowd's responses to threats. Imagine the sensational event when a group suddenly disregarded a sham alarm, or did not follow a genuine flight of one of the primates and that response proved to be a smart one and a beneficial, too, for they did not abandon their territory. Such self-possession must have gradually curtailed the episodes of group terror of what we now call *socially shared emotions*. That was presumably the real 'Big Bang' in human evolution. That does not mean that the catalysts of socially shared anxieties vanished.

In the majority of people, potentially perilous and clandestine cues may alter behavior only slightly on a model of subliminal priming so that they or other people would remain clueless about a threat. Recognizing the latter, most people will not panic, simply because we all commonly view hazards as more risky for others than for ourselves.[34] The first hint of fear when threatened might take the form of suppressed worries that would invade consciousness as Wegner's rebound "white bear" intrusions (Chap. 4a). Next, a number of those who have a greater ability to infer other's people mental states would be more eager to monitor their own health and then experience symptoms, real or bogus that would require a 'rational' explanation. And so, larval socially shared sensation would take its first step.

The propensity to 'rationalize' the baffling and mysterious is part of our mental programming aimed at providing an explanation, even a bizarre one, so that the mystery will not remain unsolved. What can be done while waiting until health authorities or government pronounce the 'truth,' and that provides immediate relief to anxious individuals? And then, how is 'truth' defined for a panicky person, other than as 'advantageous for survival'? The pragmatic notion of 'truth' is nurtured by radical philosophical skepticism. Of course, truth could be based on the plausibility that expectations are right. But that kind of truth may not be proven for many decades and is never an instrument in an emergency. Rob Rechard,[35] introduced his admirable essay on the history of performance assessments for radioactive waste with the line, "Fear of harm ought to be proportional not merely to the gravity of the harm, but also to the probability of the event … ."[35] That dictum might seem obvious if not for the fact that the need for such rating of danger was recognized as early as in the 17th century. Should then 'truth' be communicated as a series of probability computations?[16] Questionable. In the context of what Kurt Lewin[37] defined in 1943 as 'psychological ecology,' an individual's behavior is chiefly determined by 'subjective probability' (e.g. pondering over the likelihood of the ceiling in one's apartment coming dawn) as opposed to 'objective probability' of such an event based on computations by engineers. He seems to be right, since pushing the demand for truth to the limit would lead to outright subjectivism. In our social world, the demand for truth is impossible since it is beyond analytical checks. We all fear lightning because it is a concrete dangerous occurence, even though the individual risk associated with it is extremely small. By contrast, women hardly worry about the danger of oral contraceptives ('subjective probability') since they are considered safe regardless of some side effects and even death they might cause ('objective probability').[16] A desirable aid when discussing impending risks, be it auditory pollution, radiation, endocrine disrupting chemicals, carcinogens, carbon dioxide and global warming or the effects of electric and magnetic fields is not 'proof of truth' but an inference based on available ('concrete') evidence, such as graphical displays of 'risks of normal living' across a wide range of conditions with which people are familiar.[16]

Ultimately, in the search for informed opinion we always turn to science. Still, the major hazard in decision-making is not one of formal error, but one of judgment to act on or not to act on input. Scientists' judgments about risk are also influenced by emotion and ideology — or what Plato designated 'true falsehood' — particularly when they are approaching the limits of their expertise. Worried about relaxing the criteria for what constitutes scientific fact, scientists often disagree. Their scientific theories are mostly tentative, subject to elaboration and further testing and therefore, consensus building in science is a slow, error-prone, and often fragile process, particularly in cases of emergency, or when a forecast should be made regarding 'remote and improbable dangers.'[36] Therefore, science is not in charge of providing perpetual alerts. It is only responsible for its accuracy.

Since the dawn of medicine, each generation of medical students has been told a tale that all diseases in the world have roots in a devious plot of the ceremonial offering of a neatly gift-wrapped box by a pretty woman named Pandora. That devastating 'whimper' was engineered by the god Zeus to punish Prometheus. Pandora was prearranged to be a wife for Prometheus. But the latter, as his name suggests, had 'theory of mind' abilities and was thus able to guess correctly the god's wicked intentions. In a quick change of plan, the gods sent Pandora to his brother, Epimetheus. Though warned not to accept the gift from the implacable Zeus, Epimetheus found nothing wrong with the girl, and was happy to make her his wife. Warned or not, as the name implies (*Epi-metheus* means 'one with hindsight'), he would not have much success in parsing the truth of the evil intent. It is therefore surprising given the catastrophic outcome that most of the literature obsessed with the myth calls attention to the curse of the *Femme Fatale*. Less often noticed is the fact that Epimetheus was not in charge of appetitive/consummatory impulses, as manifested by his being instantly swayed by the girl and her gift box. Epimetheus's impulsive acceptance of reward against presumably his better interests is associated with faulty hedonic control mechanisms. The latter hunch is quite possible considering speculations of a positive relationship between information deficit and impulsivity and between the latter and the speed of acquisition of reward expectancies. Although somewhat whimsical, one lesson of the myth alludes to what may happen when decisions are made rashly. Its other moral is not just to remind us of the value of foresight and trust of timely good advice, but also to tell us that regardless of it, and in keeping with old convictions,[37] risk assessments, as usually practiced, will remain inherently subjective, a blend of rational (scientific) judgment with personal, social, cultural and political factors. Observing September 11 through a rear-view mirror, most of us feel more clued-up. That retrospective intelligence means that potential villains will always have an edge. An almost apocalyptic appreciation of the threat that the 'sky will fall' makes policy makers and the general public somewhat more jumpy.

Like individual anxiety disorders, socially shared anxieties are driven by the presence of deep collective uncertainties regarding the future, but they also contain elements of specific phobias of a present potentially catastrophic situation with their explicit and plentiful implicit cues. While individuals with specific phobias tend to withdraw from threat, mass anxieties on the contrary are expected to cause public swarming that would augment emotions and make contagious pathogens and toxins more perilous. Unlike specific phobias and anxiety disorders in individual patients that have been successfully researched by several groups in the US and Europe, the neural triggers of mass anxieties have yet to be elucidated; their laboratory models are virtually absent; their control is complicated. Therefore, the other message learned is that health psychologists who aspire to work in the health delivery system would need, at the minimum, to get equipped with unambiguous guidance as to how to act if epidemic disorders and panic strike. Regrettably, the required practical bioterrorism-related information is spread throughout a variety of websites. There is not much one can find regarding health psychologists' role in community, schools, or hospitals that would be easy to integrate as classroom material. The National Association of School Psychologists (*http://www.nasponline.org/index2.html*); the Center for the Study of Mental Health in Schools (*http://smhp.psych.ucla.edu*) or the American Psychological Association's (*http://helping.apa.org/daily/traumaticstress.html*) websites provide *no* prospective material on disaster control tailored to school children or health psychologists. There is nothing as useful for health psychology students as the quality of materials that are offered for physicians on disaster preparedness by the American Medical Association site (*http://www.ama-assn.org/ama/pub/category/6206.html*).

Mulling over mass anxieties where chance and necessity may so unpredictably interact, a thought could come to mind that many professionals shut out from the core of data would default into the popular notion that anything that is wise to do in emergency is hardly a function of knowledge — since very few professional, let alone lay people are able to rationally analyze the impact of all hazardous agents and events in emergency, but rather a function of *trust*.[31,38,39] Although a search for consensus among all competent researchers is mandatory,[40] trust is an ultimate arbiter and often a substitute for 'truth' for the restless and fearful. One of its responsibilities, we are told, is to reduce the headache of attempting personal investigations in all matters of vital consequences. We often surrender to the opinions of authorities, peers, and appointed experts not for a lack of character or moral obtuseness, but as a means of reducing 'social complexity.' The latter is a term of social science for a way of delegating decision-making to those — to paraphrase Putt's Law — who understand what they do *not* or should not manage, rather than to those who manage what they do *not* understand. However, reliance on trust will get you only so far — the health psychology community at large will never be able to depend completely on faith. Admittedly, health psychologists would be able to fine-tune their response to potential threats more successfully if they remedy their curriculum blind-spot for the role of infectious diseases. That would facilitate their constructive dialogue with other health care professionals in circumstances where threat-related information is deficient, and demand for promptly dealing with it is high.

SO WHAT?

Dangerous situations promising "the sky to fall" may cause lasting phobias in vulnerable populations. Other phobias develop as 'insights' that the public should acquire a different lifestyle, dietary habits and responsibilities or that some of our long adopted behaviors or habits are considered harmful. Public anxiety may appear as a vaccinations scare, suspicions over genetic crop alterations, refusal to eat red meat over fears of mad cow disease, expectations of bacteria or toxic substances spread by terrorists, the threat of globalization, and many others. No person is completely impervious to disquiet when mulling over potential threats or observing the signs of alarm in others. Although such fears may not necessarily cause mass panic, they are likely to have enormous economic repercussions.

It is only human to lose sleep in circumstances where information is deficient, whereas the demand for coping fast is high. Thus, it is hardly realistic to expect that education will provide a complete cure for all; a small segment of the population will certainly require assistance by psychologists or psychiatrists. One might wonder whether the fact that people view hazards as more risky for other people than for themselves protects society from shared disquiet from occurring on a more massive scale.

At present, the neural machinery contributing to anxiety disorders, panic and specific phobia in a single patient is actively being explored by many research groups. This chapter has presented some examples of mass phobias and a great deal of speculation, but little empirical evidence. Major gaps exist in our understanding of mass anxieties. An exploration of the various forms of mass anxiety is extremely important from both applied and theoretical perspectives. Practical panic-related information for health psychologists is considered necessary in view of the world's manifold threats. The theoretical aspects of mass anxiety must certainly represent a major emphasis of future interdisciplinary research providing a meeting ground for social, cognitive and neurobiological researchers.

6

A Complementary Point of View

The word *medicine* originated from the Latin *medeor, mederi,* which denotes treating, caring for, guarding, or looking after. That was a visible component, and perhaps the key element of what was medicine:

Dieppe[2] reminds us of an old cliché, *guerir quelquefois, soulager souvent, consoler toujours* (cure sometimes, help often, and comfort always), and appeals to doctors to return to their origins by regaining the ability to help and console. This, he asserts, is the primary goal of medicine that has allegedly been deserted in the paradigmal shift from subjective to objective, and the reliance on increasingly more sophisticated technology.

"Until the 17th century, the first priority of the professional, learned physician was to advise his (and it was "his" almost exclusively by this time) client on how to maintain health through the proper regimen which focused on ... sleep and wakefulness, motion and rest, food and drink, air, evacuation and repletion, and the passions or emotions."[1]

Health psychologists do not use much technology, if any, and would probably be perfect candidates for 'caring,' 'guarding' and 'comforting.' However, complementary/alternative medicine already profits from providing such services. Regardless of some superficial similarities between health psychologies and complementary practitioners, they differ in that the latter are mostly, if not exclusively, physicians who are entitled to prescribe drugs, but do not haste to use (standard) pharmacotherapy, whereas health psychologists recommend remedies, but are not licensed to supplement psychotherapy with drugs. The temptation to straddle the line between dietary recommendations and the expert use of drugs in psychopathology is an implicit effort to look a lot like medicine, in which only after the 17th century "did the treatment of the ill begin to replace regimen for the healthy as the learned physician's first priority."[1] In effect, professional (health) psychology seemed as though it was backtracking from the movement after World War II to allow non-medical practitioners to practice psychoanalysis. This chapter will discuss the tenor of a debate on prescription privileges, the role of placebo and some aspects of complementary practices as they reflect on health psychology.

Prescription Privileges: Good or Bad for the Profession?

The advocates of prescription privileges draw attention to the fact that dentists treat within the area of the viscerocranium, podiatrists do the same on the feet, and optometrists are allowed to prescribe a limited range of drugs for eye problems.[3] They posit that their plea was inspired by the rights granted to these practitioners. Many psychiatrists do not have imperialistic objections to psychologists prescribing some psychoactive drugs, inasmuch as psychologists are more inclined, as compared to physicians to serve in rural communities and to work with people with severe and chronic mental disorders, prisoners and the elderly. This is consistent with the age-sanctified practice whereby other professionals had to step in to help the needy. In 18th century England, clerics and apothecaries were on the periphery of healthcare. Nonetheless, they were often recruited to help the sick when there was a shortage of physicians.

Today, family physicians are overloaded. They are in charge of prescribing no less than 40% of psychoactive drugs, in spite of the fact that they are inadequately trained in diagnosing and managing psychopathology as compared with clinical psychologists, who spend more time with their patients than family doctors do, and are more familiar with their needs and views. On the face of it, the claim for prescription rights is quite reasonable and is based on the unspoken recognition of the biological foundation of contemporary psychiatry. In fact, some psychologists are already 'heavily involved' in the development of physical interventions in the treatment of a variety of somatic conditions. Admittedly, being a participant in a research team and being personally responsible for the treatment of patients are altogether different. Students of experimental psychology are routinely involved in research on electroconvulsive therapy (ECT) and a fair range of neurosurgery in laboratory animals, but no clinical psychologist would ever ask to administer ECT in a psychiatry setting, let alone practice neurosurgery in humans, even if such practice were certain to offer "financial benefits and improved professional esteem of practitioners" (Box 6.1).

Pharmacology is a medical discipline that explores the mechanisms whereby drugs work. It intertwines with physiology, biochemistry, molecular biology, and pathology. If psychologists are granted prescription privileges, clinical or social psychologists would have to do the job, as they have earned a deserved respect in psychiatry. Handling medical patients would either necessitate at least a superficial familiarity with pharmacology, and certainly various areas of medicine. Mandating new responsibilities at a time when these subjects have virtually no place in departments of psychology, at least not in its 'clinical part,' is at least shortsighted. At the outset, health psychology was *ad hoc*ish in nature and its students were free to develop themselves in whatever direction and extent its leaders felt to be profitable. It would not be a simple task for the university departments of psychology to accommodate such a new discipline, both in its implicit scientific and clinical demands, as well as in the administrative sense. By just adding pharmacotherapy to the set of professional choices would cause a transgression of boundaries set by medicine, unless clinical psychology would comply with the established standards for acquiring knowledge.

Box 6.1: Motives for drug prescription rights (based on Refs. 4 and 5).

- Recognition of biological factors underlying psychopathology;
- Dissatisfaction with cost-effectiveness of psychodynamic techniques;
- Perceived responsibility to society, such as improving service to underserved groups (geriatric population, rural population, chronic psychiatry patients);
- Other professions having already obtained limited prescription rights;
- Expected increase of financial benefits and improved professional esteem of practitioners;
- Anticipated recognition of clinical psychology (by other professionals and insurance companies) as an autonomous profession.

Psychologists are hardly undivided in their attitude to the use of psychopharmacology as propaedeuitic to medicine.[6] Some voice direct opposition to the 'pro-priviledges view,' arguing that they should continue to do what they have been doing all along. They correctly point out that drugs are misleadingly labeled as performing specific health operations for mood, memory, or circadian cycle, as they seem to do something for the intestines, skin, liver or heart. Sharing in prescription privileges assumes they maintain, at the minimum, that clinical psychologists would allocate extra time listening to patients' accounts of progress in overcoming heart palpitations, stomach upsets, urological problems, or skin disorders. Spending most of their time in hospitals and fraternizing with medical doctors will estrange them from academic psychology. And if all psychologists ultimately play the role of mini-physicians, will they be required to take care of somatic disorders of their patients? What should the health psychologist worry about: the greater chance of cardiovascular complications and dying from an overdose of a tricyclic anti-depressant or a drug with a wide therapeutic margin that sometimes causes liver damage? What degree of risk is acceptable; what is an acceptable risk and to whom? Would such a new professional be able to respond to complaints and suffering of patients with somatic symptoms if they emerge in the course of psychotherapy or pharmacotherapy? "What about the diabetic, the hypertensive, the cardiac patients?" asked DeNelsky[7] pointedly.

Another question is, would a new role for the psychologist do any good to mentally sick patients? Even if the threat to clinical psychology from an excessive reliance on pharmacotherapy and from physicians who, as DeNelsky maintains, are dominated and manipulated by the pharmaceutical industry, are somewhat dramatized, his point that for such a complex mission "psychologists would need to learn how medications affect the unusual, medically complex patient"[7] is well taken. Nowadays, by the time a physician completes a three-year residency program, there is an obligation to take in an extra dose of pharmacology to catch up with a few dozen new drugs available on the market, as well as new perspectives on the principles of their action. Thus, a possible outcome of arming a new profession with drugs is against its self-interests because it could make psychologists, as DeNelsky argued, somewhat akin to junior (biological) psychiatrists. They would need a new curriculum to measure up to that of medical practitioners and that would entail constant updating via a continuous education program. In short, to paraphrase the line of Lewis Carroll's Red Queen, they will need to do a lot of running just to keep in the same place. In the meantime, DeNelsky fears, counselors and social workers who do not aspire to use drugs would fill the vacuum of psychological and behavioral intervention.

Psychopharmacology assumes the need to deal with many iatrogenic effects that continue to plague medicine to this day. Even in the hands of trained physicians, drugs may be a menace and a source of morbidity. This is certainly a heavy burden for physicians, but if psychologists find it difficult to take care of untoward drug effects, they will send the disturbing message to a potential client that they are ready to distribute prescriptions, but appear helpless when something goes seriously wrong.[8] This is not a small problem given the number of drugs prescribed by US physicians. The scenario of potential toxicity due to drug interactions can be gleaned from the fact that according to medical statistics, 2–5% of admissions to a hospital are associated with drug-induced symptoms. Annually, 106,000 fatalities are estimated to be attributed to drug reactions alone. Some of them are likely to be caused by over-the-counter drugs.

To conclude, a special issue of the *Journal of Clinical Psychology* published in 2002 revealed a deep division in clinical psychology on the issue of prescription privileges. The editorial introduction written by Elaine M. Heiby[6] tells us with unveiled exasperation that after very vocal and dramatic prevarications of the pundits of the polar convictions, it took nearly four long years of struggle and fear to put the issue into print. This debate implies that a shift from clinical psychology to health psychology is not merely a better or rather more contemporary choice of words, but represents a deeply disparate concept, a "divide between those trained to be psychotherapists and those trained to be scientist-practitioners" that fuels the futile quest for a new 'miniprofession.' Heiby[6] maintains that in order to secure the vitality of university departments of psychology there must be a rapprochement between these two factions. Her credible analysis actually shows that a détente is only possible if the pursuit for prescription privileges for psychologists is rejected. To make her view more than a mere affirmation of faith it is desirable to show, though briefly, how demanding practicing pharmacotherapy might be. No lesser an authority than Sir William Osler (1849–1919) felt that one of the most important duties of the physician is to educate the masses *not* to take medicine.

Drug-Response Variability

One of Kenneth A. Weene's[9] clients was unhappy that her son was not responding well to Prozac while she responded so well to her medication.

Here is the dialogue intended to convince the reader that patients might gain if psychologists were to participate in pharmacotherapy:

"Oh," I responded, "you're on Prozac, too."
"No, I'm on Serzone. It's been wonderful for me."
"Tell your son's doctor to switch him to Serzone, and let me know the results. Remember that he has half his genes from you and all his mitochondria, the little factories that make chemicals in his cells" (p. 618).

The doctor must have taken to heart the instructions about the 'genes and mitochondria' relayed by the patient's mother since the patients must have improved. "Needless-to-say," assured Weene, cheerfully[9] "this simple phone intervention was successful."

Why not? Perhaps, psychologists would perform handsomely if given limited veto power over prescriptions written for their patients. It is superior to making them solely responsible for prescribing drugs. As far as this author is concerned, it is better to have prescribing physicians bristle when their authority is challenged by psychologists than to overlook a good drug they suggested. Individualization of drug therapy is more than decision-making over drug choices. Drug efficacy is influenced by a variety of factors, among them body mass index, sex, age, drug history, and diet. Psychopharmacological medication is conducted together with grapefruit in the morning, a few cups of coffee, a dozen cigarettes during the day, a glass of wine in the evening, and so on. Patients who are over 60 years of age pose still another problem. As an old axiom of geriatric psychiatry reminds, "the older people become, the less like each other they become." It is certainly correct, at least in view of the load of comorbidity, i.e. the presence of coexisting ailments, and the number of dissimilar drugs they ingest that entail patients' education. Older adults, particularly those with mental disabilities require careful dose titration and vigilant monitoring of their compliance. In short, the nature of the 'chemical behaviors' of drugs in the body can be accurately predicted, but only to a point. Drug effects comprise a complex chain of pharmacokinetic and pharmacodynamic factors; they are transported by different types of proteins, interact with one or more drug-receptor targets or other drug targets, and finally metabolized by several different enzymes, often acting collectively.

Many of us are guilty of an enthusiastic attribution to genes of just about everything in the body. Although Sir Peter Medawar is said to have facetiously branded such a view as 'geneticism,' genetics is visibly on the winning side in psychopharmacology, which has become unavoidably molecular. Lots of vital steps of the drug journey in the body, from drug distribution to metabolism, are actually under considerable genetic control that is dealt with by a new field of pharmacogenetics. A lay example of everyday pharmacogenetics is at a dinner table, when the tastes of diners significantly differ. Some of the taste is learned, but much of it is inherited. To prove the role of inheritance, people can be tested using an interesting chemical, phenylthiocarbamide, which when diluted tastes sour for nearly 70% of Caucasians, but tasteless to the other 30%. This blandness or dullness of taste is inherited as an autosomal recessive trait.

The need for prescribing for racially diverse patients adds another dimension to the unknown in pharmacotherapy. How does ethnicity or race play a role in treatment decisions on antidepressants? And how does a doctor determine a person's race in mixed marriages when only "half his genes" comes from the mother? Race is not just a social or political notion as it tends to interact with the potency and efficacy of medication. However imprecisely defined, race is the best proxy currently available for surmising different drug effects in different ethnic groups.

A symposium entitled *Experimental and Clinical Aspects of Pharmacogenetics* that took place in the course of a 1965 meeting of the Federation of American Societies for Experimental Biology opened a new area in drug treatment and research. Yet, the nature of genetic drug variability began to be sorted out in the late 70s with the discovery of hepatic cytochrome P-450 enzymes (CYP450), a superfamily of microsomal drug-metabolizing enzymes that catalyze phase I drug metabolism (*www.icgeb.trieste.it/p450*). A specific genotype may be vital in determining the effects of medication for one ethnic group but irrelevant for another.* Likewise, a specific genotype may underlie individual variability in drug response.

---

*Although the majority of people metabolize drugs at about the same rate, between 2% and 5% of the white population and up to 25% of African-American and Asian individuals are slow metabolizers of some antidepressants and antiepileptic drugs via the CYP2C19 enzyme. About 30% of people of Chinese origin may be slow metabolizers of tricyclic antidepressants. At least 5% of the Spaniards possess more than one copy of CYP2D6 and are phenotypically fast metabolizers. They may manifest no therapeutic response to drugs metabolized by this enzyme when the drugs are taken in regular doses.[10] Such genetic polymorphism can make a generally efficacious drug ineffective in some patients, and toxic in others. That is particularly important for drugs with a narrow therapeutic window. Curiously, fast metabolizers may be noncompliant because they do not experience a desirable effect of a given drug whereas slow metabolizers may be noncompliant because of the swift appearance of its untoward effects or excessively long aftereffect of medication.

Bertilsson and colleagues[11] of the Karolinska Institute in Sweden provided the earliest clues that cytochrome P450 is also related to personality differences. They phenotyped 769 healthy Swedes and established that 6.6% in their sample are poor hydroxylators. Next, they submitted the Eyseneck personality questionnaire as well as the Karolisnka personality inventory to 51 poor and 102 extensive hydroxylators. Poor hydroxylators had significantly lower score in the Karolinska psychasthenia scale and a higher frequency of extreme response. A low psychasthenia score implies high vitality, alertness, efficiency, a lack of hesitation and an ease of decision-making. Regardless of the fact that psychasthenia is an antiquated term, its instruments permitted one to suggest that debrisoquine hydroxylase could possibly metabolize endogenous substances in a personality related fashion. The 'plot' of pharmacotherapy becomes more interesting and infinitely more difficult than was thought in the past. In the future, there will be a possibility for improving the safety and efficacy of drug interventions since pharmacogenetics understands 'phenotype' as an individual who has not reached a critical age when a deficiency in a particular enzyme is not felt because its onset of expression has yet to occur. This definition explains why individual differences become problematic in attempting to apply psychopharmacology in pediatric practice on the model of adult efficacy. There are also uncertainties as to how pharmacogenetic traits are felt in the frequency of exposure, the width of the therapeutic index, sharpness of dose-response curves, or the limited availability of additional drugs that are pregnant with ethical and legal concerns. The multiplicity of these factors along with the safety concerns and the need to overcome taxonomic problems makes the tailoring of drugs increasingly complex.

Natural Remedies: "Don't Exaggerate!"

Herbal medicines are regular medicines, save for the fact they seldom comply with the standards established for product quality for regular drugs. Their safety is as good as the willingness of manufacturers to stomach high quality controls that exclude inferior products. This highly diverse class of substances may be broken down in the body into myriad metabolites, which, in turn, influence multiple biologic pathways. Although the public uses herbal remedies confident of their mystic workings, some 'all natural' products can be formulated to illicitly contain regular 'Western' medicine,[12] or contaminants contributing to poisoning (lead and arsenic), abnormal heart rhythms, and impotence.[13] Many herbal remedies and nutritional supplements come from countries where manufacturing standards are something less than ideal. In some traditional pharmacies one can buy a mixture of cockroach droppings with various herbs for about US$2 per pound, to alleviate constipation.[14] Even remedies as benign as laxatives, hypnotics, contraceptives, or antacids might be potentially unsafe. Likewise, dietary supplements do not have to undergo the mandatory testing and surveillance that are required of prescription drugs, inasmuch as adverse events associated with them are recorded only through voluntary reporting of symptoms or their users' admissions to poison centers. Many of the so-called herbal drugs stop being a representative of indigenous practices, but become an item of mass marketing disguised as herbal in a commodity-driven globalized health industry. They are marketed in response to our collective obsession, which includes naturally grown produce, free roaming cattle, poultry matured in a 'low-stress environment,' a ban on growth stimulants, tofu, and Alpine water.

Even practicing homeopathy may not be innocuous regardless of the fact that the bulk of what homeopathy recommends acts no better than Holy Water and for an analytical chemist the remedy will remain nothing but H_2O. Somehow, we remain exceedingly credulous. Homeopathy must have survived throughout the 20th century owing to ignorance as well as the opportunism of *conventional* medicine.[16] On occasion, it might cause allopathic side effects, even if only because the control over such drugs are very lax. A case in point is a 47-year-old man with multiple sclerosis whose state continued to exacerbate despite therapy. He was compelled to start using a walking stick, and then began to experience abdominal colic and difficulty in bladder control.[17] In addition, he became increasingly confused, incoherent, and occasionally violent. This did not look at all like multiple sclerosis. Sure enough, it was not. It appeared that eight months before admission, the patient started a home-made homeopathic remedy called *plumbum metallicum* for treatment of symptoms of multiple sclerosis. Many patients with multiple sclerosis use homeopathic, herbal, chiropractic, or nutritional therapies. The medicine he had taken was not available for analysis, but as the name suggests, it was prepared using lead. He continued taking this remedy intermittently until admission. In addition, during that period he started smoking marijuana for treatment of the symptoms of multiple sclerosis. He used a metallic silver pipe made in Thailand that had metallic inlays. A metallic lump the size of a match head found inside the cone contained 26%–39% lead, and the laboratory tests suggested that this would give off large quantities of lead with smoking. A measurement of blood lead concentration confirmed that the patient had lead levels ten times higher than maximal. It is of interest that all cerebellar features and some cognitive and behavioral problems that were resistant to previous therapy, responded rapidly to chelation therapy, thereby suggesting that they were contributed to by alternative-treatment induced encephalopathy rather than being associated with multiple sclerosis.

The renewed trust in homeopathy is maintained by claims that chaos theories confirm the plausibility of potency of the extreme dilution's (homeopathy) or the "paranormal" claims of healing at a distance. Some physicists advertise electromagnetic water treatment, catalytic water treatment, "super-ionized water," "oxygenated water," "vibrational healing water," and other fraudulent devises. Quantum-mechanical logic does promise to deliver a cup of hot tea when a tea-pot is placed on a cold stove. But even someone with a limited experience in tea-making would not wait for a miracle on a quantum mechanical scale to treat a patient.

Some catastrophic cerebrovascular and cardiovascular events have occurred in apparently healthy young persons following 'supplements,' such as those containing ephedra alkaloids. Recently, the *New England Journal of Medicine* published several reports prompting for greater scrutiny of these unconventional treatments. Commenting on reports about ephedra, G. Alexander Fleming[18] tells us that the notion of "dietary supplements — an innocuous and even holistic-sounding term" is a misnomer. He recommends legislating "a holistic approach to drug regulation and amending the Dietary Supplement and Education Act to close the loophole." That would be a timely undertaking. We are just beginning to learn about the numerous bioactive agents, including those ingested with foods that though present in less than picogram quantities, play a role in important physiological functions in newborns and adults. These are *nutraceuitcals* or *functional foods* that have blurred the borders between drugs and substances used for their general nutritive properties, as well as for the impediment and cure of specific symptoms or diseases. Undoubtedly then, the definition of a drug by Webster as "a substance *other than food* intended to affect the structure or function of the body"[19] (ital. added) seems to be excessively restrictive.

Activity Directed Drug Disposition

When a drug is ingested or injected into the body, it is transported everywhere by the blood regardless of the intended target site. Only a fraction of the dose appears at the areas of deficit or injury. Drug prescriptions are always fraught with the problem of the potential toxic liability associated with the use of non-discriminating agents. Therefore, drug targeting exclusively at specific organs, tissues and receptors (i.e. 'site-specific drug delivery') has been an important objective of medicinal and pharmaceutical chemists from the beginning of the century. This remains an important goal of pharmacotherapy motivated by the necessity to reduce overall toxicity of drugs, and maintain their therapeutic payback. The majority of approaches for site-specific drug deliveries capitalize on drug formulations, explore the possibility of paramagnetic drug tagging and subsequent 'dragging' of magnetic microparticles, selecting biological drug carriers or chemical drug enhances at the relevant sites. Psychologists are not participant in this research but might conceivably increase the accuracy of drug localization and resulting action within the brain by learning how to influence drug response with added 'activity' in the form of 'environmental manipulations' (muscular work or 'top-down' cognitive effort).

Almost thirty years ago, Murray Weiner and I advocated the use of such combined pharmacotherapy and psychotherapy, hoping that it would result in superior drug delivery and improved therapeutic responses. The idea, labeled 'activity-directed drug disposition'[20,21] hitched a ride on the fact, which is much better understood today, that biomolecules can bind together by the mechanism of 'induced fit,'[22,23] even if they are not optimized for binding with such target sites. Such protein's promiscuity expands the genetic limitations of the organism by allowing for a better functional enhancement and flexibility.

The term 'activity' implies a broad array of effects and metabolic responses and, therefore, can potentially be defined in numerous ways within the many environments and contexts. Yue and Cole[24] compared the effect of a training program of repetitive maximal isometric muscle contractions with force output achieved after mental training. One group of normal participants exercised during four weeks and five sessions per week to produce repeated maximal isometric contractions of the abductor muscles of the fifth digit's metacarpophalangeal joint. Predictably, their average abduction force of the left fifth digit showed a 30% increase. Another group of participants was asked only to *imagine* effortful isometric contractions of the same muscles. Spectacularly, their average abduction force increased by a robust 22%, thereby suggesting that strength increases can be achieved without engaging in repeated motions. Although force gains may result from engaging the central motor programming system, it would not be wise to recommend visualizing one's muscular contractions as a substitute for running, playing tennis, or exercising in the gym.

Dennis Feeney and colleagues[25] subjected rats to unilateral ablation of the motor cortex and tested their locomotion on a narrow beam. The rats manifested transient contralateral paresis. A single dose of *d*-amphetamine given 24 hours after injury caused an immediate and enduring acceleration of recovery. Recovery was drastically reduced by the administration of the dopamine antagonist haloperidol or by restraining the animals for eight hours, immediately following amphetamine administration. Later, a similar effect was reproduced in cats with unilateral motor cortex injury. Following injury, the cats manifested a prolonged loss of tactile placing in the contralateral forelimb. Again, amphetamine (5 mg/kg) temporarily reversed this tactile placing deficit as early as four days following the injury.[26] Fox and Raichle,[27] using the labeled water ($H_2^{15}O$) PET regional cerebral blood flow technique, have reported a 31.5% increase in visual cortex blood flow to patterned visual stimulation at 7.8 Hz. Such a robust increment may certainly affect drug distribution. Since then, a number of studies confirmed the presence of significant increments in blood flow using a variety of radiopharmaceuticals and activation techniques of different complexity. More recently, Feeney's group showed that administration of *d*-amphetamine when paired with ten one-hour sessions of speech/language therapy facilitated recovery from aphasia in a small group of patients in the subacute period after stroke.[28]

The science of psychopharmacology, narrowly defined through its academic goals, is a "scientific discipline that utilizes drugs to increase our knowledge and understanding of the workings of the mind."[29] Activity-directed drug disposition would complicate this characterization by emphasizing that psychopharmacology is a scientific discipline; that it also utilizes the workings of the mind in order to increase our knowledge and understanding of drug distribution in the brain. Activity directed drug disposition was proposed when the concepts of drug targeting were less advanced than they are now. Therefore, it is infinitely less specific than splicing into the viral genome the beneficial gene and then exposing the patient's cells to the virus. But genetic therapy has its own obstacles and is still quite a few years away from making the genes do their work in the right cells. Thus, the potential environmental effects on regional blood flow present an untapped opportunity to enhance the desired effect of centrally active drugs at their site of action without enhancing systemic toxicity. If ascertained that this and other modalities of cognitive therapy are capable of influencing physiological and physical chemical parameters that determine, say d-amphetamine disposition, the method would have significant promise.

In a more broad restatement of this position, if a doctor believes that a more rational drug targeting will reduce a patient's need for a drug by using programs that belong to the category of 'lifestyle alternatives' it would seem superfluous to demand prescription privileges and the freedom of choice with regard to treatment. When health systems of the same efficacy differ in cost, the one that does not requires additional knowledge and special training would be preferable. Considering this dictum, clinical psychologists may rather benefit from participating in studies exploring activity directed drug disposition than personally prescribing psychoactive drugs.

Medicine of Self-Deceit

To help the Israelites who feared to walk in the sand infested by snakes, Moses created a bronze serpent capable of healing those bitten by real ones (Numbers 21:5–9). It is not at all certain that individual victims survived with this remedy, but the bronze serpent must have encouraged the tribes to cross the desert. A bit later, Jesus was able to restore health of the sick by his sheer presence. His patients were not just anxious and superstitious expatriates as Moses's clients were but a more heterogeneous and demanding assembly of "lame, blind, dumb, maimed and many others" (Mathew 15:30). As we depart from remote history, our ability to demonstrate such miraculous examples of magic mass cures dwindles. Yet the tide of anecdotes is still impressively high.

Placebos

According to Dorland's pocket medical dictionary, a placebo is "an inactive substance or preparation given to satisfy the patient's symbolic need for drug therapy …"; "a procedure with no intrinsic therapeutic value." One might derive from this that placebos are not about drugs or doctors. They are about the common need to give a chance to the miracle. Here is an example of when such trust in the miracle was indeed phenomenal.

A terminally ill cancer patient persisted in requesting a novel and presumably superbly potent anticancer agent. It is difficult to refuse an experimental drug to dying patients who believe that a new agent can restore their health. The drug was prescribed, and the patient did show a striking remission. He was discharged and resumed his normal activities. As publications began to appear that Krebiozen, as was the name of the agent, is ineffective in malignancy, the man relapsed as soon as the bad news reached him and became terminally ill again. Convinced that his previous recovery was purely psychological in nature, his physician persuaded him to try a new "purified" form of Krebiozen, and injected distilled water. The patient made a spectacular recovery. Two months later the patient came across an authoritative government report showing that Krebiozen was of absolutely no value. The man died a few days later.[30] This anecdote, although rather unique in its drama, illustrates the fact that a substance inactive in a specific disorder might act as if it is endowed with a salubrious power when there is an expectation of its efficacy.

The efficacy of 'cheap or worthless' substances described under the name of 'placebo' is known since the dawn of medicine. Not a single library shelf could be filled with placebo analyses. The art of medication is based on prescriptions of numerous agents that were considered at one time or another as powerful cures, but with advancing knowledge and experience turned out to be plainly useless. "Therapy, in general," mused Shapiro, "rested on placebo foundations, despite the tendency of most historians to glamorize and sentimentalize medicine"[31] (p. 447). In a sense, the placebo often turns the weakness of medicine into its strength. Unwittingly, the placebogenic properties of drugs also work as their safety valve. They permit a practitioner to make the sick and their distressed families hopeful and comfortable. By taking the mind off a disease with a placebo, the therapist is letting the malady run its course. This promotes natural healing, irrespective of whether or not the drug was good or useless. Placebogenic effects balance some untoward results of drugs when a patient, as a fashionable joke has it, often recovered not because of drugs, but in spite of them.

Virtually any vegetable, plant or substance difficult to obtain, or of an arcane source was once used as a therapeutic agent. They derived their supernatural qualities from their form, color, material, novelty, and origin. They could function as devices designed to avert evil (i.e. apotropaic) or aid in other votive and symbolic functions. Pepper, aloes, spices were all some time ago powerful drugs. When the potato was first introduced into Europe it was sold as 'medicine.' For many years, regular remedy had to taste bad, leaving a persistent nauseating aftertaste or better still, abdominal pain, so as to be considered different from a nutrient, and thus trusted as 'the real thing.' Many foods, particularly those that are associated with health benefits have a bitter taste. As carnivores, humans are better able to detect bitter compounds, including extremely toxic bitter poisons in micromolar amounts. Although there is no direct relation between toxicity and bitter taste thresholds, bitter quinine is detected at 25 μmol/L concentrations and bitter toxins are detected at even lower concentrations. By contrast, agents that did not taste bad or cause discomfort when ingested, or did not irritate when topically placed were not noticed by a patient and therefore were not considered particularly helpful.

In the past, the composition of 'effective' drugs had to be excessively complex in order to make a good impression. One Hebrew alchemist recommended the following prescription:

"Take a bat and burn it, and pound it with sulfur, and mix it with the juice seldonia (L. cheldonia is a weedy plant of the poppy family), and put in a vessel up to six days, and then distill it, and this water has many uses"[32] (p. 214).

This abominable concoction is apparently prepared on an ancient principle that the remedy should be derived from the same ill spirit that caused the malady. Its curative properties reside in the patients' convictions that the medical man is capable of establishing the nature of demonic forces. Urine, too, was in demand for the treatment of sore eyes, particularly the urine of a faithful wife. When it was not notably effective, the blame (surprise!) was not placed on the 'remedy' but necessitated the proof of virginity. The current high incidence of rape of young girls in South Africa is also explained by a common belief in Africa that sex with a virgin cures AIDS (so-called "virgin cleansing").[33]* As a science, medicine cannot publicize irrationality as treatment. That does not mean that such practices cannot be defended (not proven

---

*Not surprisingly, urine is the only bodily fluid that is not high on the list of disgusting substances. In fact, in cross-cultural comparisons of what is considered disgusting, only in India did urine occupy second place after feces. Neither in West Africa, the Netherlands, United Kingdom nor Athens International Airport did items of disgust provided by the opinion poll include urine at all.[34]

to be desirable!). Every medical student is taught that to speak the truth is one of the most important deontological principles in medical ethics. The redeeming feature of such deviation from truth-telling is that the act of prescribing a presumably inert substance, or recommending a therapeutically-nonspecific regimen, becomes a sign of responsibility, 'stating an obligation,' assuming authority and therapeutic bonds; something comparable to the 'prestige suggestions' of psychotherapists. Doctors and nurses, like everyone else, have a *prima facie* duty not to lie, but they are not duty-bound to avoid intentional deception.[35] The bioethical principle dubbed as the 'double effect' prohibits doing a bad act for the sake of superior consequences, but accepts a good act in the knowledge that untoward consequences will result.

What in medicine is defined as 'side effects,' in combat is branded as 'collateral damage.' Yet the 'bad act' is not synonymous to an unethical act. Many painful acts in medicine are delivered on the conviction of improving health. Admittedly, placebo drugs are in the category of the 'bad act,' but their prescriptions are given by a desire to shield patients from what is happening to them. Back in medical school, a professor of pharmacology used to moralize that when in doubt, leave a patient with a prescription. "Truth is mandatory," he was in the habit of pontificating, "but occasionally deceit is salubrious, even though such fake treatment is sure to make health care excessively expensive in the longer run."

The etymology of the word 'faker,' as Merriam-Webster tells us, denotes someone who "seeks to deceive by ascribing great value or efficacy to cheap or worthless products." Apparently, it originates from the word 'fakir' (Arabic *faqir* — poor) or closer in time (*faker* in French), for an impoverished itinerant wonder-worker. The counsel of my late professor is still acceptable since "For the most part in the history of medicine, beneficence has far outweighed any other duty, including that of veracity"[36] (p. 403). Disease is a lonely condition. In the state of loneliness and helplessness, a sick person who desperately wants to get better would accept any promise of improvement. The more a cure is needed, the more a useless agent might parade as remedy. It will remain in the toolkit of healers until the medical profession learns more about the mechanisms of drug action and the way to use chemical agents in a more tailored fashion. By deliberately misleading a patient, a contemporary physician might employ symptomatic medications for short-term benefits to gain time for a better therapeutic answer.

Hróbjartsson and Gøtzsche[37] conducted a systematic meta-analysis of clinical trials in which patients were randomly assigned either placebo or no treatment. Overall, they identified 130 trials that met their inclusion criteria with relevant data on outcomes: 32 studies with binary outcomes (involving 3,795 patients), and 82 studies (involving 4,730 patients) with continuous outcomes. As compared with no treatment groups, placebo had *no* significant effect on binary outcomes, both subjective and objective. There was a significant effect of placebo for the trials with continuous outcomes, but the effect decreased with increasing sample size, indicating a possible bias related to the effects of small trials. Admittedly, small trials with negative outcomes have not been located nor do they have a chance of being accepted by editors. Finally, the pooled standardized mean difference was significant for the trials with subjective outcomes but not for those with objective outcomes. Pain, obesity, asthma, hypertension, insomnia, and anxiety were each investigated in at least three independent trials. Only the 27 trials involving the treatment of pain (including a total of 1,602 patients) showed a significant effect of placebo as compared with no treatment. This solid study demystified the belief in the powerful clinical effects of placebos. The authors conclude that using placebos outside the aegis of a controlled, properly designed clinical trial cannot be recommended, and when it is practiced, such 'benevolent deception' should be guarded by several straightforward rules.[36]

Placebo as Deception Paradigm

Commenting on the study by Hróbjartsson and Gøtzsche, John C. Bailar III compares placebos with the Wizard of Oz, who 'was powerful because others thought he was powerful.' That is an ultimate proof of deception taking a ride on gullibility and preconception. What is its machinery? De la Fuente-Fernandez[38] and colleagues at the University of British Columbia in Vancouver explored the possibility of the presence of placebo-released endogenous dopamine in Parkinson's patients. They examined six patients under two conditions, a placebo-controlled blind study in which the patients did not know when they were receiving placebo or the active drug (apomorphine), and an open study without placebo. Using positron emission tomography (PET) to estimate the competition between endogenous dopamine and $[^{11}C]$ raclopride for binding to dopamine D2/D3 receptors, the study obtained evidence of the placebo-induced release of endogenous dopamine in the striatum. A significant decrease in striatal raclopride binding potential was found when the patients received placebo as compared with baseline observations in each patient. The magnitude of a decrease was comparable to that of therapeutic doses of L-DOPA or apomorphine. Patients who perceived placebo benefit also showed greater PET response than those who did not. This was in keeping with well-known observations suggesting that good adherents to drug treatment and those who believe in it benefit more than do others from placebo.

The study leaves us uncertain of whether the 'believers' gain from placebo because they have an enhanced sense of control over the events of medication, or whether they simply show a typical conditioned response since they had enjoyed the effect of anti-Parkinson's medication (L-DOPA) in the past, and were therefore more optimistic anticipating it. The word 'optimistic' alludes to still another possibility associated with the fact that dopamine is implicated in reward. The release of dopamine could have maximized positive expectation, confidence and trust. Unwittingly, the expectation of the impending therapeutic progress might have engaged the nigrostriatal system, as well as other limbic or neocortical structures which were not explored under the chosen protocol. There is no acceptable, subject-independent yardstick for assessing the 'accuracy' or intensity of expectations or beliefs. One can be confident, though, that Parkinson's patients were eager to re-experience the familiar therapeutic effect of L-DOPA.

Placebo is similar to religious experience in its being anchored in expectations of a miracle with presumably preconceptual and immediate affective outcome. On the other hand, it is a rational attribution of success to the higher authority. Nina P. Azari and colleagues[39] used [15]O PET in a group of self-identified religious subjects in order to glean the neural correlates of religious experience. If religious states (reading Biblical Psalm 23) engages emotions, there must be, they guessed, certain activation of limbic brain areas, whereas if religious experience is a cognitive attributional phenomenon, neocortical brain areas associated with reasoning are more likely to be activated. They noticed that during religious recitation, religious subjects activated the circuit composed of the dorsolateral prefrontal, dorsomedial frontal and medial parietal cortex, mostly on the right side. That tells us, as they assert, that reading the Psalms reflects the *cognitively* elicited neural network. Yet, the religious state is also yearning, need, enthusiasm, compliance, reward, conflicting goals, uncertainty of one's worth, trust and the like when the foregoing *non-cognitive* factors collectively (but apparently in different combinations in different individuals) determine whether our attention will surrender to expectations. More specifically and in terms of reading Biblical Psalms, the preponderance of affect is that of *awareness* of being looked after and *awareness* of a sacred or divine presence. Therefore, a very private religious insight represented in Azari's study as though it is a universal group occurrence might impress one as somewhat strained.

In general, when a person is made aware of taking a centrally active drug, that awareness will elicit a system of cue-monitoring and uncertainty, which are integral parts of what we call the hope of healing. When a person does not know what cues to look for, his experience reminds one of religious attributions that are made in anomalous or ambiguous situations. One might relinquish any search when expecting a miracle to occur. Unlike placebo, spiritual expectations are driven by hope and uncontested reliance. Nor do they have to be motivated by previous positive treatment (drug) experience. Given that exploratory or bogus surgery has long been noticed to heal by modulating bodily symptoms in accord with expectations, one might wonder whether some paradigms of perceptual deception might serve as an interesting alternative to studies of an individual placebogenic potential (and thus hopefully profile the candidates with a better placebo effect).

In the past, my students and I used one compelling illusion known as the ventriloquist effect.[40] The latter exploits an irresistible tendency to hear in the direction of visual regard which underlies a blatant misattribution of speech. Using the ventriloquist effect it was possible to prove that preconscious auditory signals in the space perceptually neglected following brain damage become available to consciousness when a dummy speaker is placed in the attended space. The ability to alleviate the signs of inattention by such a simple trick seemed remarkable therapeutically since patients with hemispatial neglect following right hemisphere lesion are terribly disabled by not attending to auditory and visual stimuli presented in the left hemispace. In the spirit of Aldous Huxley, one might guess that telling normal people that they ought to make out more than they consciously know they hear, would be close to what happens in a placebo scenario. The question seemed so intriguing ecologically and socially, and so relevant to the understanding of placebo phenomena that it was tempting to explore the neural machinery that is recruited for expectation. That may sound like reducing the problem to the bare bones as compared to reading the Biblical Psalm. Nonetheless, its advantage is in providing better control over input conditions, and also circumventing such major confounders as timing and the pharmacokinetic/pharmacodynamic properties of drugs, or prior experience with drug effects.

Brain Image of Deception

Individuals with hemispatial neglect tenaciously and detrimentally to themselves act as though they live in only one side of extra-corporal space. The question is whether normal individuals would behave on instruction as though their space perceptually shrank so as to become slightly imbalanced. Francois Lalonde asked normal individuals to solve an impossible perceptual task of pointing at the side where the sound was louder in an acoustic environment (actually, sound was perfectly bilaterally balanced since subjects listened to CD-recorded scanner noises through the headphones). Preliminary behavioral trials showed that although all participants admitted perceptual difficulties, there was a surprising rate of false 'detections.' They confirmed that a person who accepts as true that one of two identical free-field sounds is louder, easily succumbs to the biasing instruction in spite of the contradictory objective evidence.

With this study done, it was now possible to use functional brain magnetic resonance imaging (fMRI) to explore whether the neuronal network recruited by instruction to search for spatial imbalance ('placebo') would overcome ambiguity, and concerns over the likelihood of errors. In that study conducted with Lalonde, Choyke, Tang, and Sunderland (Geriatric Psychiatry Branch, National Institute of Mental Health), each subject naïve with regard to MRI technology was positioned in the scanner. The study was carried out under two conditions designated as placebogenic and one perceptual control (Fig. 6.1a). In the opening 'guided' session, a subject was told to be 'sensitive' to the centrally positioned cues (codified by arrows) displayed on the monitor that indicated louder sounds, as opposed to an image of diamonds signifying balanced sounds. The subject had to press a hand-held pushbutton in response to each 'recognized' imbalance. In reality all subjects were exposed to acoustic noise produced by switching B_0 gradients, a maneuver similar to that of placing a subject in a gigantic loudspeaker (Fig. 6.1a). Next, each participant was assured to be fully trained so as to be able to make a spatial commitment on the basis of sounds alone and given the 'blind' testing session. In it, the subject had to identify the side of louder sounds whenever a centrally positioned circle appeared on the monitor. Finally, in a control task, the sound intensity was ensured to be identical and the subject had to acknowledge the presence of a visual signal by pressing a hand-held pushbutton.

We hypothesized *a priori* that the trust in sham guidance would elicit mostly parietal activation and only some prefrontal activation (a case of

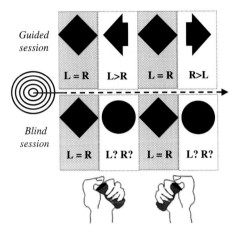

Fig. 6.1a Deception paradigm modeling placebo. Each subject was given two pushbuttons, one for each hand. They had to respond by pressing the pushbutton on the side that was judged as louder. To obviate the installation of special sound-generating equipment, the study used acoustic noise produced by switching B_0 gradients (concentric circles on the left), a maneuver similar to that of placing a subject in a gigantic loudspeaker. In the upper 'placebo' or 'guided' conditions the centrally positioned cues (arrows) directed attention to the left or right side (thereby training each subject to 'detect' a bogus imbalance). The diamonds indicated to the subject that sounds were balanced, as they were, indeed, all the time. It was hoped that the implied spatial validity of the cue would cause misallocation of sounds on the model of the ventriloquist effect. In the 'blind' conditions, a centrally positioned circle preceded 'imbalanced' sounds and subjects had to make spatial commitments without visual guidance, on the basis of previous 'training' they all completed. To control for brain activity elicited by motor responses to cues, the pattern of activations was examined in a perceptual task where subjects were asked to press the pushbuttons in response to the presentation of the left or right arrows when sounds were said to be balanced (not shown on the schematic).

limited personal investment in decision-making). By contrast, a blind session would activate wider areas of the prefrontal and posterior parietal cortex. In keeping with these expectations, Figure 6.1b shows that selection of louder sounds on imagined cues in the guided task was associated with some prefrontal and parietal activation. By contrast, the blind task elicited a significant activation of a large region of the right prefrontal cortex, cerebellum and right superior parietal association cortex that is a marker of the spatial aspects of audio-visual behaviors. Note that in both tasks, much as in a placebo paradigm, having accepted an explanation of specific input conditions and treating them as if they were true, a person committed to the possibility indicated

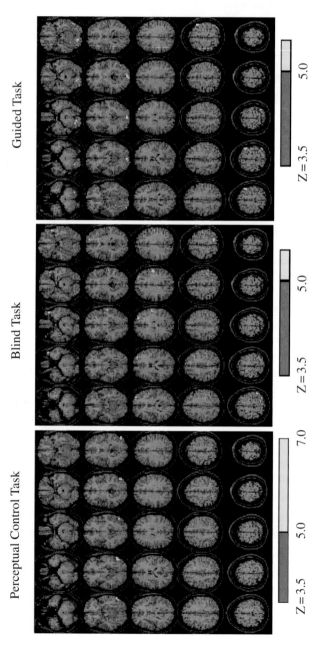

Fig. 6.1b Brain activation under three perceptual conditions. Grand average functional MRI data ($n = 6$) on the grand averaged, spatially normalized high-resolution MRI from the same subjects. Fusion with high-resolution T1-weighted structural scans allows an easy visualization of relevant anatomical regions of the processing network. The Z-score mapping simplifies the determination of regions of high activity. A Z of 3.5, rather than 2.0 or less, was chosen so as to limit the number of false alarms. The sacrifice is that the system is then geared to the detection of a relatively large effect. The orientation of images is according to neurological convention, the right hemisphere is on the viewer's right. An acquisition protocol was based on the BOLD contrast method (TR/TE/flip 3000/40/90°, 26 contiguous axial slices, 5 mm thick, 64 × 64 matrix, FOV 24 cm). (Unpublished study by Lalonde and colleagues.)

by the stimulus and was searching for corroborating evidence. This effort increased the credibility of perceptual confirmation favoring the bogus hypothesis at the expense of viable alternatives.[41]

In the blind test, however, the listeners were left to their own devices to find the perceptual effect and that uncertainty elicited a broader processing network in the prefrontal cortex, anterior cingulate and the supplementary motor areas, also on the right side. Amazingly, though that the network elicited in response to a bogus task was generally similar to that activated by the pious experience.[39] Both are nurtured by the same insecurity and compelling wish to have a winning choice. To paraphrase Bettoni,[42] placebo, like hypotheses does not have to 'correspond to' reality but merely be 'viable in' reality. And viable it often is.

That study was conducted with a small number of subjects and in an effort to minimize variance it was intentionally limited to men. More work is needed before the map of conflict monitoring on bogus input is refined. By way of stipulation, we must tirelessly remind ourselves of the dictum of René Magritte, *L'image n'est pas l'object.* One can only guess whether the network is recruited in response to the perceived ambiguity of the situation, the high probability of errors, the cost of error paid by a highly adaptive system where vision dominates audition, or the desire to succeed in a difficult perceptual task. It must have entailed the comparison of environmental cues against internally established criteria based on a prior audio-visual experience, self-monitoring, self-doubt, previous training, and an action on ambiguous input in the hope of guessing correctly. The other problem in fMRI (PET) research is the problem of *epistemic observation*[43] created by the cataloguing of cognitive characteristics, the degree of anxiety and depression, or immune variables and their correlations with the site and size of signal intensities of 'functional landscapes,' even though the majority of the cognitive processes are not precisely localizable, or their localization changes in time, or that there may be a dissimilar fractionation within the functions of the anatomical site in question. We do not experience the limitations of our sensory machinery, which is only a small fraction of other systems, whereby the organism transduces energy in the environment into information useful for survival.

Finally, an additional methodological problem shared by all such studies is in the impossibility to ascertain the attainment of the requested target state. In a study of this kind one cannot ascertain whether our subjects really 'detected' imbalanced sound or just passively complied with instructions, and thus to a degree, 'fooled the deceivers.' In a way, reduced prefrontal and cingulate activation in the guided task might suggest that the subjects passively complied with the guidance. The presence of sustained activity within neuronal ensembles is not synonymous with 'competence' and may not necessarily show either a decline or a greater efficiency of those regions in function maintenance. There is good evidence that brain areas that maintain tasks that are less predictable or poorly rehearsed could show greater activation. By contrast, activity returns to resting levels once the task becomes routine or expertly executed. In functional imaging studies, like this one, researchers must trust participants' reports that a required emotional or perceptual status has been achieved (no doubt a source of inaccuracy, given people's differences in both meticulousness and insight). Here, our paradigm fails in comparison with placebo, albeit only when symptoms are alleviated by the inert remedy. It is not surprising that much of our laboratory data may be easily overinterpreted and misconstrued.[44]

Alternative (Complementary) Health Practices

> "Virtually anything anyone might do in the company of another person may now be defined as psychotherapeutic. If the definer has the proper credentials, and if his audience is sufficiently gullible, any such act will be publicly accepted and accredited as a form of psychotherapy."
>
> *Thomas Szasz*[45] (p. viii)

Although the best of psychology remains strongly committed to neurosciences, its applied health direction gradually evolves into 'alternative psychology,' which threatens to become part of unconventional (alternative, complementary or integrative) medicine. Alternative medicine is an umbrella term, whose operational definition is that of an occupation based on practices of restoring health that are outside the established range of conventional medicine. It "represents a heterogeneous population promoting disparate beliefs and practices that vary considerably from one movement or tradition to another and form no consistent ... body of knowledge."[46] It is thus an alternative to science and has parallels to mysticism and intiution. The rapid popularization of the complementary area has spawned a voluminous literature with anecdotal claims of cures for just about any named sickness. A short-list in Table 6.1 is familiar to the lay public and independently licensed practitioners in many US states. Its greater part is a disjoint hodge-podge of quasi-scientific and spiritual connections, which use silly paraphernalia and

Table 6.1   Five main loosely defined categories of unconventional medicine.*

Category	Type
'Spa therapies'	Aromatherapy, Herbal Medicine, Juice Therapy, Homeopathy, Hydrotherapy, Kneipping
Nutritional approach	Copper Effects, Naturopathy, Environmental Medicine, Fasting, Lepore Technique, Macrobiotic Therapy, Metabolic Therapy, Orthomolecular Medicine
'Energy' therapies	Bioenergetics, Energy Medicine, Hellerwork, Magnetic Field Therapy, Manual Healing, Negative Ions, Polarity Balancing, Psychic Surgery, Pyramid energy
Musculo-skeletal practices	Alexander Technique, Applied Kinesiology, Bodywork Therapies, Cupping, Chiropractic, Craniofacial Therapy, Reflexology, Rolfing, Shiatsu
Mind/Body-control therapies	Art Therapy/Sound Therapy, Autogenic Training, Biofeedback, Guided Imagery, Hypnotherapy, Psychotherapy, Relaxation Response, Magnetic Passes, Meditation, Past Lives Therapy, Yoga

*Note: An excellent essay on the topic of this and other fads is in Ref. 49.

irrational therapeutic procedures. It advocates the need to shift orientation from 'curing' to healing people in their entirety. It is a hoarding occupation, all is accumulated, and nothing is ever rejected. The description of all available therapies from A to Z with some explanations and comments would easily require a handbook format.[47]

Table 6.1 does not include practices that explicitly appeal to specific ethnic or religious groups since we shall not deal with the therapeutic benefits of religion, as it is more complex than just faith. One cannot deny that they may well be helpful since they are ministered to their own people, and are thus reassuring as the presence of supportive social bonds.[48] Therefore, some physicians advocate the necessity of unconventional techniques on the grounds of sociocultural and anthropological correctness to many immigrants who would otherwise be reluctant to submit to Western practices. It is not at all gratuitous that the fast growing population of patients coming from Asian and Middle Eastern cultures prompts some prominent representatives of the intellectual elite to marshal articulate arguments in favor of building on the cultural, religious, and ethnic diversity of patients (Chaps. 3 and 7).

However, an appeal of the Eastern tradition and its narrative are esthetic qualities. It is erroneous to treat them as paradigms of medicine regardless of occasional salubrious effects.* As Peter Atkins[51] put hit in his uncompromising prose:

> *"I know that people sometimes say that there should be a peculiarly Islamic science, or that more of the Eastern traditions should be blended into science, just as some say that there should be a feminist science to displace what some perceive as its predominantly male component. I think that is dangerous nonsense. Of course, there should be local interests in science, such as the study of indigenous herbal medicines, but science is so successful in its current mode that there is not the slightest need to contaminate its procedures by politics"* (p. 26).

The extent to which local shamanistic practices have clinical efficacy is a matter of ongoing debate. Whatever the outcome, they belong to other aspects of healing in the religious context known since the time of the prophets, which are not relevant to the theory and practice of medical and/or health psychology. It would be futile to convince the true believer in the irrationality of indigenous treatment practices whereas nonbelievers might not be receptive to the language of murkiness. If some of these practices are endorsed that would be rather worrisome.†

---

*The same is true *a propos* the pressures to understand the medical needs of other ethnic minorities. For an absurd example, consider the fact that until the 1960's, the Wari Indians, who dwell deep in the Amazon jungle just outside Santo Andre in Western Brazil, used to roast and eat the flesh of their dead. The Wari do not practice their anthropophagic funereal rites any longer, even if they admit of missing them. Conklin,[50] who extensively studied the tribe, thinks that this custom illuminates a universal effort of dealing with grief. Understanding that requires, in her view, overcoming Western misconceptions about anthropophagy. However politically correct, 'understanding' and empathy are not identical to helping the bereaved within the perimeter of their beliefs.

†In some cultures, a physician is not regarded as the person to whom one goes for the prevention or treatment of disease. There are countless national and ethnic differences as to what is considered healthy. The most common methods are practicing folk medicine, poultice, geophagy, eating or avoiding special foods, and magic, including voodoo practices. In Europe, the tendency to spit in public was banished when tuberculosis was rampant. However, the habit of noisily clearing the throat and spitting right on the floor can be encountered everywhere in China, even in movie theaters or restaurants. Chinese medicine regards phlegm as a sign of a natural imbalance in the body, and spitting is part of a health maintenance routine directed at immediate restoration of health stability. In order to build a new image of Beijing before the Olympics, one thousand anti-spitting centers were set up around the city, with microscopes showing the dangerous bacteria in sputum and banners bearing slogans analogous to, "Keep fit. Don't spit."[52] Surprisingly, the therapies emphasizing unity with the eternal are in vogue. Healing life force or esoteric energy therapies, such as Japanese Reiki,[53] "therapeutic touch" (often practiced by nurses),[54] or "the laying-on of hands,"[55] which elude every efforts of scientific detection of their efficacy, belong to these categories.

Alternative Distant Healing

A healer is assumed by some to be so powerful as to be able to transmit 'positive healing energy' to a patient at another location. Published accounts of successful alternative treatment typically involve small sample sizes and widely varying circumstances, making it difficult to ascertain the reality of the claims. One study[56] attempted to examine the efficacy of this low-budget cure on a common and easy to score problem, that of skin warts. That was a daring experiment. Unlike other variables such as depression, anxiety, or self-esteem, the effects on warts are easy to compute in terms of their size and number. A total of 84 patients with warts were randomly assigned either to a group that received 6 weeks of distant healing by one of ten experienced healers or to a control group that received a similar preliminary assessment but no distant healing. Both the patients and the evaluators were blinded as to group assignment. It appeared that the mean number and size of warts per person did not change significantly during the study. Actually, their number slightly increased in the healing group and decreased in the control group. Likewise, there were no significant between-group differences on the depression and anxiety scores. In another study,[57] those who 'received' prayer to treat alcohol problems did not demonstrate clinical advantage in the treatment of alcohol abuse. If anything, those who reported at baseline that the family member or friends were already praying for them were found to be drinking significantly more at six months than were those who reported being unaware of anyone praying for them. Ancient Greek warriors were more courageous, too, when convinced that their favorite deities were fighting their battles.

Not persuaded by the futility of such trials, some practitioners are serious about verifying the claim of miraculous telehealing even in cases such as AIDS.[58] In the latter study, 40 patients with advanced AIDS were pair-matched for age, $CD4^+$ count, and a number of AIDS-defining symptoms, and then randomly allocated to either 10 weeks of distant healing or a control group. Distant healing was given by self-identified healers representing many different healing practices and spiritual traditions throughout the US. At six months, a blind medical chart review found no significant differences in $CD4^+$ counts. However, the 'treated' patients acquired significantly fewer new AIDS-defining symptoms, had lower illness severity, and required significantly fewer doctor visits and consequently, fewer hospitalizations. Clearly, there was a robust placebo effect that needs to be ascertained. The study was concluded, however, with an optimistic declaration of the utility of distant healing, although recommending distant sex as an ultimate AIDS preventive measure would have been infinitely more profitable.

My Mother Taught Me about My Roots: 'Do You Think You Were Born in a Barn?'

Many a myth has grown up around complementary birthing practices. Since the programs of future health trajectories are patterned already *in utero* and around the time of labor (Chap. 2), perhaps, it does make sense to invest in reducing the risk of childbirth. With the growing openness to complementary and alternative therapies, the emphasis is on the women's preferences and convenience in choosing options for their babies' births. There are diverse rituals intended to increase the sovereignty over childbirth, generate positive attitudes, short- and long-term *'salutogenic'* effects for expectant mothers. But what could be more 'natural' than normal vaginal childbirth?

Operationally, natural birth means almost anything different from delivery in bed, and something short of delivering baby completely 'naturally' and unassisted. The list of options varies from waterbirth, birth by squatting, sitting, and standing, clinging to a rope, kneeling, semi-reclined on a mat, to birth supported by all four extremities and such odd procedures as women biting off the umbilical cord of their babies at birth. In birthing places designated as 'alternative,' expectant mothers become patrons who are able to order services in the spirit of a natural way of life and vegetarianism, or a 'good life' with an extra dose of luxury for those with adequate income. That is no longer a fringe movement founded by the divisive British physician Grantly Dick-Read (1890–1959). In Switzerland alone, the rates of waterbirth have steadily risen and stabilized at around 40–50% of spontaneous births. The 'Mayan-birthing' or stool-birth is also a sought after technique. Its rates reached the peak of popularity in 1993 (23%), 5 years after its introduction, and then dropped to 10% of spontaneous births.[59]

Admittedly, the foregoing styles of delivery have long been tested by natural selection in different cultures. They are as reliable as any physiological function. Some Hmong women, who came to the US from Laos, prefer to deliver by squatting and go through labor alone.[60] Occasionally, they can be held from behind by their husbands, who massage their bellies, when they assist delivery. This practice is similar to that in contemporary rural Brazil where traditional midwifes are old, poor, and uneducated women who learned to attend births by themselves or by helping another similar practitioner. These midwives do not perform shaving pubic hair, vaginal exams, and artificial rupture of the membranes. In a country where medical help is costly, where people do not trust health institutions, expectant mothers quite naturally seek medical help from people they know. Like Hmong women, they refused episiotomy and early cord clamping.[61]

Back to the Stones

It is not clear why the currently popular sitting or squatting posture is credited to the Maya. We know little about Mayan obstetrical practices, other than that a figurine of the Aztec birth goddess, Tlazoteotl, portrays the squatting posture of delivery. A relief on the Temple of Esneh that shows Cleopatra's delivery in a squatting position is closer to our culture. Biblical women, too, delivered in a squatting position as is suggested by the macabre instruction of the Pharaoh of Egypt:

ויאמר מלך מצרים למיילדות העבריות אשר שם האחת שפרה ושם השנית פועה: ויאמר בילדכן את העבריות
וראיתן על האבניים אם-בן הוא והמיתן אותו ואם בת היא וחיה

> And the king of Egypt spake to the Hebrew midwives, of which the name of the one was Shiphrah, and the name of the other Puah: And he said, When ye do the office of a midwife to the Hebrew women, and see them upon the *stools*; if it be a son, then ye shall kill him: but if it be a daughter, then she shall live. (SHMOT; A 15–17; ital. added)

Note that there is no word for the 'stools' in the Hebrew text. The Pharaoh who instructed Shiphrah and Puah actually referred to women sitting on האבניים (i.e. ovnaim, the stones), thereby suggesting that Hebrew women might have used a design made of two stones with a hollow space between them. Egyptians were aware of the bricks used by their Hebrew captives for birthing and very likely used similar devices themselves. The reference to the birthing stool might have been introduced by a translator erroneously or intentionally. During the Egyptian Pharaonic era, from 3000 BC to AD 200, obstetric furniture was hardly known. Birthing stools were a later invention, since such stools were in use by the Greeks, as can be derived from the birthing procedure on a relief of a votive tablet of 4th century BC (found at Oropos, now in the National Museum, Athens).

Christianity adopted many of the Greek customs, and translating the Pharaoh's order exactly, would be misunderstood by the reader. The familiar image of Madonna sitting on a block of marble or a low stool with the child on her lap is apparently a birth position to call attention to the painless birth. That was reminiscent of Cleopatra's newborn almost half her size, which must have symbolized either a miracle of her having remained alive after delivery of a colossal baby and/or her painless delivery.

That is not the only version of the Nativity. Some portray the Virgin on a box-like seat with no feet, with or without a back, which was a basic piece of furniture in Greece, or lying on a mattress, thereby suggesting that either a mat was a place of birth or she was exhausted by the miraculous delivery. The Christ-baby humbly born on the straw is portrayed by Amico Aspertini's (c. 1500) *Adoration of the Shepherds*. That Renaissance illumination is especially important since in the early Middle Ages illuminated manuscripts were produced in monasteries and were thus based on the early Catholic doctrines of the Nativity. The Virgin Mary placed baby-Jesus in a manger, which held feed or fodder for livestock in a stable, presumably because there was no room for her at the inn (Luke 2,1–6). But that may be an odd excuse since the owners, unaware of the divine occasion, could have been simply reluctant to offer their house. Apparently, the manger was not an improvised cradle for lack of more sanitary conditions, as Luke's gospel has it, but a normal circumstance for any delivery at the time. Blood was forbidden for the Israelis as inherently impure so that the stable, like the 'stones' in a remote place, may have been an acceptable location for delivery.

In rural Brazil the process of delivery is also delegated to the stable. In remote areas of Nepal, in deference to local customs,[62] approximately half the children are delivered in animal sheds even though these babies are at a significantly higher risk of dying than are those born in the home setting. A common explanation for using the shed is that the family is eager to avoid irritating the 'household deity' by celebrating delivery in living quarters. Perhaps a more realistic reason given by those who prefer the animal shed is that it is easier to clean following delivery. The strain and pushing required to deliver a baby is often associated with defecation. The contemporary expletive 'Holy shit' may be a spillover of the fascination attributed to feces produced in the course of birthing. In India, cow dung is referred to as 'bricks of gold' whereas in ancient Mexico real gold was called 'god shit.' That is why defecation or rather its products were used for divination and were a part of ancient remedies.[63] Whether sanctified or not, defecation was a regular event in delivery and a real piece of obstetric furniture could be an improvement over the

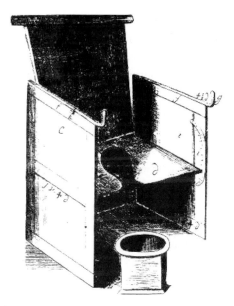

Fig. 6.2 Early 18th century birthing stool (Van Deventer, Hendrik. Operationum Chirurgicarum Novum Lumen Exhibentium Obstetricantibus, Leyden, 1733). The birthing chair was the next step following squatting births. Sitting was more comfortable than squatting and provided women with support during the delivery. The shape of the birthing stool shown here would require the least additional cleanup work. They were a prototype of contemporary indoor sitting toilets, something more advanced than the primitive devices called 'privies.' Images from the History of Medicine, NLM (*http://wwwihm.nlm.nih.gov/ihm/images/A/29/360.jpg*).

Biblical stones (האבנים). Obstetric stools may have inspired the design of the present sit-on toilet. This coprological digression hopefully illuminates the fact that the birth-stool must have been a widely popular innovative item and reasonably safe medical device at that. A drawing and a detailed description can be found in Dr. Raynalde's *The Woman's Boke* (sic) of 1545. Gradually, the 'birth-stool' has become a symbol of old and illiterate midwives before it was reborn as a 'natural' craze of modernity (Fig. 6.2).

Why is There a Tendency to Change?

A question, parallel to that of the subtitle is why the above-mentioned 'elective' practices were not met with forceful resistance? Why were they left to patients' good judgment? The answer is that what we consider normative is in fact an 'alternative.' Francois Mauriceau (1637–1709) must have been the first to introduce the oddly novel and widely opposed procedure of delivery in bed. The continuing arrival of man-midwives and physicians into the profession must have accelerated the evolution of the science of birth care, and made bed delivery a common practice.[64] Amusingly, the invention of the bed was just one of many innovations that sharpened the boundaries between midwifery and professional medicine, when physicians were endowed with powers to modify, mend and overhaul anything they considered unhealthy. Still, the acceptance of delivery by a woman lying on her back had to wait until the late 18th century with somewhat bolder efforts of operative deliveries from the perineal floor. With the coming of an obstetrician-scientist of the 20th century who practiced his art in the hospital (and that was almost exclusively a 'he'), pregnant women were handled as potential patients, so as to protect them from any eventuality. Their delivery position was no longer a whim or a practice based on cultural preferences. As everything else in the hospital, it was an issue of medical regulations.

In Western industrialized countries, physicians deliver the overwhelming majority of babies. By and large, there is a high level of patient satisfaction with obstetric care.[65] Why then do women seek alternatives? Are they seduced by the idea of a return to nature? A common explanation of the popularity of alternative birthing is that the freedom of choice concerning delivery, and personal relationships with the midwife rather than the doctor (and that midwife is almost exclusively a 'she') creates a relaxed ambiance, which is lacking in standard delivery procedures. A great deal of data indicates that certified nurse midwives provide a safe and viable alternative to maternity care.[66] The unavoidable display of medical technology in delivery rooms presumably causes a considerable unease for anxious expectant mothers. Women in midwifery care seem to require relatively fewer medical procedures in labor and a shorter length of stay. Perhaps, they have more unsutured tears but overall, there are no significant differences in perinatal mortality between midwifery and standard (obstetric staff) care.[67] Although maternity care is still overwhelmingly dominated by male physicians the role of the nurse-midwife is increasingly more visible.[68]

Why would a woman fear being admitted as though she were a patient even just for the time of delivery? Startlingly, doctors came to realize that women attended by midwifes are less exposed to hospital-acquired infections, which commonly plague neonatal nurseries with large numbers of neonates. Jeffrey A. Fisher[69] forcefully explained why a doctor for whom

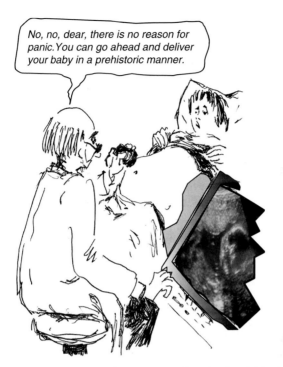

Fig. 6.3 Ancient natural deliveries have become somewhat of a gimmick in that they are seldom followed up by infant-rearing practices common in Third World cultures, such as extended nursing (e.g. breast-feeding for two-three years) and a greater proximity to mother for baby-mother bonding). Ironically, women who wish to deliver naturally or at home seek rigorous medical advice and diagnosis utilizing all electronic equipment and qualified personnel who work within a health care system. Indeed, imaging techniques (e.g. ultrasound or MRI) allow us to minimize brain injury and discover the presence, if any, of brain hemorrhages or white matter disease.

"the sights, sounds and smells of the hospital" are part of an everyday routine, would be terrified of hospitalization:

> "It is simply because, far more than anyone else, they are aware of the danger lurking there. They know too well that in those gleaming, high-tech institutions, where medical miracles are performed every day, roam the ghosts from the ward of the past, from a time we thought we'd never have to see again. They know that although in the 1990s the typical hospital patient admitted with organic disease such as cancer, heart disease, stroke or diabetic complications, the pendulum has increasingly began to swing back to the 1930s. They know that hospitals are in jeopardy, of once again being overwhelmed with untreatable infectious diseases such as pneumonia, tuberculosis, meningitis, typhoid fever and dysentery. And they know

that just by being in a hospital they are at risk of contracting one of these deadly illnesses" (p. 10).

To that one might add that hospital-acquired pathogens also tend to be more virulent.[70] That is a sufficient rationale to predict that the attempts to experiment with 'natural' birth are not just a passing obsession or a caprice to adopt a more active posture and added self-control.

In the US, birthing is considered to have the potential of a 'worst-case' scenario and all women are expected to be 'patients' unless they decline to go to the hospital; in Europe, many opt for home birthing, with the Netherlands leading the nonconformism. The overall picture that seems to emerge, even though many studies are not easy to interpret, is that no significant differences exist between licensed out-of-hospital midwives as compared with physicians or certified nurse-midwives in hospitals on outcomes, such as birthweight, Apgar scores, and neonatal and postneonatal mortality. Research into this subject is still in its infancy. After some enthusiastic reports of natural delivery practices, and the benefits of the sitting position, there were a few more balanced accounts of advantages and disadvantages of alternative childbirth practices.[71,72] Thus, a woman who cannot resist experimenting with the 'natural' position of delivery has to be told that 'back-to-the stones' squatting or even semi-recumbent positions are physically demanding and that maintaining such positions over a considerable length of time might be a disagreeable experience. Yet, it is proper to assure an expectant mother that in completely normal pregnancy the upright posture in labor is *not* harmful to either mother, fetus or to the progress of labor, inasmuch as despite marked differences in socioeconomic conditions and care facilities, the mortality and morbidity rates in developing countries are by and large comparable with those in developed countries, save for low weight babies.

In sum, until the onset of the 16th century, men were not allowed into the birthing chamber but for a difficult or life-threatening situation. We now see the same trend, albeit in reverse. Traditional female midwives began to take control over birthing whereas male doctors are seen as an emergency reserve. Actually, midwifes are winning the territory. Dr. James Owen Drife, professor of obstetrics and gynecology at the University of Leeds, asked with humorous self-depreciation: "How do you face extinction with dignity?" His personal achievement, envied by many, is that a group of distinguished female colleagues made him an Honorary Woman ("No surgery or hormones, you understand ...", he says, "I shall wait a few more years before setting up the Medical Men's Federation, dedicated to promoting the interests of the new minority"). The advantage of obstetric care with the current reclined bed becomes immediately apparent if the laboring woman has prenatal risk factors, high risk of rupture of the anal sphincter or complicated delivery that requires a transfer from an obstetric chair to a conventional delivery table. Another problem is the potential need for neonatal resuscitation (e.g. the requirements for bronchial intubations). A physician may thus need to be literally at her bedside fully armed with medical technology. In such cases, the 'contemporary bed' wins hands down in the comparison with holistic philosophy, reformist ideas of a return to nature, or a feminist passion for independence. Thus, the advance of women-controlled models of delivery and midwifery would hardly reverse the modern tradition of 'male mid-wifery' and the reliance on physician-assisted delivery.

Why Do Unconventional Practices Prosper?

The Edwin Smith Surgical Papyrus, so named after the American egyptologist who purchased the scroll in 1862 in Egypt, introduced the famous tripartite approach, that of diagnosis, 'verdict,' and treatment. When deciding upon the latter, ancient Egyptian physicians were guided by three principles: (a) "an ailment which I will treat"; (b) "an ailment with which I will contend"; and (c) "an ailment not to be treated." Contemporary physicians continue this tra-dition, meaning that they state the limitations of their knowledge and might doubt their ability to cure even when a patient is accepted for 'management.' By contrast, 'integrative' practitioners accept a case regardless of 'where,' 'how,' 'why' and 'when.'

Nearly all individuals are 'symptomatic' at one time or another in their lives. But only a small number of them will ever pay a visit to a physician. The rest are at the mercy of denial (or idleness, or patience), and ultimately they feel better either in spite of their self-neglect, or because of it. As Bernard Shaw[73] famously pointed out, "When men die of disease they are said to die from natural causes. When they recover (and they mostly do) the doctor gets the credit for curing them." Ancient physicians were appreciative of the enormity of their ignorance when called to treat a disorder or predict its outcome. Ever since Hippocrates's *Decorum*, "Physicians have given a place to the gods. For in medicine, that which is powerful is not in excess. In fact, though physicians take many things in hand, many diseases are also overcome for them spontaneously"[74] (p. 36). Centuries ago, Amboroise Paré humbly declared, "I dress the wounds, and God heals them." This stipulation is a part of the faith healing principle practiced by Christian Science today.

The healing power of the organism is based on the endogenous processes of self-monitoring and self-repair, whose molecular foundation only recently became an arena of active research. Whatever their nature, a presumably formidable symptom may simply go away of its own accord (a feature of life that every quack comes to count upon). Much of the success of healing is thus determined by patients' patience (no pun intended) to physicians' opportunism in exploiting this natural healing power of the body. Alternative practitioners do not need the counsel of clinical health psychology since they shrewdly wait until the natural powers of the body and mind take over and the sheer presence of a practitioner will be fixed in the memory of the patient as that of an able healer who provides the treatment. The practitioner thus easily wins over the patients by addressing their well-being or by 'looking after' rather than treating the disease. Perhaps, unconventional medicine is a concept of help that shifts the focus from curing diseases to affecting the memory of the sick by being at hand in the course of healing. Given that unconventional medicine is highly controversial and unsupported by evidence, one might demand: Why are people willing to pay a great deal of money for 'unproven' medicine when scientifically-based medicine is available at no extra personal cost? And who practices CAM?

Who Practices CAM?

On January 23–24, 2001, the National Center for Complimentary and Alternative Medicine (NCCAM) co-sponsored an extraordinary conference in London, England, entitled: "Can Alternative Medicine Be Integrated into Mainstream Care?" (*www.altmed.od.nih.gov/news/pastmeetings/012301*). Charles, Prince of Wales, sent a videotaped message to share his conviction that health care treatments should maximize the contributions of the "well-tried" traditions that emphasize "the body, mind, and spirit of each individual," instead of simply "looking at the clinical problem and ignoring the whole person." The title of the meeting was surprising. Not many believe that there is a confrontation, and those more enlighten of the previous clashes were also aware that the war of medicine with alternative practices was long lost. In a formal affirmation of a need for 'medical pluralism,' the US Congress created in 1992 the Office of Alternative Medicine based in the National Institutes of Health, to assure that alternative medicine be phrased and researched as a regular medico-biological field. That is a gracious, albeit Sisyphean, goal. One might wonder how long it would take to validate the short-list of techniques summarized in Table 6.1 and organize a credible study of thousands of claims of shamanic healing, spiritual healing and numerous cases of miraculous surgery, when clinical psychology and biological psychiatry have yet to evaluate the efficacy of over 250 available systems of psychotherapy.[75] In the meantime, 'integrative' models of health care, however marginal, have received a hefty economic and liberal legal admission. Although the outlook for alternative medicine is contingent upon the validation success, its presence within the framework of NIH is already advertised as a harbinger of the new status of integrative medicine that may lead to its incorporation into mainstream healthcare delivery.

Some trust that after centuries of struggle with 'irregular practitioners' academic medicine is getting increasingly more lethargic in defending its bastions and are experiencing some sort of 'battle fatigue.'[16] There may be other incentives. Many practitioners and educators feel that they can score points in heaven by living a life that is more lackadaisical rather than being martyred in a futile struggle against profitable big business. Though alternative medicine does not enjoy the same level of publicity as the glamorous conventional practice, it also suffers less from damaging criticism when something goes terribly wrong. Being an academically thankless endeavor, it does not expose itself as readily to relentless scrutiny, and therefore avoids a clear defeat in the open. However, a patient rejected by conventional medicine, but recovered on complementary recommendations is always a source of embarrassment for the former.

The reason for some to practice alternative medicine is consistent with the expectation of risk theories that extreme events requiring expert knowledge are rare. As mentioned above, if the case is not especially threatening, it does not matter whether a physician's diagnosis and treatment are right or wrong. Thus, in the ocean of trivial everyday symptoms, being an expert provides a little increment of accuracy and quality of treatment and even less of an incentive to arrive at (and pay for) an accurate diagnosis. Many physicians take over complementary and alternative medicine and blend it into their practice. These medical 'mixers' consider longer visits for difficult patients, but mostly have complementary medicine as a reminder "to become more consumer-savvy and to 'placate' public dissatisfaction with such perceived mainstream health care problems as the impersonality of medical technology or the absence of robust patient-physician relationships"[16] (p. 193).

It is sensible to recall that by the end of 18th century the French government experienced pressure to examine the claims of the Viennese physician Anton Mesmer (1734–1815) that his sensationally successful treatment was more efficacious than simply curing patients. Acting on the model of 'science by committee,' Louis XVI endorsed in 1784 a commission of several internationally renowned scientists, such as Antoine Lavoisier, 'the founder of modern chemistry,' and Benjamin Franklin to investigate Mesmer. They filed a binding report to the Academy of Sciences that Mesmer's techniques were based on myth. Still 'magnetizers' were practiced in Europe and the US for most of the 19th century, and then evolved into the industry of magnetic devices.

With the advantage of hindsight one might admit that no damage to public health was done or rather each category of medicine did damage of its own to its own kind of public. One of the difficulties encountered in defining complementary medicine (the most recent and by far the most complex of all methodological and technical problems that determines the daily practice of practitioners) is a *special kind of consumer*, as was mentioned in Chaps. 1 and 3. These consumers are people who prefer lengthy in-depth consultations with the therapist, or patients who have difficulties communicating what really bothers them. Most of these patients are *mesmerized* by the more refined bedside manners of alternative physicians, their more pleasing, tolerant and satisfying communication with patients than medical physicians. These people are 'culturally inventive,' with at least some college background, arguing for personal and psychological growth, wary of environmental, and who are interested in esoteric spirituality, the foreign and exotic. Commensurate with their holistic orientation, as well as their beliefs in the dominance of mind and spirit in health, 55% of this group are more likely to chose complementary medicine when they are sick (as opposed to 24% of the general population).[76] With regard to symptoms, those who choose alternative over mainstream therapies suffer from those diffuse chronic symptoms that were dealt with in Chap. 3. Undeniably, many patients favor alternative therapies merely because their physicians were frank in acknowledging their limited ability to remedy the patients' conditions, as still mysterious, and thus implicitly encouraged 'doctor's shopping.' This explains why patients who saw their physician more frequently might be disenchanted enough to use unconventional medicine (0 visits: 7%, 1–2 visits: 22%, 3–6 visits: 35%, 7 or more visits: 44%).[77] Keenly aware of the fact that the strength of alternative practices is in their placebogenicity, unconventional practitioners never talk down to their patients.

Reflections on the Lineage of Complementary Medicine

Intriguingly, *ars medendi* — the art of medicine, or *medeor* (to treat) — seem to share their origin with the word *mead, medu* — fermented honey beverage. Honey must have been one of those early ultimate remedies across many geographic areas and cultures that were given to avert sickness or to treat and care, thereby establishing what is known as *ars medendi*. Otherwise, every culture or subculture, until very recently, had its own kind of medicine that evolved vertically, so to speak, with very limited horizontal cross-fertilization since medicinal views were built on philosophy and religion. Ever since the age of medieval or Renaissance alchemy, European medicine advanced in a 'non-ecological' direction, with alchemy as its chief inspiration. That does not mean that drugs from geographically remotes places did not reach Europe. However, what trade and plunder brought to the Western shores from the ecological medicine of other worlds was adopted relatively slowly and often painfully. It took decades to accept coffee, tea, chocolate, potatoes or tomatoes, which were a part of the empirical reality of other cultures, and internalize them within the prevalent pharmacological and dietary customs. Were these acquisitions useful? Undeniably. Reflecting on the role of natural remedies, Stephen E. Straus, the first Director of the National Center for Complementary and Alternative Medicine (NCCAM), disclosed in his statement before the Senate Appropriations Subcommittee (in March 28, 2000):

> "A number of practices once considered unorthodox, have proven safe and effective and been assimilated seamlessly into current medical practice. Acupuncture is routinely applied to manage chronic pain and nausea associated with chemotherapy. Some of our most important drugs — digitalis, vincristine, and taxol — are of botanical origin. ..."

But is it a sensible explanation behind a desire to become more familiar with complementary medical practices? Acupuncture is seemingly useful, too, and so is ECT, of which we know very little. The necessity to learn more about both modalities would have to come from the same budget. All drugs of the Third World, as well as those of ours were of 'botanical origin' since there was no other kind, because other drugs were difficult or very expensive to produce in quantities, or because they were impure under the most rigorous manufacturing conditions. That does not inspire many to practice the animistic and cosmological medicine of the past, or to embrace the stance that is admittedly magical, or reexamine the virtues of alchemy.

Why then has the mood changed in recent years from rejection to semi-acceptance of these drugs and practices? Has medicine changed, or was too much expected from it in the past that the turn to embrace complementary medicine was an act of desperation? Is it the common ebb and flow of the public love-hate relations with innovation and technology that is impatient to bring back an old and 'pure' world of organic foods, pure spring water and unpolluted air? Or is it our voracious appetite for miracles that still remain at the level of Homeric Greeks? As in a multiple choice exam, one might concede that all of the above certainly matter. Still, what has lowered the bar of tolerance to alternative practices in an age of science is something else. That 'something' is a gradual realization that society is unable to support the public health service at ever increasing levels. Through the eyeglasses of cost, it is clear that we had better look for a grain of scientific truth and wisdom in complementary medicine, or else ... And thus, what was once rejected as irrational has become cost-effective and desirable.

In an effort to enlist the support of the US House of Representatives, Herbert Benson lobbied in November 1997 for the recognition of mind-body therapies as a decisive factor in a new healthcare strategy. "Consider for a moment," he lured his audience,

> "that I were here today discussing a new drug and the scientific evidence indicated that this new drug could successfully treat a wide variety of prevalent medical conditions — conditions that lead to 60 to 90% of visits to physicians. Furthermore, consider that it could also prevent these conditions from occurring and recurring and that it was safe, without dangerous side-effects. And, consider that the new drug was demonstrated to decrease visits to doctors by as much as 50% and that this decrease could lead to annual cost savings of more than US$54 billion. The discovery of such a drug would be front-page news and immediately embraced. *Such scientifically validated mind-body belief-related therapies have been shown to produce clinical and economic benefits,* but as yet have not been so received." (ital. added) (*www.apa.org/ppo/benson.html*)

Such assertions are propagated at an era when the cost of medicine is expected to increase over time as a percentage of the gross domestic product from 13.9% in 1999 to 16.6% in 2007. In dollar amounts that is a trillion dollars more than we are spending now (*Health Care Financing Administration (HCFA)*; *www.hcfa.gov/stats/nheproj/ tables/t01.htm*).

Benson's 'economic argument' was well taken. Straus recognized that US healthcare consumers are expected to spend nearly US$31 billion in

2000. This sum is greater than the cost of all US hospitalizations, but that is precisely why such a bottomless market is so attractive. It would entice the pharmaceutical industry to 'complement' their traditional pharmaceutical lines with herbal products; some medical schools would offer selected courses on complementary medicine; the managed care, insurance carriers, hospital providers, and major academic medical centers would gain economically by providing the idiosyncratic integrative practices at a lower cost.

In a classic plea of a political campaigner, Benson argued that research funding should reflect public fear of a disease or the economic impact of diseases, rather than the likelihood of real scientific advances:

> "Mind/body, self-care interventions reduce costs of medical care by reducing visits to doctors up to 5% … In contrast, when patients use an alternative therapy, such as acupuncture, they do not give up penicillin and surgery. Alternative medicine is cost additive."

In the same testimony he declared that 'mind/body therapies' are not to be confused with 'so-called alternative medicine,' as he put it:

> "Therapies such as the relaxation response have scientific documentation of their therapeutic utility. In contrast, alternative treatments are without scientific foundation. After all, if alternative therapies were scientifically established, they would not be alternative."

To be fair, complementary medicine does not require expensive diagnostic tests before learning what is ailing their patients. Benson is right, however, that if inert substances work — as they occasionally do, as was mentioned above when one believes in their efficacy — then 'mind healing' is an acceptable healthcare arena and should be explored. If successful, it is certain to boost the field of health psychology as it is capable of outperforming medicine in terms of the excitement in the public eye. The problem is that many Western patients may not be as lucky as promised by using mind power to maintain sanity and somatic health. Mao Zedong is said to have quipped that in revolutionary wars, violence is inevitable: "You can't make omelets without breaking eggs." Quite sensible for an omelet eater, but quite wretched if you are an egg. Nobody knows the real cost of misery if the concept of mind/body healthcare is implemented to save money, and patients would obtain medical help with a significant delay to alter the course of their disease.

All this is not to deny Straus's conviction that many useful drugs can be found in the tropical forest. Non-human primates (East African chimpanzee populations, as well as bonobos and lowland gorillas) use a variety of non-nutritional plants and nutrient-poor bark seemingly to control parasite infection and provide relief from related gastrointestinal upsets. Intriguingly, both bitter pith chewing and leaf swallowing of the same plant species that apparently included recreational drugs tend to occur among neighboring groups of the same ape species. Local traditions of plant selection appear to be transmitted when females of the same species transfer into non-natal groups. This and other fascinating observations of *zoopharmacognosy* indicating that apes and humans with similar illnesses select the same medicinal plants provide insight into the evolution of medicinal behaviors in modern humans and the possible nature of self-medication in early hominids.[78,79] The concepts of herbal medication with such ancient roots must be very conservative, and decidedly reluctant to depart from learned lessons and established traditions. If in our enthusiasm we agree to return to the style of drug selection and design of the past, we would have to wait no less than the decade or two needed to deliver a successful agent to the shelves of apothecaries.

The term 'drug' reflects an old craft-based practice in storing and preserving vegetation selected for its medicinal, social or nutritional value. It must have originated from the word 'dry' since crude medicine was made of dried berries, and crushed leaves and flowers that patients had to slurp as potion distilled from herbs with the help of water or alcohol and sold as medicinal drinks. Some were used on the skin as dyes and ointments, others were burned in pipes to inhale with the smoke (e.g. tobacco, marihuana). Dried organs and bones of exotic animals, as well as their dried excrements, were valuable ingredients of numerous remedies. Such unhygienic cures as Hippopotami droppings had been recommended to heal fevers and epilepsy since antiquity.[63] In all probability, Ngabhi Diamini, the Speaker of the Parliament of Swaziland, must have learned something of the profligate ways of Nature's defenses from hippos. According to Ralph A. Lewin,[14] the Speaker was asked to resign after being caught stealing cow dung from the royal herd, which he believed to have had special powers. Grocers, tobacconists, and druggists were more or less similar occupations since, initially, apothecaries were just storehouses (the first one in Europe was apparently opened in the city of Utrecht, Holland in 1267), and following this custom, 'drug stores' in the US still have their products under the same roof with food items. In turn, druggists, alcohol merchants, chemists, and pharmacists were also overlapping professions. All of them, including those in the liquor industry could claim the honor of the same lineage. As we all know, alcohol was considered a remedy in its pure form and a basis for extracts beneficial for a number of ailments. Much later, the success of proto-pharmacology necessitated an industry of fast-drug products. They must have been formulated as an easy to swallow pellet, occasionally sugared to increase their palatability.

The history of drug formulation in the form of tablets could possibly be traced to one of Europe's antique pharmacy symbols, that of the Gapers. There are a few commonly understood earliest symbols of the medical profession and of pharmacy. The Aeasculapius' staff has become the symbol of physicians; the pharmacists took the Hygieia's bowl and snake bowed over it, even though the snake as an old symbol of wisdom and placebo could easily be used by physicians. The barber post is another omnipresent sign by which barbers advertise their business. Its red-white-blue pole does not denote a French origin, as some believe. It is the symbol of the surgeon/barber where blue stands for venous blood, and thus illustrates the goal of bloodletting, white color symbolizes the dressing applied, and red is the color of iatrogenic complication, when an artery was pierced. The post did not merely have a symbolic value: it was sorely needed to support many a patient since the most common adverse event during bleeding was fainting. The Netherlands is the only European country where druggists adopted an idiosyncratic symbol of their profession, the 'gaper' ('yawner') positioned at the entrance of their shops (Fig. 6.4). Commonly, these were loudly decorated men's heads made of wood, papier-mâché or plaster that portrayed oriental or dark colored men with mouths opened widely as if at the midpoint of a yawn, as well as an overhanging tongue. The race of the gapers was easy to explain. In the Netherlands, 'kruiden-dokters' (herb doctors) and 'kruiden-verkopers' (herbalists) are said to have hired well-built Moorish-looking abettors in exotic Oriental garb as symbols of vitality that must have prompted the onlookers to purchase the advertised miraculous remedies. What would the Dutch gapers protrude the tongues for?

The stuck-out tongue is a sign of strength and aggressiveness in Hindu mythology since it is associated with the cult of Kali (the black woman), who stuck out her tongue to lick up the blood that hit the ground ever since she went on a violent rampage killing innocents as well as demons. The Maori is another culture where protruded tongues and intense gaze are a part of the martial stance to scare enemies. On the other hand the gapers did not look like

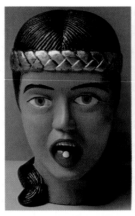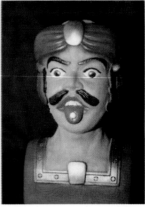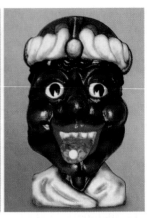

Fig. 6.4 In the Netherlands, kruiden-dokters (herb doctors) and kruiden-verkopers (herbalists) often positioned the images of the gaper ('yawner') at the entrance of their shops. The name 'gapers' is erroneous unless one has ever seen a yawner with a mouth full of food or a pill. A rare example of a woman gaper is shown here along with traditional gapers. Men manifest exophthalmos typical for the majority of gapers and rather suggestive of some gastrointestinal disorder. Reproduced with permission of the Netherlands Drugstore Museum, Maarssen, the Netherlands (*www.museum.com/jb/museum?sub=drogisterij*).

a symbol of superior health. Rather, in the tradition of Renaissance iconography, the dark skin of some heads was an emblem suggesting that the gaper must be outside of the world of health and cleanness. They could be suspected of suffering from *morbus gallico* or other infectious disease and thus were in need of assistance. Accordingly, their tongues, an ancient mirror of inner health, would be protruded as a testimony of fitness. Of course, the gaper might be a trivial 'yawner.' But why would symbols of pharmacy need to display a yawn? Also, anybody who witnessed yawning might recall that it is associated with the eyes being closed whereas all gapers had widely opened eyes bordering on painful exophthalmos. In addition, one would have a problem forcing the tongue out while yawning. Clearly, these heads cannot symbolize sleepiness or display the signs of torpor.

An alternative idea is that the Moors rather certified the sophistication of the business and the credentials of its owners. From the end of the 7th century, Islam in its Arab, Ottoman, or North African and Spanish variety, adopted an assortment of Egyptian and the Judeo-Hellenic medical and pharmaceutical traditions. Somewhat ironically, the Dutch, who were relentless slave traders, were not immune to the medical wisdom of the plundered people, inasmuch as their pharmacists were skilled in storing, and preserving drugs; their apothecaries were capable of manufacturing syrups, ointments, and other preparations used by the sick. A possible clue to the puzzle is suggested by the fact that some gapers are shown with a pellet or two located on the tongue.

The French word dragée is a name for the sugar-coated pills or small colored candy beads for decorating cakes. Sugar traveled a long way from the Far East through the Nile delta to Europe. One of the first refineries for producing the crystallized sugar from the imported sugarcane was opened in the early 16th century in Antwerp, and since that time it has become an important apothecary item. The gapers must have proudly exhibited those still novel drug formulations after 1638 when the pharmacists in Amsterdam had to be members of the *Collegium Medicum* and the use of pharmacopoeia became mandatory.

It is not improbable though that the contemporary term 'drug' originated from the medieval verb *dredge*, meaning to search, gather, or pull out or up. That is precisely how different roots were collected, including that of the famous mandrake (*Mandragora·officinarum, Atropa Mandragora*). The mandrake is a plant with an ancient medicinal history and enduring popularity as an 'alternative' remedy and recreational agent chosen for altering states of consciousness, relieving depression and anxiety. It is known to have served as an adjunct to shamanistic healing in dynastic Egypt. The traditions surrounding the mandrake were a fashionable theme for writers on occult, medication, and botany for several centuries. Much folklore grew around the sexual effects of the root and it is still in demand. What is relevant for the present section is that there is another mandrake, *Podophyllum peltatum*. The alcoholic extract of its dried fruit is known to be an excellent emetic. Ingested on the conviction of a purchase of the hallucinatory or aphrodisiac plant *Mandragora officinarum*, remedies based on the 'counterfeit' *Podophyllum peltatum* mandrake could elicit violent vomiting that requires emergency hospitalization.[80] In a word, regardless of theoretical considerations and anecdotal therapeutic effects, the trend of excessive reliance on herbal medicine, although ascending to ancient practices, can be pregnant with a variety of untoward effects, including death. Even an honest conviction of 'knowing' why a given agent does the job, or at least that it is a real remedy, may not guarantee that in the end it will not be a disappointment. Therefore, alternative drugs should be scrutinized as doggedly as regular medical practices and drugs.

So, is it the lesson learned at the portals watched over by the gapers? Possibly. It may sound incongruous, but the frugal Dutch must have also known how to keep their human cargo healthy. However, most gapers, even well preserved by time and inclement weather conditions in the Drugstore Museum look unhappy, as though they were terribly unwell, so as to stick out their tongues on the request of doctors to check on their health. They might thus advertise the pills as a recommended remedy. Around the year 1600 a 'Gaperstraat' ('Yawnerstreet') was known to exist in the Provincial Town of Hertogenbosch, where a beer was brewed by the "De Gaper" Brewery. The latter apparently was not just a bar. It might be safe to assume that many individuals who frequented it were so drunk as to be unable to stagger to their families and needed urgent detoxication. Could then the pills on the gapers' tongues be promoting either the vomitory or nausea suppressants?

In the past, physicians and apothecaries must have handled numerous cases of poisoning. Modern pharmacology itself was facilitated by the need to provide an antidote against toxic substances, such as animal venom or to produce potent poisons on demand. The nature of poisons ingested recreationally, accidentally, to commit suicide, or murder was hardly possible to determine. With the advent of alchemy of the flamboyant German physician Paracelsus (e.g. antimony, mercury, and powdered magnetic iron oxides) the potions prescribed by doctors were nearly as dangerous as the poisons of one's mortal enemies. It is uncertain how many of these adverse events (including deaths) were caused by raw herbs or legal drugs. An ingestion of a chemical emetic was thus a needed maneuver in acute poisoning barring the stroking of the back of the throat with a finger. Does it mean that Dutch drug stores were not only a place for the herbals, but a center for the management of urgent medical problems and care in cases of acute poisoning? Is it possible then that Dutch 'gapers' actually portray the misery of retching?

Many explanations have been put forward for the weird and wonderful symbols of Dutch pharmacy. The present view is counter to the popular explanation that the Moors were needed to advertise drugs from the colonies for their healthy look. The Dutch were enterprising travelers who were keen to take advantage of Oriental sophistication in medicine and pharmacopeia. It thus seems that the gapers advertised 'alternative' detoxicating institutions, 'Gaper's Bars,' when Oriental medicine was infinitely superior to European doctoring; when a drug such as mandrake was reputed as a potent painkiller, muscle relaxant, and narcotic, often used together with opium and henbane, and hemlock before surgery in a practice recorded since the time of the famous Arab physician Avicenna. That is all our remote history. Gaper's bars all but disappeared. Their message in the current age of excitement with alternative medicine is that for the majority of drugs, alternative drugs included, there is a limited period for excitement with their efficacy. Health practitioners might close the shutters on those drugs whose worthlessness is recognized, when their side-effects are encountered or when a more efficacious or potent remedy is found. To the considerable relief of environmentalists, the success of the anti-impotence drug Viagra, for example, has drastically reduced the demand for alternative remedies based on deer antlers and seals penises. But tonnes of other alternative remedies are bottled every day. It would be fair to admit though, that society cannot let medicine produce anything it wishes to do, and provide funds for everything it cares to create. New technology is substantially more expensive than alternative natural preparations, and thus for the present, harvesting herbal medicine will have to be endorsed as a cheaper alternative compared to developing novel drugs. Besides, the costs are passed on to the consumer who wishes to experiment with these agents. That leads to the conclusion.

Coda: The Gods Must Be Crazy

"Asclepios learned the art of medicine from his father Apollo the physician and took his residency under Chiron the Centaur, whom he quickly surpassed in herbal and surgical skills. Unfortunately, he became too skillful and began to anger the gods."

Nora, J. *JAMA*. 275:1386, 1996

This 40-word poem accurately submits the origin of problems with contemporary medicine. If the gods were jealous about the procedural superiority of Asclepios, they must be increasingly furious with contemporary physicians for their excessive reliance on technical skill. They must have sent the gift of 'complementary' medicine to exercise the wide range of traditional practices or treatments that seemed quite benevolent and devoid of scientifically sound methodology. Indeed, if we try to understand complementary medicine sympathetically from its historical roots and the Eastern forms of consciousness that nurtured it, we find it seductive and engaging. Its concepts are broadcasted in language which does not impart the conflicts, animosity, and irrationality of our medical history. However, many of its modalities are completely opaque and will remain such for years to come, so as to resist the need for their scrutiny; others were carried with the previous tides of globalization to alien lands and are more recognizable. Still others are reminiscent of the discarded soda bottle in the Kalahari Desert that descended on a Kalahari bushman in the famous movie of the 80s, *The Gods must be Crazy*. That bottle was one of the strangest and most beautiful things the bushman had ever encountered. But ultimately the gift was the source of conflicts in the tribe. In a series of comic and pathetic episodes that "evil thing" had to be returned to the Gods to reinstate order to its original state. A gift of this kind might be a handy one if you had no other container for water when marooned on an isolated island. However, a similar gift landing as you walk down a street is unlikely to please. The Gods must clearly be crazy or oddly benevolent to package complementary medicine and give its practitioners the opportunity to increase practice revenues, and boost their market shares by proactively responding to consumers' ignorance and mainstream medicine infatuated with technology.

Complementary medicine has its own politics, sponsored by the loyalty of its patients' lobby, and powered by the investment of those who have made it their career. The lobby of alternative medicine was sufficiently sophisticated, so that in 1998, the US Congress elevated it from the 'Office category' to the status of National Center for Complementary and Alternative Medicine (NCCAM) and came up with the money for its administrative authority in designing and managing its own research portfolio. When describing the state of integrative medicine in their paper, quoted above, Eisenberg and Kaptchuk[16] had to admit, somewhat ruefully, that the recent increased awareness of alternative medicine represents both a historic continuation of the tradition of US medical pluralism and a dramatic reconfiguration away from antagonism toward a postmodern acknowledgment of diversity. Although a "cease-fire, if not a complete armistice" has been achieved, the climate of debate is currently determined by the worries of reaching a proper balance between the supposed consumers' benefits and our needs as the community that has to educate the young, to do expensive research and to struggle with deceptive practices.

Among the things that are difficult to swallow with the legitimacy of alternatives is: What is the role of science and scientific evidence in their 'complementarity'? Since a "proof is accepted if it obtains the endorsement of the leading specialists of the time or employs the principles that are fashionable at the moment,"[81] the Juvenalian question (*'Who judge the judges?'*) might be, Who are the referees? and who gets to deliberate on their verdict? This is a precarious definition of proof since expert opinions are not data. Shall we expect hard data to come? And what would be their impact if they are difficult to interpret or inconclusive? If the mystery of natural drugs seems more appealing than the hard evidence of conventional help, the question is, Will consumers acknowledge the accomplishment of improved performance based on science? To what extent will alternative medicine be assimilated, 'co-opted,' or even truly integrated into a new single system before we know? Then, will the medical profession seek to absorb only scientifically proven therapies or will it begin to include therapies that provide marketing advantages (e.g. homeopathy, polarity healing, and the healing power of touch, as well as other bogus maneuvers, based on 'energy manipulation' and telehealing)?

SO WHAT?

This chapter was meant to provide a taste of the current interface between health psychology and alternative medicine. The reemergence of the latter occurred within a polemical context of therapeutic success and marketability of (as of now) 'complementary' and 'integrative' practices. Alternative medicine has its own politics, sponsored by the loyalty of its patients' lobby, and powered by the investment of those who have made it their career. Those who envisioned the latter as providing the solutions to numerous practical problems in health psychology are bound to be disappointed.

Although most of that polemical context remains, the current state is that of an effort to subject complementary and alternative methods to rigorous and sound epidemiological study evaluations before they are offered as legitimate. In addition, alternative explanations for unexpected or unexplained findings should be explored, and additional confirmatory information provided before one embraces any new therapeutic or prophylactic modality.

It was reaffirmed that the homily that 'nothing succeeds like success' is nowhere truer that in complementary medicine. It thrives in the absence of the quality of the evidence, which is a basic requirement for any field of medicine. Nothing can be as misleading as undeserved triumph. It is difficult to say how long the popularity of alternative medicine will last since it is an occupation that, using Freidson's[82] words (out of context), "seeks to sustain or create public belief about it without having any necessary bearing on the objective prerequisites for the occupation's real work" (p. 187).

Given that very few practitioners have a righteous commitment to alternative medicine the question is, What is happening at the meeting point between psychology, medicine and complementary medicine? The majority of 'straight' medical practitioners (using chiropractors' terminology) seem to stay within the confines of their profession. For psychologists the impact of complementary medicine is uncertain. Psychology is irreversibly science by virtue of its methodological sophistication, with tendency to examine itself and reject what is substandard. It is likely that people will view with suspicion an appeal for tolerance and benevolence of contemporary consumerism as a valid credential for entry into the profession and be seduced by its tools.

7

---•---

Holistic Philosophy and a Recipe for Causative Goulash

When asked where it hurts, a patient is very likely to point to the anatomical origin of the pain. Not surprisingly, most health professionals specialize in diseases of particular body parts, systems and organs. Giovanni Batista Morgagni (1682–1771), professor of anatomy in Padua, formalized the medical response to such complaints from the 'surgical point of view' by arguing for the necessity of operationally identifying the locus of abnormality 'by the sound of its cry.' Any part of the body giving off the 'sound' was understood as representing a 'system,' regardless of how small it is. Medicine, much like biology, has a limit on how close it could profitably scrutinize some units of the system since for a very myopic distance from the target, biology ends and physics begins. This method of scrutiny of the bodily functions and their aberrations by deriving their nature form studying its increasingly smaller elements and guessing how those parts influence each other is called in modern parlance 'reductionism.' The 17th century French philosopher, Rene Descartes (1596–1650) laid down the current reductionistic concept of illness. His stance was that (somatic) disease is akin to a machine that is broken down. A modernist representation of Descartes' view is the popular Fritz Kahn portrayal of the human body as an "industrial palace," or a chemical plant (*Der Mensch als Industriepalast*). Descartes' views were to become the foundation of what is known as Western medical science. By de-emphasizing the 'wholeness of the body,' physicians were granted an epistemological foothold which helped reduce the impact of the precarious 'noise' of beliefs, fears, mores, traditions, and other factors potentially contributing to illness, thereby increasing the chance of detecting the real signal of diagnostic and prognostic utility. Excessive tinkering with 'noise' would have unduly expanded the field of view of practicing physicians, and postponed for centuries the coming of scientific methodology.

Admittedly, the allusion to a failing organ is often erroneous, but diagnosis is always a hypothesis that has to be tested by the outcome of medication or, however miserably, autopsy. The more specific the hypothesis tested is, the closer it is to the level of 'organ' or 'tissue,' the easier it is to be falsified. The concept of the wandering uterus in hysteria or Plato's attribution of sexual desire to a peripheral organ (again, uterus) rather than to the whole woman, typify those splendid reductionistic absurdities that exposed inadequate theories. Yet for many, reductionism has become a target of hostilities and wanton abuse, when the acknowledgment of being a member of the 'R-club' almost equates to 'coming out of the closet.' All later efforts of a post-Cartesian world view were directed at apologizing for the controversial analogy between the body and machine and at pointing out the limitations of the asphyxiating authoritarian scientism, which does not allow for phenomena such as self-healing.

The notion of wholeness as tantamount to *complete health* has a longer lineage. As an equivalent to functional and anatomical integrity, it was spelled out in the New Testament. Those who wished to be cured had just to touch Jesus's garments, "and as many as touched were made perfectly *whole*" (Mathew 14:36). On another occasion a girl who was "grievously vexed with a devil was made *whole*" from the very hour that Jesus spoke with her mother (Mathew 15:28). Yet, a complete theory of 'wholeness' (a word all holistic writers are fond of even though it makes better sense in connection with wheat grain than with human health) in European medicine can be traced to the name of Paracelsus, one of the most original thinkers of Renaissance medicine, mentioned above. In a somewhat opaque language for the contemporary reader, Paracelsus decomposed wholeness by looking for the origin of illness in *'active principles'* such as the influence of the stars (*ens astrale*), the influence of poisons (*ens veneni*), natural causes (*ens naturale*), the spirit (*ens spirituale*), and finally, the will of God (*ens dei*). Medicine recognized very early that to include all these components amounts to a delusional stance. At least, one component such as natural causes (*ens naturale*) is all it hoped to master. Charles-Édouard Brown-Séquard in France deserves credit for helping to find the binding glue for *ens naturale*. According to his conceptualization, one way of understanding the 'broken machine' was by guessing how the 'bad' organ was capable of affecting the 'whole' of numerous remote tissues. That, he believed, was caused by bad reflexes from the sick organs, such as the uterus, nasal mucosa, heart, genito-urinary tract or stomach, which could send sick signals to remote parts of the body ('reflexively'). The departure from the unknown and semi-fantastic into the realm of 'nerves,' has armed the theory with a credible attribution of symptoms. With time, it also created a host of useless remedies and an army of miserable patients. This mishmash of the rational and the irrational has become a distinguishing mark of many therapeutic pains of holism throughout modern times. By the turn of the 20th century the theory was brought into disrepute, only to be later restored under the name of 'reflexology.'

The lineage of contemporary holism can be traced back to the seminal book, *Holism and Evolution* published in 1926 by Jan Christian Smut, who can safely be given most of the credit for creating the holistic movement. In it, an area under scrutiny was pronounced to be merely an artifact of disproportionate attention that creates the "luminous center." This is surrounded by "smaller or larger dimensions, in which the luminosity trails off and grows fainter until it disappears." According to this view, "the hard and abrupt contours of our ordinary conceptual system do not apply to reality."[1] The notion of 'cause' was thus challenged as relevant to only a limited portion of the 'luminous center,' whose shapes are artificial, and gradually lose their meaning the more complex their boundaries and the farther they are from the epicenter of luminosity. Many scientists working with complex systems, such as irregularities of heart rate, global atmospheric circulation and earthquakes fields, express their intellectual debt to holism. It has become an indisputable magnet in postmodern philosophy and induced, or at least prepared, greater upheavals than any other field or factor in areas such as fuzzy logic, fractal mathematics, self-organized criticality, and stochastic resonance. However, the meaning of holistic methodology outside of these areas has never been explicitly stated, and therefore, one has to put together various perspectives on the term to understand what it means.

To those engaged in researching diseases, holism showed none of the advantages experienced by physics and mathematics. Consequently, in health sciences, holism has remained a metaphor, a sort of password to denote quite dissimilar academic and professional trends. Even an admonition of the great French physiologist, Claude Bernard[2] that "in organisms ... all components are interdependent and influence each other" was driven by pragmatic necessity. He admitted that "when we break up an organism by taking the different components apart, it is only for the sake of convenient experimentation and by no means because we consider them as separate entities"[2] (p. 154). In experimental settings, the notion of wholeness was mostly a nuisance and had to be placed outside the relevant parentheses of research equations. It was abundantly clear that many biological processes are dependent on a large number of interrelated variables. Very few experiments can be set up so that variables can be controlled at the will of the investigator. Thus, other than the declaration of the futility of tinkering with 'totality' in experimental paradigms, Bernard's ideas have made only a marginal contribution to the attitude of wholeness. Some of its proponents discuss holism in the context of the cosmic unity of organic and inorganic matter, which borders on ecocentric Vernadsky-type philosophy. This endorses the holistic infatuation with the 'cosmos of life' as the 20th century equivalent of the preaching of wandering prophets, which stops short of demanding that the patient's microcosm be viewed in its equilibrium with the macrocosm of influences emanating from the far-away stars — something akin to the Paracelsian *ens astrale* and *ens spirituale*. In medicine, 'wholeness' has become synonymous to a rebellion against the perceived inhumanity and coldness of rational doctoring. It spearheaded an anti-reductionistic debate, and was most enthusiastically welcomed by those who were less likely than others to be engaged in research. Kurt Goldstein,[3] one of the major proponents of the holistic approach to human nature conceded facing a 'difficult epistemological problem':

This outlook is similar to the exclusion postulate of Claude Bernard mentioned above. Yet, Goldstein's authority made holistic ideas particularly vocal in such

> *"For us there is no doubt that the atomistic method is the only legitimate scientific procedure for gaining facts."*

areas as neurology and psychology, whose practitioners were frustrated with intractable problems of mind and cognition that were then inaccessible to experimental analysis, and whose practitioners objected to 'mechanistic' views about brain performance as the leading paradigm for explaining both normal functions and their aberrations following local brain lesions. His 'organismic orientation' (which is essentially the same thing as the 'holistic view') was the disposition intended to inject a spirit into the 'machine model' of brain and mind.

In psychology and 'integrative' medicine, holism took a minimalist approach as a principle of healthcare. It recommended healing a patient from a biopsychosocial perspective which meant that all items of an impressive smorgasbord, such as the number of children in the family, social class, race, location of the household, income, education, leisure life, personality, emotional and financial security, promoting caring and empathy, mutual trust, positive state of mind, optimism, and knowing not only what symptoms are, but also what the patient's dog wishes, are tied up together to achieve therapeutic goals. This trend, which is increasingly popular in the nursing and medical press, was designated as *clinical holism*.[4]

The following sides with those who maintain that, by gratuitously overstretching the claims of complexity, one sends a signal of knowing little and being prepared to learn even less; that an imposition of holistic solutions to problems that can be approximated by their 'chunking' is intellectually dishonest. It is equivalent to the position that if everything is relevant then everything is redundant, or to the Nietzchean conviction that "if everything is possible, nothing is true."

Coping with Complexity: 'Risk Epidemic'

Using a special compartment, Kenneth G. Libbrecht[5] of the California Institute of Technology was able to synthesize snowflakes. Crystals are simple structures and what he was able to achieve confirms the obvious. All snowflakes were constructed on the same theme set by the hexagonal structure of ice. What he was unable to produce is revealing. Although he used presumably identical microscopic ice crystals, no two snowflakes appeared alike. This might be surprising for anybody who has faith in the predictability of the laws of physics. Yet, the combination of randomness, complexity, and humidity variation even in the climate-controlled chamber, made the flakes somewhat dissimilar in detail. This is an example of a system with interconnectedness and sensitivity dependence.

Holistic writers allude to interconnectedness within and between the systems and look for their interpretations 'beyond the mechanistic models.' An organism might be conceived of as composed of dissimilar 'tiers' of tissues that blend into one another, interact with each other, and vary in their functions and morphology through the seasons of individual history. The more 'tiers' the organism has, the more its genetic programs are open to environ-mental modulators and act in concert with environmental factors.

A popular way of making rational decisions in predicting behaviors of complex systems is by grappling with two sources of uncertainty, epistemic doubts (lack of knowledge about fundamental laws, say, of pathogen-organism interactions) and aleatory uncertainties, such as sampling errors, measurement inaccuracies, subjective biases, data misclassification, and expectation errors.[6] A host of such uncertainties is encountered when dealing with pharmacodynamic and pharmacokinetic effects, the placebo the effect, psychoneuroimmunology, and even more so, in spontaneous remissions of apparent terminal conditions. Systems with many degrees of freedom are known to exhibit chaotic behavior. Thus, a relatively small change of some quasi-casual factors may be expected to lead to non-linear effects, such as a large increase in the severity of response (e.g. in the direction of either a dras-tic aggravation of health problems or, indeed, to a recovery from disease), particularly in systems with sensitivity dependence. This conforms to the admonition of "assigning zero to events that are not 'impossible,'"[7] or of being careful when dealing with log-normal probability distributions, so as not to discard low probability events occurring in the 'tails' of bell-shaped curves, particularly when an outcome is potentially vital.

Among quantitative nonprobabilistic approaches, chaos and catastrophe theories might be particularly useful for describing the transition from a regular baseline to abrupt, acute or paroxysmal events (e.g. stroke, fever, psychotic episodes or epilepsy). The presence of chaotic dynamical systems does not preclude all forms of prediction, but they are almost impossible in the realm of psychopathology (e.g. see Chap. 3, in passim). The property of com-plex processes of settling down to specific final states ('attractors'), allows considerable latitude for predictability for some limited trajectories of disease evolution. Therefore, the various stages of progression from health to disease, as well as its phases, can be studied and often expected, despite the presence of chaotic dynamics and attractors, as though they were quasi-linear and pre-dictable. When Koch's requirements (discussed in Chap. 1) were impossible to satisfy, and many diseases evolved as 'catastrophe' cases without warning, they were considered non-infectious and subsequently complex multifactorial entities. Numerous exclusions from the dictum 'one germ — one disease,' as well as the limited applicability of the principle 'one gene — one disease' were used to expose the notion of monocausality as an example of the 'greedy' version of reductionism.[8] One way of dealing with that epistemic problem in the medical setting (when adhering to the holistic world view) is to examine everything conceivably relevant to morbidity when the world of environmental stressors is enriched with "the psychological and attitudinal environment as well."[9] All of them may be potential risk factors (meaning a list of amendable attributes that predispose one to a specific malady). Such multiple sources of influence were very tempting excuses when dealing with the unknown origin of the pathophysiology of the majority of disorders, and when such cause escaped detection. Such relationships with 'distributed' effects are designated 'statistical causality.'[10] Why is statistical causality so compelling?

The notion of factors acting together or as an elaborate chain has become the most pervasive dogma of medicine. It is a cliché of practicing medicine to find a diagnosis in order to be capable of choosing the right medicine. However, scientists are seekers of deeper certainty and are fascinated with the infinite correlations that imply the presence of some relevant empirical connections. This multicomponent organization is often likened to the popular Russian dolls, each nesting inside another in a hierarchy of figurines decreasing in size.[11] Physicians hold fast to the principle of 'medical uncertainty,'[12] that posits that 'there is always one more thing that might be done,' and that more risk factors might be considered since the absence of an effect or a negative response coming from a diagnostic test can never be accepted with *absolute* certainty. Epidemiologists caution that the ecologic study design should be reserved for generating hypotheses rather than estimating risk. Yet regardless of such admonitions they are often used in that capacity. When a simple self-limiting illness is 'overdiagnosed' as a life threatening condition, or when innocuous substances are mislabeled as harmful, such errors of judgment are considered infinitely less flawed than assuming the opposite, i.e. mistaking an ill person for a healthy one, or classifying a toxin as a safe agent. When cost is not a factor, medicine tends to be trapped in the 'medical uncertainty' principle because physicians may not know much of what is going on with their patients or do not know enough to make a comfortable decision. Consequently, there may be too little understanding between the two styles of exploration. Thus on certain segments of its history the field may progress blindly along the line of least resistance to some 'bottomless truth' until it is halted by a discovery that makes all circumlocutions irrelevant. John-Arne Skolbekken[13] marshaled convincing evidence that many 'risks' are so designated by being companions of potential factors, their components or modulators.

Much of his argument can be illustrated by the controversy over the dangers of cholesterol, and the claims for the success of cholesterol lowering trials (*http://bmj.com/cgi/content/full/316/7149/1956*).

With the advent of molecular biology, the number of risk factors for some diseases threatened to reach the threshold of a landslide, since each 'factor' may not be a *prima facie* representative of an actual underlying process and may be fragmented and multiplied as one learns more about the system scrutinized. If the word 'enzyme' were to be used as a replacement for cholesterol then its assembly scrutinized with the black box or 'problem box' methodology would require a set of environmental factors, multiple peptides and amino acids, each controlled by a different gene. If some components are reciprocally wired, a deficit in one of them will benefit the other, albeit at the disadvantage of the chain. The whole synthesis is a process of incredible complexity. Given that the enzyme is the final product, each step or component in its creation would be akin to what is understood in epidemiology as a 'risk factor.' One can only marvel at how molecular biologists manage such a multistep assembly line and successfully so, unshaken by these numerous 'risks.'

In the more intimidating ethical, litigious, medical, economical, and sociological ambiance of the last decades, medical journals in the US, Britain and Scandinavia have shown a rapid increase in the use of the term 'risk.' Predictably, the most rapid increase has been contributed by epidemiological journals. Skolbekken[13] designated the phenomenon "risk epidemic" (Fig. 7.1).

The Fallacy of Factorology

The process of sorting out factors and their clusters is antithetical to the notion of holism, since such an analysis means, both mathematically and intellectually, that a finite group of components may adequately describe or predict a specific pragmatic goal. And yet, more than anything else, that process has contributed to the endorsement of holistic concerns of the intervening variables, probabilistic 'mediators,' or 'moderators,' thus obstructing the proposal of simple, albeit not necessarily sufficient, cause-effect assumptions. It was easier "to say that the cause of disease is multifactorial, to remain ignorant as to the mechanisms of the etiology of the disease, and consequently to focus on inappropriate markers to attempt to prevent or treat the disease. It is all too easy to confuse factors which play a role in causing the disease …"[14] (p. 590). With

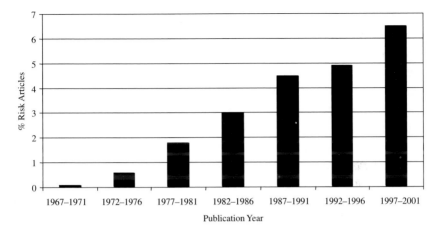

Fig. 7.1 An epidemic infatuation with the term 'risk' in the medical literature. It shows that the number of articles dealing with risk has risen from about 1,000 in the first year covered by his analysis[13] to over 80,000 in the last (1987–1991) and keeps on rising, as shown in his gracious update. Courtesy of John-Arne Skolbekken of the Norwegian University of Science and Technology.

time, the view that the causes of illness are input variables that are expected to predict an outcome after some smart juggling of the data evolved into a self-limiting "black-box paradigm of chronic disease,"[11,15] implying that researchers should be satisfied by processing input variables and meticulously assessing output variables. This principle exempts physicians from establishing what may be the 'absolute' or obligatory factor. For example, neurodevelopmental aberrations are a result of multifactorial processes that can easily impact at any stage of life. However, the establishing of a 'root cause,' such as, say, intrauterine infection with cytomegalovirus, has the advantage of postnatal antiviral therapy that might improve the prognosis of infected neonates since those who survive symptomatic intrauterine infections require comprehensive therapy and home-based early intervention programs to reduce the severity of abnormalities. The proliferation of factors with no improvement of the understanding of maladies has become quite unproductive, scornfully designated as factorology,[16] and has subsequently drifted away from the concept of the 'causality' of illness. Such disrespect is a reflection of the serious confusion and lack of clarity about the systematic status of 'cause' in empirical investigations that has been contributed by holistic methodology. Therefore, a key objective of contemporary medico-biological research is to narrow the list of factors to those most relevant and to eliminate the burden of imposters contributed by the philosophy behind the provision of healthcare.

Historically, the problem presented by the physician, in which he requested the help of other health researchers, was to identify the 'true' underlying disease and then to establish its 'exact' cause. Since for many diseases the diagnosis might be uncertain, the manner of study employed was the description of as many symptoms as possible, and guessing the likely cause for each of them. Consider an example of such a prototypical multifactorial disorder as hypertension. This has a variety of life threatening effects that have their own causes thereby adding to the complexity. Two decades ago our pathophysiological portrayal of hypertension seemed knotty. We were taught that genetic predisposition contributes about 30% of the blood pressure variance. But then, psychological stress, poor nutrition (monosaturated fat, chronic high sodium intake, inadequate potassium and calcium intake), obesity and smoking were conceived as preconditions or factors that determine the severity of hypertension and with it, the development of diabetes mellitus, insulin resistance, arteriosclerosis, increased vessel resistance, cerebral infarction, intracerebral hemorrhage and cardiac infarction. Perhaps this factorial approach to disease was woefully incomplete at best and therapeutically inadequate at worst, since each factor was not necessarily a member in a system whose manipulations were sufficient to affect health outcome, but health psychologists and physicians have behaved as though all of them belong to the same causal pathway or the "causal network instantiation."[17] The fact that factors could reside at different locations of the 'proximal-distant' continuum of the impact of pathogenicity, with their specific causes, at least in specific ethnic groups, has not been openly articulated.

One could go on and on by adding to the above listed factors a few 'negative' conditions, such as not exercising, not drinking in moderation, avoiding siestas, being unscrupulous about keeping doctor's appointments, snoring at night, adopting a self-image in a society that does not endorse it, and other contemptuous items from McCormicks's[18] register. Although listed with a dose of flippancy, all are impeccable, even if are never sufficient, attributes. These features are treated as 'facts,' even though the basis for inclusion of some of them might have been suspicions, false beliefs, trust, or flimsy correlations so that ultimately their relevance to the real world is lost. As the standard quasi-philosophical joke goes, a comparison between a violin and a shoe might classify them within the same family since they have a number of shared characteristics: both have a smell, cannot see, are hollow inside, neither have a square form, and so on. This 'accept everything' attitude, looks like a corollary of Paul E. Meehl's principle: "Reward everything — gold and garbage alike."[19] Arranging these factors is a process that involves judgment about their order and interrelations rather than firm data as to how many factors are really needed to cause a disease. This approach is not particularly specific for hypertension. With the majority of clinical problems, one may not know when to stop looking for additional factors, thereby implying that all relevant factors have been identified.[20]*

Health psychology is keen on dedicating its efforts to modulating secondary, 'life-style factors,' or even tertiary factors (comorbidity, personality, situational and occupational variables, etc.). But such risk factors are relevant to therapeutic intervention only to the extent that they precede the outcome, and when the weight of such factors and their interactions are known. For example, racial oppression may be one of those factors that "does enter the casual chain eventuating in the pathological symptom ..., but it is a factor shared in a very large number — let us say the vast majority — of 'normal' persons; and it does not exist in a greater quantitative degree in the patient than it does in the rest of us"[19] (p. 247). As was shown in Sally Satel's[22] book *PC, M.D.* such attribution is also harmful by making vulnerable people hopeful that a change of social attitudes or fight for them will improve their health when in reality, learning to alter their own destiny would certainly be more profitable. By peddling victimology, such beliefs can only delay the deployment of badly needed medico-biological solutions.

Finally, attempts to deal with the constructs as complex cultural, emotional, socioeconomic and ethnic factors as variables are fallacious. Their "seductive fallacy," as Meehl[19] observed in a different context,

"consists in *assuming*, in the absence of a respectable showing of causal connection, that the medical, psychological, or social aberrations that define him [a person, a mental patient] as a patient *flows from* his conflicts, failures, frustrations, dissatisfactions, and other facts which characterize him as a fallible human being, subject like the rest of us to the human condition" (p. 246, ital. in orig.).

---

*In the Indo-European tradition, counting over the number "three" is excessive. The word '"three" originates from the Latin prefix "trans" (meaning beyond), the French "tres" (meaning very), and the Italian "troppo" (meaning too much).

In conclusion, the awareness of the multiplicity of factors that are potentially involved in disease may not signal therapeutic benefits, and as a natural
defense against information overload, professionals either ignore most of the
data,[23] or insist on adherence to 'beneficial factors' thereby imposing a regime
of surrender of the patient's autonomy, dignity, and self-respect.

The Utility of the Swiss Army Knife

The true Swiss Army Knife, the SAK, patented in 1897 has become
immensely popular with the military for folding into a pocket-size gadget
with multiple blades and a corkscrew. There are reservations about its contemporary pet versions that evolved into a gift doodad featuring a dozen specialized tools from magnifying glasses to fish scrubber and toothpick, and
even a 'chair' that was derisively proposed by a cartoonist for the New Yorker
magazine. If that is what you own, you must have overpaid for the blade, or
even worse still, you have purchased a dozen excuses for having a blade with
no cutting power and short life span. On a hunting trip, very much like in
medicine, numerous helpful, but insufficient tricks do not justify omitting a
single, decisive measure. We have all learned that hard way that in using
antibiotics, one should stick to the dictum of Theodore Roosevelt: "The
unforgivable crime is soft hitting. Do not hit at all if it can be avoided; but
never hit softly."

Sociologists have long noticed that people who tend to be reliable when
dealing with adversity may show a precipitous decline of their initiative in a
group whose members share responsibilities. A detailed description of the
response to shared responsibility is beyond the scope of this discussion, but
it has been repeatedly noticed that even people who are normally in command of their life tend — in complete agreement with the volunteer's
dilemma — to relinquish their accountability for personal safety and delegate it to others when they believe the burden of responsibility is shared.
Holistic principles are a case of conceptual *diffusion of responsibility* that
allows for a failure in a complex case by maintaining that a simple ('muscular') solution is unjustified because there are too many contributors to the
problem to ignore.

The diffusion of responsibility is often practiced when a therapist is confronted with a hierarchy of probabilities of pathological outcomes. Their utility hinges on the ability to scale therapeutic or preventive success vis-à-vis

restrictions imposed by health strategies. Such 'intervention-value' ratios are never computed since risk factors do not occur in isolation. Thus, the 'causes' of disease do not transcend the 'cataloging stage,' thereby representing an account of a meager understanding of 'how things are.' The missing strategy is adding input parameters only when there is a specific model or an algorithm. Consider again the role of low birthweight and prematurity discussed in Chap. 2. Fetal injury was suggested to be a risk factor for later obesity,[24] as well as result in a reduced number of nephrons in the kidneys, thereby impairing their capacity to effectively regulate blood pressure with advancing years. This marker is so robust that Linda S. Adair and Tim J. Cole[25] wondered whether a birth cohort of Filipino infants born between 1983 and 1984 to a different culture will show a pattern similar to that described in the US and UK. They conducted a study based on bimonthly home visits from birth to 2 years postpartum of 2089 infants and then followed-up these children in 1991, 1994, and 1998 when the index children were, on average, 8.5, 11.5, and 15.5 years of age. Their study confirmed that children who were relatively thin at birth and grew more rapidly were at >2 times higher risk of having high blood pressure compared with boys with similar growth rates who were not malnourished in utero. As a consequence, they recommend that prevention of hypertension of Filipino adults aged 60 and older should be delegated to prenatal and early postnatal periods.

Some factors that account for infants' low birthweight were discussed previously (Chap. 2). In reality, they are more plentiful, such as mother's age, education, marital status, birth order, length of interval from previous pregnancy, maternal birthplace, number of prenatal visits, and socioeconomic status, to mention just a few. Even maternal perception of exposure to racial discrimination during pregnancy and the dwelling in violent communities have been considered factors associated with very low birthweight.[26] So what is it in the mountain of risk factors that made an individual more prone to hypertension in adulthood associated with impaired fetal growth?

The control of blood pressure is achieved by structural vascular, neural (sympathetic nervous system activity), endocrine, and renal mechanisms with predictably compensatory interdependent changes. When correlations between all factors are presented to make a point, the point is seldom compelling and therapeutically significant. Martyn and Greenwald[27] felt that progress is achieved if and when "specific hypotheses are formulated and tested" rather than when correlations are computed on collected data. In their determination to follow this logic they hoped, in their own words "to put our money where our mouth is." They maintain that in fetuses with impaired growth there is a parallel deficit in synthesis of a rubber-like macromolecule in the walls of the aorta and large arteries, *elastin*, that leads as the name suggests to permanent changes in the elastic properties of these vessels. That may not be the only adaptation of the fetus in response to influences that retard its growth, but it is an interesting hypothesis to test, inasmuch as the thickening of the capillary membrane is part of the pathophysiology of hypertension as well as experimentally induced and clinical diabetes. Another possibility is a decreased capillary density.

Insofar as a large part of the pressure gradient takes place in the microvascular network, its abnormality may be a key defect leading to hypertension in adulthood. Ordinarily, when pressure is applied tangentially to the wall, a tubular vessel can withstand a much higher pressure than the one that is clinically considered as hypertension. According to Laplace's Law, the tangential tension is proportional to the product of the tubular radius and distending pressure. Thus, assuming that the vascular bed is sufficiently branched, a small body size is protective against high-pressure injury. However, a possible outcome of low birthweight and prematurity is a reduction of the density of arterioles and capillaries, i.e. so-called microvascular rarefaction. This is potentially an important characteristic of various microvascular beds in many forms of hypertension, and fetal decrease of small blood vessel growth is a possible structural anomaly underlying hypertension.[28–30] The density of the capillary network is proportional to the metabolic needs of the cells, so that the capillary surface area roughly corresponds to the volume of mitochondria (1 μm^3 of capillary blood corresponds to about 3 μm^3 of mitochondria).[31] With increased body size, rarefaction must be compensated for by an increment of blood pressure. Assuming that a premature child is immoderately fed and evolves into a corpulent adult, one might wonder whether rarefaction contributes to the higher rate of hypertension in the black community. Perhaps, but that has yet to be elucidated. Rarefaction further implies that hypertension originates very early, and may show clinical signs with a considerable delay. In the long term, capillary abnormalities lead to a gradually increased capillary resistance, which could affect bodily and cerebral blood flow.

In sum, although increased peripheral arterial resistance is the hallmark of essential hypertension, the preceding is not intended to defend the primacy of vascular (microvascular) remodeling. Hypertension has a strong genetic component even though the genes with large effects on blood pressure have yet to be found. Blood pressure is so redundantly controlled that the disorder is treated as a complex multigenic characteristic, affected by individual and environmental factors and numerous feedbacks that are also presumably under genetic control. The foregoing argument simply illustrates the need to break down the 'disorder' into several syndromes and continue the search for specific genetic, molecular movers that make an individual more reactive to ancillary environmental factors. Among such *core measures* is obstetric care that can be steered towards improving *prenatal* health rather than toward changing lifestyle and nutrition of individuals with hypertension. This would require a considerable investment, which could be offset by almost US$15,000 for each of 270,000 low-birth infants. The treatment of these infants would otherwise incur enormous costs, since many of them will have significant comorbidity with advancing years. Occam decrees that in theory, as well as in diagnosis and treatment, 'It is vain to do with more, what can be done with fewer.' Those who are unenthusiastic about the SAK metaphor, may exploit a paraphrase from the famous Principle of Parsimony ('Occam's razor'): holistic principles should not be applied without necessity.

Gresham's Law in Medicine

Let me return to atherosclerosis and coronary heart disease since these are familiar textbook examples. They are easily defended within a typical holistic paradigm because their handling requires taking into account the role of genetic liability, gender, age, diet, blood pressure, diabetes mellitus, occupational variables, pollution, cigarette smoking and obesity. With the advent of a social theory of coronary heart disease, the A-personality factor and other life scares and environmental stressors have also become increasingly popular. As mentioned earlier, the role of cholesterol and hypercholesterolemia has received maximal consideration in atherogenesis.[13] Although central to current health policy, this concept was repeatedly criticized as based on false premises, scientific misrepresentation, and fallacious data. Stehbens[32,33] compellingly argued that serum cholesterol levels display a poor correlation with atherosclerosis and that coronary heart disease is a nonspecific complication of many diseases including atherosclerosis, and therefore cannot be equated with coronary atherosclerosis due to differences in pathology and pathogenesis. Does the falling death rate from cardiovascular disease in the world imply that the outlook is getting better because the public is finally convinced of the role of lifestyle factors? Not at all, since it could also be explained by a dramatic effect on the survival of those who were earlier diagnosed with having infections and treated with antibiotics.[34] After decades of infatuation with cholesterol, the dominant hypothesis now is that infections and proinflammatory cytokines are important 'mechanistic' links between various risk factors.

The role of infection in the etiology of atherosclerosis was recognized by the end of 19th century. Yet it was neither popular nor influential. As Javier Nieto[34] pointed out, "The multifactorial-degenerative model of atherogenesis was further strengthened, at the expense of almost total abandonment of research on the putative atherogenic role of infections." And again:

Nieto's review illustrates the paradox that proximal factors may be for some time treated as irrelevant, since 'mainstream' researchers keep themselves busy combing distant variables.

> "The past and recent reluctance to admit the possibility of the infectious theory of atherosclerosis is more dramatic given the extraordinary preventive potential that it could offer"(p. 944).

Original ideas are often better accepted when they are *not* excessively novel. Consequently, the proximal (ultimate) or *"differentiating"* casual agents[19] have the misfortune of being pushed to the sidelines or "driven out of circulation" by the interest of health professionals and public fear in the myriad of less relevant issues, thus fragmenting both public attention and research funding organizations. The following example brings home the point. By 1985, over 270 factors were considered as contributors to cardiovascular disease. Faced with that number of risk factors one might hazard a guess before exploring the list, that only a few of them are 'precisely known' or supported by laboratory or clinical data; the rest being 'expert' opinions based on values, analogies, and anecdotal findings. Although conventional coronary risk factors explain very little, or only part of the variation in the incidence of coronary heart disease, health psychology professionals churn out numerous papers, in which they show how social and psychological factors cause stress, and then how to reduce the risk of death from coronary disease by changing one's lifestyle, abstaining from smoking and eating proper food. Part of the problem is that epidemiologists tell us that up to 90 percent of coronary heart disease can be prevented by the optimization of known cardiovascular risk factors.[35] The sheer volume of these factors camouflaged the role of inflammation and infection that were considered to have atherogenic effects more than a century ago. Psychologists who work with patients cannot easily see, on a daily basis, the factors that large-scale epidemiological studies have found as relevant for translating their knowledge into local action. When they do, at least two barriers appear to lie between these goals and their execution. The understanding of who will be in change of the care. And what specifically one should take under control.

The state of mind that sets off this practice is centuries old. It was recognized by Sir Thomas Gresham, the master of the mint and adviser to the royal court of Queen Elisabeth I. He noticed that people faced with a choice of two currencies of the same nominal value but of dissimilar quality (e.g. silver and golden coins) preferred low-value coins thereby ultimately driving the high-value coins out of circulation. The stipulation that "bad money drives out good money" is known as Gresham's law.[36]*

Today, the assertion that atherosclerosis is an inflammatory disease caused by infectious microorganisms is no longer controversial. Inflammatory changes found in atherosclerosis were attributed to both viral and bacterial pathogens. Among them, Herpes group viruses, especially cytomegalovirus and herpes simplex virus type 1 (HSV1), have been associated with atherosclerosis. In the last decade, of all potential candidate organisms, *Chlamydia pneumoniae* (*C. pneumoniae*) has become most strongly implicated in atherosclerotic lesions of various major arteries. It is implicated in atherosclerosis, coronary heart disease, and myocardial infarction. Its role is supported by seroepidemiology, pathology, and animal studies. The pathogen has been retrieved from atherosclerotic tissues; the level of raised plasma titers has been correlated with the severity of symptomatic atherosclerotic disease; the incidence of *C. pneumoniae*-responsive T cells in peripheral blood appears to increase in

---

*Gresham's law strikes one as nonsense, but the forces obeying the law are also at work when a political agenda is not favorable to the promotion of specific opportunities. The costly refusal of Japan's Samurais to use guns in the 17th century was prompted by the same logic. The armor with which Samurais engaged in mortal combat was so exquisite that they were prepared to hinder their fighting efficiency than to sacrifice their decorative attire by using ugly, but deadly guns. In distinction from the 'research program' of Imre Lakatos (1922–1974), the spell of Gresham's law does not require to level a fight for the program. Rather it could be a myopic disregard of all conflicting evidence. By contrast, in the Lakatosian 'research program,' its 'hard core' is being actively sheltered by the negative heuristic that maximizes its 'confirmation' with auxiliary hypothetical patches.

patients with coronary heart disease. Recently, *H. pylori* genomic material has been found in the coronary arteries of myocardial infarct patients. *H. pylori* and chronic dental infections have also been linked to coronary heart disease even though their causal relationship has yet to be elucidated. Ultimately, the final verdict will be made by successful intervention trials with antibiotics and a vaccine capable of protecting against infections that lead to community-acquired pneumonias and periodontitis. Although adequately powered clinical trials are still wanting, preliminary evidence from clinical trials suggests that treatment with some antibiotics may improve outcomes after ischemic events, and may reduce the risk of developing a first-time myocardial infarct.[37] Once a successful theory is recognized, its merits seem so obvious to the next generation that its success is assumed to be due solely to its excellence.

In fact, in science, the acceptance of a novel finding can be a lengthy process. A number of researchers continue to comb the old and barren soil for diet and personality factors in coronary disease. A PubMed search of the term 'coronary heart disease' meshed with *C. pneumoniae* generated a total of about 190 publications. An even less discriminating mesh with 'infections' harvested 631 publications. By contrast, coronary disease meshed with the term 'diet' yielded a robust 2209 papers published in the period from 1966 through 2000. During the same period, 1271 studies have been devoted to the role of personality in coronary disease. These results show that even though they are not techniques of statistical decision, they allow qualitative evaluation of the problem posed. The role of personality in cardiac disorders still feeds a good platoon of psychologists. This style of research is likely to go on despite the fact that primary prevention can avert more than 100,000 premature deaths each year in the US alone.

There are, however, some grounds for optimism. The European Atherosclerosis Society Workshop on the Immune System in Atherosclerosis held in March 2001 had a narrow mandate to examine the status of atherosclerosis as an infectious/immune-mediated disease. One of the chief conclusions derived from a recent summary of the meeting[38] is a strong restatement that the process of plaque formation is chiefly determined by inflammatory processes; that any infectious agent, especially multiple chronic infections (even as 'trivial' as chronic bronchitis, as well as periodontitis), can contribute to and accelerate atherosclerosis; that 40% of subjects having myocardial infarction or cerebrovascular accident are not exposed to any of the traditional risk factors for atherosclerosis. Finally, in keeping with Koch's postulate, experimental animal models seem to support the atherosclerosis-infections association. Despite the seemingly strong support behind this line of research, the authors of that summary felt it desirable to make a guarded statement that this association does not discount the traditional risk factors, such as smoking and diabetes. True, they are right, in some cases. Those who maintain a low-fat vegetarian diet, stop smoking, engage in stress management training, and do exercises of moderate intensity showed a regression of coronary stenosis, as opposed to control patients who showed signs of its mild progression.[39] That may well be an outcome as seen in some epidemiological studies. However, given that it may not improve endothelial functions or the predilection to plaque recoil, one has a simple dilemma: to obtain immediate help from the medical practitioner or to use self-help as recommended by holistic medicine. Let us take some comfort from the hope that, if one needs to kindle a campfire, it would be amusing to exercise the techniques of our ancestors when there is a box of matches in the backpack.

In a truly competitive contemporary research environment, an active academic-style researcher cannot survive on a low budget on the cutting edge of knowledge. Conducting a second-tier research program that has no applicability and a low chance of funding is inherently dicey, no matter what authors of such projects tell us in their defense. Consider an example from psychiatry of such a chronic syndrome of unknown etiology as schizophrenia. Until very recently, the dominant model conceives of schizophrenia as a neurodevelopmental disorder. It is undeniable that different chemical agents and physical stressors acting in critical periods of brain development could disrupt the processes of neuronal maturation and contribute to behavioral teratogenicity (Chap. 2). Yet two potential etiological factors, such as perinatal trauma and intrauterine environment, show a relatively meager yield of publications during the last decade (107). Schizophrenia presumably develops over years, distinctly emerging in late adolescence or later. During this tempestuous period in life when one's hormonal and physical changes become perceptible to the self and visible to others, and sexual, emotional, and volitional identities are being consolidated, one tends to disengage from the control of parents and siblings. Thus, although neurodevelopmental aberrations were not dismissed by research psychiatrists, the focus of interest in the field shifted some time ago to the then-fashionable stress models. Schizophrenia was therefore pictured as stress-related developmental anomaly.[40]

Stress is a familiar ground for dumping difficult problems. James Parkinson felt in 1817 that fright and shock precipitate a specific disorder his name was later linked to. Much of what is commonly written about schizophrenia also converges on the initial and delayed organismal reactions to chronic social and psychological stressors. But stress is present in response to novelty, intense mental activity, chronic effects of defeat and immobility, mating and disruption of sexual activity, and increment and decrement of aggressiveness. It appears in diverse disguises, in the cognitive, physical, and psychosocial domains, as well as in merely imagining adverse scenarios. Although schizophrenia researchers still circulate the term 'stress' as a cliché for a catalyst of the psychosis from comorbidity to misfortune, it was inevitable that an interest in the classical notion of stress as an environmental trigger of schizophrenia would decline. Meshing the term 'stress' with 'schizophrenia' gives us only 17 studies published during the last decade. So if stress is still in a neuromythology area, why some people are much more vulnerable to emotional stresses than others? An answer might be provided by examining depressed individuals rather than schizophrenics, where the scenarios of stress may be less trustworthy. One prospective-longitudinal study[41] found that individuals with the short allele of the promoter region of the serotonin transporter gene manifest more depressive symptoms and suicidality in relation to stressful life events than individuals homozygous for the long allele. In a commentary on these findings in the same issue of *Science*, Dan Weinberger of the National Institute of Mental Health was cited as defining the result as 'the biggest genetic fish yet netted for psychiatry.'*

After decades of frugal research funds and computational limitations on the earliest days of psychiatric genetics, a renewed interest in the presence of genetic liability[43,44] is reshaping the direction of psychiatry research. That *zeitgeist* is partially reflected in the robust 487 references collected in PubMed for the key word 'genetic liability' meshed with schizophrenia. Although chromosomes with susceptible loci are gradually beginning to

---

*A search for schizophrenia gene(s) is infinitely more demanding than examining a long laundry list of potential neurodevelopmental stressors. The major reason for the difficulty is the potential presence of numerous small-effect susceptibility genes, let alone the possibility that schizophrenia(s) is not a genetically distinct entity. Finally, in this model, too, the 'stressor' might be required just to push the schizogenic process over the threshold. It is futile to model psychopathology by including all of its risk factors and stressors (and how does one establish that all relevant events and processes have been identified and included in the equation?). The utility of such over-inclusiveness is conceptually questionable, not least given the fact that it is biased by personal insight and preferences. Efforts to reach 'completeness' invite numerous and immeasurable errors. Contemporary methodology therefore employs simplified models, with defenses against potential errors contributed by compromises and simplifications.[42]

emerge (e.g. chromosomes 6p21.3, 8p, 13q and 22q), finding the risk conferred by each locus, and the type of interaction between loci is still a daunting task. Thus far, scientists have been able to sift through a limited number of genes for their roles in neurotransmission and brain development (e.g. abnormal forms of serotonin 5HT2A receptor, dopamine D3 receptor, catechol-O-methyltransferase, a calcium activated potassium channel, KCa3 and others), and that number is probably more than they have been accustomed to doing. Weinberger and his colleagues narrowed in recently, among others, on the gene for the brain-derived neurotrophic factor (BDNF), the same member of the neurotrophic family essential for the differentiation and regeneration in the central nervous system that presumably influences emergent phenomena such as learning and memory and regulates numerous other developmental events from emotions and hyperactivity to weight increment. Given that BDNF promotes the function and survival of the hippocampal neurons, Michael Egan, Terry Goldberg and associates in Weinberger's group looked for subtle cognitive and physiological differences between persons with the two BDNF alleles. Their participants are being assessed on a number of tests comprised of those that tap learning and memory, activate regional cerebral blood flow (rCBF) (from BOLD fMRI), and quantify neuronal integrity (by measuring *N*-acetylaspartate, NAA) in the hippocampus. They revealed that persons with one or two *met* BDNF alleles (instead of the more common *val* allele) were inferior on memory tasks, had abnormal rCBF in medial temporal regions, and showed reduced levels of *NAA*. Thus, functional BDNF gene polymorphism might set in motion processes bordering on cognitive impairments akin to schizophrenia.[43]

The bacterial origin of insanity is another idea with a respectable history.[45] It has been entertained ever since it was discovered that neurosyphillis is caused by a pathogen and thus by implication, psychoses might well be conceived of as treatable infections. However, the thought that a bacteria or virus might actually be at the root of schizophrenia seemed almost preposterous. Undeterred, experimenters went hunting for this oddity, mostly inspired by Fuller Torrey, who plucked the viral idea of schizophrenia from near oblivion. In recent times, the ideas that schizophrenia is associated with exposure to some unknown pathogens (retroviruses?) have made a respectable showing. A familiar precedent is that of HSV1 mentioned above, which maintains latency following infection and resides in infected neurons and tissues, somehow evading the immune attack by limiting viral gene expression.

Exploring this direction, Karlsson and co-authors[46] identified retroviral sequences in the cell-free cerebrospinal fluids of 10 of 35 (29%) individuals with recent-onset schizophrenia or schizoaffective disorder. None of the 22 individuals with noninflammatory neurological diseases and of the 30 individuals without evidence of neurological or psychiatric diseases had such markers. The recognition that such studies mark one of the promising new lines of attack on this hitherto intractable and inexplicable disease is reflected by an increment of recent publications on the topic (132 publications in the last decade). The 'schizo-virus' if isolated, would be a phenomenal discovery changing the face of psychiatry.

Some time ago there was a considerable flow of ideas and applications from family studies in schizophrenia. However, there is not a shred of evidence that family climate is schizogenic or that early childhood experience or dysfunctional families could cause psychopathology of this kind and magnitude. Thus far, psychologically reproduced phenocopies of schizophrenia, or any other psychopathology for that matter, remain unknown save for the somewhat reduced rate of social contact in rats temporarily isolated from their mothers. One might have expected that fatigue would have set in with this kind of research. Not so. There is still an insatiable appetite for this marginal factor. By combining this field in the Medline, one can find 178 sources devoted to various aspects of familial factors. Even if that number is inflated, it begs the question as to why the circulation of 'family relations' has been continuing for so long. Familial issues and the role of schizogenic mothers have become something of a professional backwater. One may posit that the anti-psychiatry movement of the 50–60s contributed numerous popular beliefs in adverse effects on the development of early traumatic experience, exposure to inadequate parental models, and fixation on early childhood learning experience which, although largely discredited, had deeply penetrated the theory of schizophrenia. Children are often considered to be of "such exquisite psychological delicacy," remarks Meehl ironically, "that rather minor, garden-variety frustrations, deprivations, criticism, rejections, or failure experiences are likely to play the causative role of major traumas" (p. 253). For a few, whom Meehl branded as "ideological parent haters," the role of family is still plausible.

The Principle of Goal Displacement

In a scenario borrowed from Todd and Gigerenzer's[47] précis, a man is rushed to a hospital in the pangs of a heart attack. The doctor needs to decide whether the victim should be treated as a low-risk or high-risk patient. In the latter case he should receive the most expensive and detailed care. Although this decision can save or cost life, the doctor must decide how to proceed, using only the available clues, each of which is, at best, an uncertain predictor of the patient's risk level. In the foregoing and many other cases, doctors do not have unlimited time to ponder over the diagnostic problem, or the ability to delve into an unlimited database of knowledge. But the limitations of knowledge would matter very little were it not for the pressure of 'need' (motives, empathy, or fear of a law suit). The latter adds a powerful reason to worry about the quality of decisions to be made. In addition, the 'need factor' sets up an 'aspiration threshold' and provides a stopping rule for the termination for a search for an optimal solution.

Health psychologists seldom encounter emergency cases, but the need to help nonetheless creates urgent situations caused by alarmed families or troubled patients. When the worldwide burden of tuberculosis was as ruthless as the contemporary AIDS epidemic, there was nothing to offer a sick patient other than holistic treatment, such as life in villages, sanatorium care, graded exercise, heliotherapy and photoactivity, fresh air, high altitudes, and perhaps, a bit of invasive treatment in the form of collapse therapy (pneumothorax) on the medical side. That has brought about many admirable changes, such as improvement of housing conditions, installations of drainage systems, alterations in eating habits, advancement of the value of cleanliness, encouragement of physical fitness, and the establishment of a new cult of outdoor living. It may even have planted the seeds of the sexual revolution by making women's garments skimpy, and by forcing the guests of sanatoria to trim their beards. By the middle of the 1950s, it had become evident that the therapeutic benefits of all these wonderful innovations were not too significant to count. Only with the advent of the streptomycin-PAS revolution as well as a serendipitous discovery of isoniazid, sanatoria and numerous other integrative practices were doomed. These drugs were efficacious, potent and infinitely cheaper than the high-class accommodations for those dying in Alpine sanatoria. Still, low-potency holistic remedies, such as high-calorie foods, and spring water were irresistible for quite some time even though they did not add to the benefits produced by effective drugs. It took years to abandon the spa philosophy that coexisted with antibacterial treatment, a process that was pretty much completed by the 1970s.

Although 'atheoretical' discoveries are capable of proving themselves as opposed to 'theories' even if they may not be sufficiently compelling to command universal acceptance, discarding old practices or treatment routines is difficult to displace. Looking for current publications in English by meshing the terms 'tuberculosis' and 'sanatoria' in PubMed, one will have only 20 sources to collect. However, admitting other languages, including Russian, would increase the yield of the 'tuberculosis-sanatoria' mesh to almost a 100, half of which were published after 1980. Only gradually do successful paradigms become dominant. Like the stock market, medical strategies are largely a game of confidence. Cash-strapped, Russian health authorities preferred their traditional remedies of enforced sanatoria as well as surgery. Aaron Wildavsky[48] designated this gravitation to the irrelevant as 'Goal Displacement,' since "Every program needs an opportunity to be successful; if it cannot succeed in terms of its ostensible goals, its sponsors may shift to goals whose achievement they can control. The process subtly becomes the purpose."

Uchtomsky's 'Dominanta' in Science

The story of dyspepsia and *H. pylori* is an excellent modern blueprint of how new discoveries might fare when they tend to refocus the interest on causative pathogens at a time when life factors and host variables firmly occupy the first seat. The presence of pathogens of potential gastrointestinal disorders has been known since the late 30s (see Ref. 49 for a review). However, prior to 1983, peptic ulcer disease, dyspepsia, and chronic gastritis were attributed to such factors as smoking, gastric acidity, stress, alcohol consumption, and later, conceived of within a more comprehensive biopsychosocial framework. The role of bacteria in peptic ulcers became impossible to ignore after Barry Marshall and J. Robin Warren[50] from Western Australia demonstrated the presence of 'curved bacilli' in biopsy specimens from 58 patients with active chronic gastritis, duodenal ulcer, or gastric ulcer, thereby suggesting that this pathogen may be an important factor in the etiology of these diseases. Despite the logic of the paper (especially when viewed with the benefit of hindsight), the bacterial theory of chronic gastritis was met with great reserve. Today, their article seems to be profound, but only a decade ago scientists did not see it that way. Contemporary iconoclasts are no longer enthusiastically tarred and feathered. They are simply disregarded:

Marshall's claim was bacteriological and he had to fulfill Koch's postulates. However, reproducing infection in studies on human volunteers was ethically disagreeable whereas a search for an adequate animal model was predictably lengthy. In fact, *H. pylori* is a strict human pathogen, and therefore, understanding the pathophysiology of its gastric colonization based on

> *"Real discoveries of phenomena contrary to experience are very rare, whereas fraud, fakery, and foolishness are all too common. Thus, a closed-minded 'I do not believe a word of it' is going to be correct far more often than not"*[51] (p. 167).

animal models remains imperfect. In order to recruit incredulous colleagues one often has to stage a feat of self-inoculation with the suspected pathogen. Such daring experiments prove little when their results are negative. Professor Max von Pettenkofer (1818–1901), the founder of modern hygiene, was so eager to prove that the cholera bacillus does *not* cause cholera that he swallowed a good dose of its culture, and miraculously remained completely asymptomatic. These experiments were heroic no less when they were positive since a 'successful outcome' might carry a significant risk of death. In a similar act of self-sacrifice, Marshall, too, emptied a drink loaded with *H. pylori* but *did* suffer the desired ending in the form of indigestion, nausea, vomiting, headache, putrid breath, bloating, and irritability. These phenomena represent an adequate spectrum of medically unexplained symptoms, except for the fact that Marshall knew their cause. With this self-inoculation experiment, the clutch was released from the wheels of recognition. In 1989, Marshall's gastric bacterium was officially acknowledged and named *H. pylori*. Yet the beliefs in the psychosomatic origin of dyspepsia and gastric ulceration were still nurtured by the discovery that dyspepsia may occur in the absence of organic findings of endoscopy or the presence of asymptomatic infections. Paradoxically, although iconoclastic programs drive science, they can only survive with a wide consensus in the field.[52]

In medicine, consensus building is promoted by 'consensus conferences,' which recruit believers and unify treatment paradigms. By 1996, the majority of gastroenterologists had adopted *H. pylori* eradication therapy. Still, there was a lack of appreciation of the role of the new culprit by general practitioners. Approximately one-third of primary care providers have never prescribed *H. pylori* eradication therapy.[53] Since chronic gastritis is a precursor of gastric cancer, whose rate is surpassed only by lung cancer, a timely eradication of *H. pylori* could have significantly reduced the overall risk of gastric malignancy. Health psychologists were not brought into the process of consensus building since the goal of such a process is to establish the validity of a common instrument. Although health psychologists presumably work toward the same common goal of making a person healthy, *they do not share the same tools.* As a result, the term '*H. pylori*' meshed with the term 'behavioral medicine' or 'health psychology' yields a little over 50 papers during the last five years. Assuming that consensus building is *sine qua non* for doing science, Gresham's law in science might be construed as a gradient of paradigms, caused by the inevitable time shift of two independent tendencies, a centrifugal drift of pioneering programs, and a delayed movement of the majority toward consensus. That does not explain though, why some scientists and research groups adopt new strategies, while others persist either in digging in old, depleted mines or in developing nonprofitable paradigms regardless of compelling opposing findings. This persistence may be defined after Russian physiologist A. A. Uchtomsky as 'dominanta,' i.e. a behavioral response that shows extraordinary persistence, and has the paradoxical property of being able to strengthen and solidify in the face of contrary evidence.[54] Uchtomsky formulated the concept of 'dominanta' as a principle of neuronal activity responsible for the mobilization of motivational resources and attention.[55]

Cantor's Law

The history of medicine teaches us that the more readily a physician recommends a holistic palliative, the less is known about the disease. Let us assume that two professional groups agree that 'B' contributes to the emergence of disorder 'A.' Both groups, acting from different perspectives try to limit the role that 'B' plays, hoping to eradicate 'A.' As years go by, it becomes apparent that 'A' is actually caused by an 'ultimate' (or proximal) cause, 'C' (e.g. infection, a metabolic error, or a neurotransmitter deficit) whereas a set of 'B' factors is not etiologically necessary, even if minimally contributing to the disorder. The crucial problem for choosing the remedial strategy, when 'A' is shown to develop following 'C,' is to prove by treatment that the set of causes labeled 'B' will be therapeutically relevant only as palliatives whereas success in controlling or eradicating 'C' would alleviate the disorder altogether. The group which provides weak protective or therapeutic recommendations exposes the limitation of its professional credo. Indeed, when all other diagnostic efforts fail, one way of establishing a diagnosis and/or causality is by seeking a drug that might alleviate the morbid condition. Assuming that the drug is specific enough, the diagnosis is considered established by the success of therapy. For example, based on this logic, Cochran and colleagues[56] expected that atherosclerosis would be treatable with antibiotics. That was a good guess, even if the antibacterial treatment of atherosclerosis has yet to make its first steps, and even if it is to be yoked with anti-inflammatory treatment. The price for refusing to recognize the real culprit is a delay in the identification of causative agents and ambivalence in developing specific therapeutic measures. As Cochran and colleagues[56] opined, in controlling disease it might be more prudent to enact epidemiological and environmental anti-pathogen interventions before an agreement regarding the etiologic agent is reached:

Indeed, in July 1885, the anti-rabies vaccine saved a lucky Alsatian boy mauled by a dog before the vaccine was tested. Yet despite the strong therapeutic evidence for vaccination, not

> "Had this approach been more aggressively and systematically pursued, ulcers, for example, could have been cured and a bacterial cause implicated decades earlier" (p. 440).

everybody was converted to Pasteurism, despite the strength of evidence.[57]

In medicine, 'truth' is a matter of wide compromise that is facilitated by the 'early adopters'[58] who are receptive to new ideas. However, receptiveness is not necessarily associated with quality of research. The 'early adopters' may well be among the population of bandwagon riders, whereas the 'late adopters' may be single-minded diggers of the same firm turf. Thus, the early adopters are more readily condemned for being excessively opportunistic or ready to renounce their previous line of research or wash their hands of responsibility for established therapy. By contrast, a compliance of the 'late adopters' of the use of novel medication, say, in order to eradicate *C. pneumoniae* or *H. pylori* while insisting on the therapeutic utility of lifestyle changes, would be blamed for being 'right for the wrong reasons,' i.e. for making a Type III error.[59] As an example, Electroconvulsive Treatment may be considered a good remedy designed on a completely erroneous hypothesis.*

Although not bigoted about *H. pylori*, some researchers keep proposing other precipitants and complimentary aspects which allow dyspepsia to

---

*The strategy of inference guards against two types of errors. Type I error means erroneous rejection of the *null hypothesis*, i.e. elimination of the possibility that the event or effect happened merely by chance. Type II error means erroneously missing the event or effect.

become manifest. The significant age-adjusted association with peptic ulcers of such psychological measures as depression, social alienation (anomia), and hostility or the worsening of recent-onset dyspepsia and endoscopically visible duodenal ulcer in patients with low socioeconomic status, low level of education, depression, stressful life events, or psychopathology at baseline[60] are suggested to confirm their reality. Environmental factors such as mental or physical stress could compromise intestinal functioning by causing an inhibition of proliferation in the intestinal epithelium and an increase in intestinal permeability. The mechanism through which stress exacerbates intestinal epithelial injury remains unknown. Yet, it might allow further introduction of potentially harmful antigens, microorganisms, and toxins into the systemic circulation, normally hampered by this protective barrier between the intestinal lumen and the body's interior. On the other hand, there are a number of unknowns in *H. pylori* action and biology. Persons with antral gastritis have increased acid output, a propensity to duodenal ulcers, and a decreased risk of cancer. Those who develop a more widespread *H. pylori* infection that involves the body of the stomach and sometimes the antrum as well (pangastritis) are more likely to develop chronically decreased gastric acid output, gastric ulcers, and gastric cancer. What determines either of these outcomes has yet to be elucidated. In the final analysis some environmental cofactors may be pinpointed. However, understanding the host–pathogen relationship requires considering first the virulence markers, genetic profiles of the population at risk, age at first infection, previous and current co-infections, the locus of the infection within the stomach, and the simultaneous presence of several *H. pylori* strains that compete for microniches in the stomach. Only then should the stressor and host's socioeconomic circumstances be taken into account.[61] The fact that *H. pylori* colonizes the stomach, perhaps in over half of the world's population, and that it is found in 30–40% of asymptomatic individuals, does not erode its role in causation of gastrointestinal disorders. There may be a significant lag between time of infection and irreparable damage eliciting clinical symptoms. One-third of the world's population may harbor such a pathogen as *M. tuberculosis* without any clinical manifestation of tuberculosis, although the pathogen *is* an assured cause of tuberculosis. The actuality of factors in the host or in the environment, which are necessary for the graduation of latent (quiescent) signs into the clinical syndrome, does not discount the need to postulate its cause.

By acknowledging the role of the pathogen, but clinging to an obsolete routine of dealing with the etiologic or pathophysiological factors of low relevance because of their potentially *contributory* role is reminiscent of Gresham's law.* The dynamics at work here is the dread admitting an old myopia, an uneasy feeling that a year was lost barking up the wrong tree. In this case though, a researcher is under the spell of Cantor's law of conservation of ignorance,[63] which signifies a low level sensitivity to the change of fortune in research programs or disproportionate interest in low-risk agendas, which are better understood by the public and peers and easier to communicate.

Risk Modifiers and the Wisdom of Hetty Pepper

The question of why not all people are afflicted by illness even when sharing the same causative agents gradually evolved into a new problem, that of risk modifiers. For epidemiologists and sociologists, two models of causation are relevant.[14] One does not blame the victim, says the victim of infection by a pathogen when onset occurs in the course of normal activity. Disease onset, as Morley C. Sutter[14] explained, may not be "primarily determined by the chosen activity of the victim (other than being alive) and is caused by unexpected invasion by a microorganism or exposure to a particular agent in the environment." Examples of diseases of this kind are allergies, duodenal ulcer, or flu. The other model compares diseases to accidents, for which *the victim* is at least partially responsible due to taking part in a certain activity: "Subsequent to the decision to engage in that activity, the probability of having an accident obeys stochastic processes, wherein multiple factors operate to produce the disease"[14] (p. 585).

A popular parable about Mrs. Smith tells us that she had a bad fall when crossing the street. Interviewed by a policeman, some people had dissimilar perspectives on the accident.

"She seemed rather careless and rushed when crossing the street," reported one witness.

---

*The losing battle fought by the doubters of the infectious origin of tuberculosis is another illustration of the law. The discovery of the bacillus and the success of its eradication with drugs have made numerous pathological and pathophysiological theories useless. In spite of that, many authorities had a difficult time abandoning their conviction that phthisis is contributed by dampness of the soil, bad ventilation and deficient food.[62]

"Her attention has wandered lately," offered the husband.

"Her vision is bad," proposed her daughter.

"What if she had a lethal plan?" pondered a psychologist.

"Traffic is very bad these days," complained a few occasioned pedestrians.

"Her osteoporosis is rather advanced," recalled her family doctor.

"She stepped on a banana skin, dropped by some jerk," volunteered an urchin.

The moral of the parable is that all of these factors seem to be relevant and that all were present as 'non-modifiable' variables (advanced age, race, frailty, recurrent falls, previous occupational exposures, infections and others) when "the decision to engage in that activity" was made. But the parable is modeled on a paradigm of "Why," discussed by Otto R. Frish, that was meant to let the policeman arrive at the 'real' cause of trauma. When we inquire about "Why" or "What" happened to a specific person, we do not usually intend to ask, as was plainly put by Paul Meehl,[19] "What is the complete, detailed casual analysis of all the casual chains that converge upon his diagnosably aberrant state as we now see it?" (p. 248). Meehl went on to clarify that there is nothing wrong with such a question, except for the fact that when searching for answers to questions on etiology of disease, one is eager to establish what "this person [has], or what befell him ...," so as to make him unusual as compared to those who do not develop this kind of pathology or to find the '*differentiating* casual agent.' A given cause, does not inevitably lead to a specific effect. An example offered by Meehl is that of disease, such as phenylketoneuria (PKU) (where the genetic mutation is the 'cause' or the '*casua vera*'[64,65]). It may not lead to a disorder in the absence of phenylalanine in diet. Thus, a specific dietary intake becomes the differentiating causal factor. Penicillin may play a similar role in allergy that otherwise could have been triggered by other differentiating casual agents.

In effect, the debate about causality of diseases revolves around two major propositions. One refers to *cross-sectional causation*, which is limited to factors that are relevant to the present-state symptoms and complaints. The other is *longitudinal causation*, which might refer to the major etiological cause with the inclusion of all relevant or modifying variables throughout the course of the disorder. Mrs. Smith might have been afflicted by unrecognized Alzheimer's disease, and simply got lost in habitual surroundings on her way home. Thus, the fumbling with all "incidental ecofactors"[66] leads to the devaluation of all of them. As the appreciation of such factors increases, their inventory tends to grow since none of them is ever rejected at the price of the complete exclusion of others. By the time the policeman agrees on some '*differentiating casual agents*' in the original list, such an agent might be either confusing or sheer rubbish. Evans[8] defined such 'incidental ecofactors' collectively as the *third ingredient*.

To remind the reader, the term was inspired by O'Henry's story about a humble shop-girl, Hetty Pepper, who had the misfortune to be fired from her job at a thirty minutes' notice. As the story goes, with a last dime and nickel in her purse she was able to buy just a bit of beef for her evening meal. Another hungry girl, Cecilia, living in the same decrepit apartment house, was peeling two potatoes, the only thing she had planned for her mealtime. They put their modest victuals together in order to boil a semblance of a stew. But what kind of a stew would it be without the *third ingredient*, an onion. In the Cinderella-like happy ending, Hetty did receive a desirable taste enhancer, a "pink, smooth, solid, shining onion," whereas Cecilia had an added bonus of a handsome, wealthy man. Evans[8] gives a long laundry list of 'onion factors' that may not cause disease, but could certainly determine its severity and length. Ironically, all of them are mostly host susceptibility factors (e.g. immune history and present immune status, comorbidity, or living habits) and pathogen factors that may be further broken down into numerous components. Collectively, most of what was compiled by Evans is so ubiquitous that these components of *longitudinal causation* can hardly be eluded by anyone who just stays alive.

The list of conditions and events which complicate illness may also be so confusing because of the uncertainty between the terms 'hazards' and 'risk factors.' A hazard is any event, or a set of circumstances, which may have an untoward outcome. The *probability* of the hazard causing some effect is the risk of the result. Ionizing radiation is certainly hazardous and elicits very strong public reaction even when the actual risk (based on dose-rate assessment) can be low.[67] On the other hand, driving a vehicle is an agreeable activity, but on a typical weekend in Israel, more people die or are injured in traffic accidents than in terrorist attacks. According to Evans, for infected individuals, both hazards and risk factors determine whether the sick become manifestly ill or die, and in the latter case, when they die. A closer look at risk factors that might influence the occurrence and severity of clinical disease among infected persons according to Evans indicates that many of them are mere *precipitants* or *aggravating factors*. They are somewhat akin to the 'frame' or the 'contextual set-up' that may or may not team up with some potentiating events or do so to a different extent, thereby shortening or aborting disease-free intervals, but they do not *cause* a disease. Their role might be illustrated by the example of epilepsy, which is a chronic disease with specific causes. In adults, epilepsy manifestations may be infrequent ('disease-free intervals'), and the diagnosis may occasionally require special activation procedures needed to elicit its clinical and/or electrographic signs. However, outside of the controlled environment of the hospital, precipitating circumstances may appear in the form of pregnancy, sleep deprivation, or regular sleep, alcohol ingestion, fever, trauma, infections, hyperventilation, sex, eating, viewing TV and the like.

The onion factor is a temporary ploy, an attempt to provide a cover-up for ignorance when one cannot explain why an acknowledged cause doesn't always lead to morbid conditions. The role of the onion factor is in providing external disturbing 'pushes' to the system. It should not be confused with causality or the ultimate or 'real causes,'[64] or the minimal conditions that produce disease.[68] Like a liquid chemical that often requires just a 'seed' to fall into the fluid to initiate its crystallization, some environmental triggers, although innocuous, can set in motion events that reach the border where clinical manifestations begin. The presence or absence of such seeds is not the same as causality. In the classical example of Professor Pettenkofer's failed attempt to get cholera after swallowing a horrendous dose of the pathogen, we are not in doubt (now) about the culprit of the disorder. Causal inference does not demand an inescapability of disease. Even for cholera there are some other factors that determine morbidity.

The allusion to the onion factor of pathology could be likened to 'Kitcher's knot.'[69] In his example, a telephone cord is wound around a pair of scissors. The scissors may be released very simply, if the way to free them were guessed correctly. But someone who does not know the smart way out may struggle for hours in attempts to unwind the scissors. As in Kitcher's knot, multifactorial explanations (in etiology rather than in pathogenesis) are 'possible but not desirable' since they retard etiological elucidation.[65] The reality of the trajectories of host-pathogen events that are complex, and delayed from the outcome, and thus are likely to intersect with many other conditions and pathways, is important but not crucial. So far, scientists are busy accumulating data on potential risk factors even though the complexity of their effects grows exponentially with the number of postulated variables. Despite the tremendous success of molecular reductionism in medicine, they have never entirely lost their appeal. It is seldom appreciated that the risk factor is essentially used as *cause* albeit one that is titrated on the scale of relevance. An example is a downgrading of dietary factors from risk variables or causes to 'onion factors.'

It is clear now that the downturn in coronary disease observed in the Western world since the 1960s is associated with the introduction of powerful antibiotics in the early 40s and 50s, which gradually curbed bacterial infections with atherogenic potential. Due to the lengthy latent period of clinical manifestations of atherosclerosis, this effect must be felt two-three decades later. That is precisely when the salubrious results were observed. The decline of cardiovascular mortality was noticed at a time when the rates of smoking and dietary fat intake were still high, but just about to recede. Figure 7.2, borrowed from Nieto's review,[34] conceptualizes the temporal relations between different lifestyle and healthcare factors as well as antibiotics. It shows that diet, hypertension control, improved medical care, and a decline in smoking are actually onion factors whose role was overemphasized. The actual help has come with the ability to get hold of the 'sufficient determinants,' which were missed due to the [unexpectedly] long delay in their action. Thus, every time a disease is recalcitrant, health psychology is inclined to raise the flag of such 'third factors' (causes) as lifestyle, perception of illness by the patient, social network, and various other socio-economic and psychosocial stressors. In reality, if the finding reviewed by Nieto on the possible contribution of infections to atherosclerosis and coronary heart disease are accepted, then antibiotics would be a better choice for cardiology than the excitement with the statins, let alone the infatuation with fat-fighting, inasmuch as pneumonia caused by *C. pneumoniae* is probably more frequent than it is described, and it harms many asymptomatic or mildly symptomatic patients.

Collectively, the 'third factors' have become the last bastion of biopsychosocial philosophy. It is as if we were searching for the cause of pregnancy, but avoided discussing the ultimate opening stage of egg fertilization simply because the state of intrauterine conditions and numerous hormonal variables are also relevant for its success. In such cases, the proponents of the principle of monocausality might be willing to say, "Fine, you can have it," and include all the supplemental or modifying factors in the equation. However, this position is hardly intellectually compelling. In the above-mentioned story, Hetty Pepper called attention to the point that has eluded many. It is the

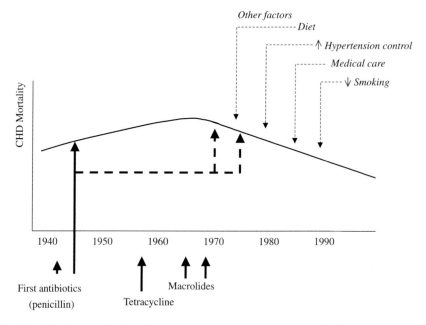

Fig. 7.2 The hypothesized relation between the introduction of antibiotics and the decline in coronary heart disease mortality in the last third of the 20th century. The introduction of the first antibiotics (penicillin) reduced the prevalence of common infections with putative athero-genic effects, which, due to the latency period of the clinical manifestations of atherosclerosis, had a noticeable impact on coronary disease mortality 2–3 decades later. The introduction of tetracycline in the 1950s and of macrolide antibiotics in the 1960s may have contributed to these trends because of their effectiveness against *C. pneumoniae* infection. After Nieto[34] with permission.

meat rather than the onion that counts when cooking a good stew, after all: "it's us," she says, grimly, to herself, "it's *us* that furnished the beef."

Kill Buddha and "Hais cuaj txub kaum txub"

Holism has pointed out that breaking down the complex biological system into its components may not help to elucidate the way the system operates. This admonition was voiced at a time when the only credible way of learning about such systems was by isolating its 'organs' and then guessing what they do in the complete and living body. Such an approach posed a great number of questions ever since the first efforts to map 'mental faculties' by conjecture, by electrical stimulation of the brain, and examining its functions after physical and chemical lesions. Challenged by these difficulties, scientists were prompted to notice the presence of interactive, parallel, distributed, 'constellational,' multifaceted, and nonlinear mechanisms that govern cognition and behavior. In addition, however, some took refuge in postulating the presence of complex interactions of the organism with the 'larger whole.' A holistic notion of environment was not used to provide a preprogrammed algorithmic solution capable of protecting against various deleterious agents and situations or translated into a sound experimental or prescriptive therapeutic guidance. Nor were holistic predictions submitted against real data since the latter's predictions and hypothetical statements cannot be falsified.[70] With this, holism exported science into the realm of a Kantian 'noumental' world that resides beyond grasp and intelligibility. Holism is guilty of a growing obsession with ever more complex models that are as inscrutable as nature itself. With numerous adjustable parameters, these models are usually unfalsifiable, so that the opportunity to learn from a wrong prediction is short-circuited. Consequently, dialogue between the holistic and reductionistic approaches gave way to contentious monologues that have resulted in an unannounced armistice. Only recently have neuroscientists and research psychiatrists found ways of asking some questions as they are related to human consciousness, normal and aberrant mental functions. Although these problems seem intensely intractable, their pursuit is governed by reductionism, which still remains the way of "the making of science and technology"[71] since winning a battle means that one has "only to bring the enemy to where we are sure we will be the stronger"[57] (p. 73).

Whereas for Western science, fact becomes acceptable ('a truth') after it has been interpreted within the lore of a universal rule, Eastern science does not look for a plausible theory as a lead to a new experiment, since any effort at explaining or interpreting inescapably engages the self ("I"), which distances the observer from the 'truth.' Nor do Eastern scientists reputedly structure their writing according to a linear logical structure or commit themselves to a final conclusion. One of the didactic tales that is frequently used by Buddhist teachers is the familiar story of *"The Blind Men who met with an Elephant."* It is meant to tell us of the great truths of cosmic existence that can never be grasped by those who approach them from a single point of view. As an example,[72] Japanese scientists are looking for diversity and complexities by scrutinizing a piece of information from a multiplicity of angles; the logic of their search is that of the net that is not strongly woven and is expectedly leaky.

Because nature is so entirely connected, they tend to define something amalgamated, fluid, in-between, and elusive, something that may obey the assortment of rules. The rationale of this philosophy is that science is a system of knowledge; it cannot conform to the one-rule despotism of hypothesis "on which Western science strongly insists." "Is it true that there should be one science?" muses Tatsuo Motokawa,[72] and answers with an emphatic negative. Although he made courteous, but guarded nods to the power of Western science and its success, he swiftly recovers from the balanced view by instructing the reader that "[Western] science may need some modification in the near future, and it is good to remember that there are *other types of sciences* in the world" (p. 501, ital. added). His view of the 'right methodology' is based on the notion of 'open system,' which requires imagination and a special state of mind and body. This approach is familiar for the Western scientist, albeit in the realm of art and poetry. That system is within the perimeter of Zen Buddhism. To make it grasped more easily by the novice, Tatsuo Motokawa[72] turns to a seemingly irreverent testimonial by a Zen master, "When we meet Buddha, we kill him!" What the metaphor of murder actually means is that the mastery of the ultimate truth requires that the Zen practitioner overcome the temptation to enter a 'closed system' of trusting the potential deception; that what one accepts as truth is not *Buddha-The Truth*, since "The absolute truth does not lie in a closed system: We have to open the system: we have to destroy the rigid shell of what 'I' thinks is the truth and thus destroy the shell of 'I' " (p. 503). Operationally, sacrificing Buddha seems to be much too whimsical a pragmatic principle for coping with the unknown. As one might gather from the multilayered intertextuality and meandering of Montaigne's *Essais,* the Europeans, too, were capable of experiencing the poignant "Que sçay-je?" ("What do I know?") intrusions into their reflections, and temptations to surrender to complexity. Yet, Faust has answered that the mastery of truth (universal knowledge) was tragically futile, and his alternative was to "march undaunted to the goal," rather than being dissolved into oblivion.

As with any charismatic yet vast doctrine, holism was destined to fragment into several factions and directions, such as ecocentric holism, anthropocentric holism, systemic, organismic, universal cosmic holism, the 'open hierarchical system holism' of Koestler, and others. With the influence of new-age cultures, holism has become synonymous with alternative medicine. Curiously, the contemporary rally of holism is explained by its humanistic appeal. Leaving out the ontological and epistemological problem, nurses opted to cater to the psychological, social, economic, and spiritual needs (i.e. holistic requirements) of their patients, i.e. something that was not formally mandated by their occupation. In the realm of medicine any theory has to produce an adequate evidence of its benefits. Holism has become a core of nursing philosophy and its practice because neither was repelled by the differences between Western and Eastern new-age philosophy. The mysterious 'wholeness' that provided us with such metaphors as 'scenarios' for algorithms, or 'perspectives' for possibility and probability, has become a therapeutic medium and organizing principle of care. For science, however, such conceptual distances are very difficult to overcome.[72]

Holistic practitioners are inclined to dole out their services to each individual as inherently special. As discussed in Chapter 3, physicians are primarily trained to 'smudge' individual differences, identify the resemblance and commonalities, and then act on individual cases as representing the 'rule.' These alternative strategies actually reside on a continuum, which is famously summarized by such anthropologists, as Kluckhohn and Murray:[73]

Every man is in some respects

1. like all other men,
2. like some other men,
3. like no other man.

The clinical version of holistic orientation is the disposition to deal with the last proposition whereas in the nomothetic spirit of scientific psychology, medicine almost entirely concerns itself with the first, unless proven in need to consider the second or the third rules to achieve a therapeutic end. The inspiring African notion of *ubantu* declares that all people are connected. That is not only a moving humanistic principle, but a sound medical standard. Kluckhohn and Murray's stages are not equidistant and the transition to the state of 'like no other man' represents a qualitative jump so that physicians tend to look for a broad reductionistic law justifying the tumble to the second and third propositions. The politically endorsed cliché that "We aren't dealing with groups, we are dealing with this individual case," was branded by Meehl[19] as the "vulgar error."*

---

*When Jean-Jacques Rousseau[74] *confessed*, "I dare to think I am not made like any of those who exist. If I am not better, at least I am other," (p. 5) his calling might alert a cardiologist, only because of his assurance in the same paragraph, "I feel my heart." Slight deviations put everybody into the category 'like all other men.' The difficulty begins when social inadequacy suggests discrepancies in quality rather than a degree, and thus a need for upgrading a case to stage 2 or 3. "It is clear," wrote Eliot Slater[75] in 1943, "that people can be more or less neurotic as they can be more or less intelligent. But there is an important

A defiant reluctance to participate in diagnostic procedures and/or follow treatment is a recognized form of protest of underprivileged patients with multiple social problems and chronic diseases, or severe and stigmatizing infections. The Hmong people of Laos seemed like 'no other men' when they came into contact with the regular procedures of contemporary medicine.[76] They believed that "the world is full of things that may not seem connected but actually are," so that "no event occurs in isolation; and that you can miss a lot by sticking to the point." For a medical professional, speaking on the same wavelength as these patients required a unique ability to depend, as the Hmong had, on "*hais cuaj txub kaum txub*," which means, "to speak of all kinds of things." That is not a regular frame of mind to adopt since Western physicians are trained to accept symptoms when they are plausible, consistent, specific, repeatedly observed by different individuals, in different places, times, and circumstances, i.e. they are 'like in all other men' in their and similar cultures.

Holism is intrinsic to the way people feel about their mental state when confronted by the unknown. The answers to certain questions will forever be unobtainable, and perhaps, *hais cuaj txub kaum txub* is relevant when pondering the problems bordering on '*qualia*' (an ambiguous term to designate the introspectively accessible, phenomenal aspects of our mental lives, the limitations of our consciousness by the things perceived and learned about the world), the mind-body problem, or how qualia relates to the physical world both inside and outside the head. Our metaphors, like that of the Hmong and the Wari are bounded by what we know. Thus, someone who holds doctorates in both psychology and cultural anthropology would be able to make use of spiritual tools, utilize arcane procedures, beliefs in deities, help of the community — or any combination of these factors. Such cross-cultural knowledge could certainly open the door to imagery and fantasies, but it could also lead to a methodological misconception, that a problem cannot be understood unless *hais cuaj txub kaum txub* is included in the equation. That is certainly not a practical way to a compassionate practice of

---

practical difference. For whereas differences of degree of intelligence are much more striking than differences in quality, the opposite is true of neurosis, when we are more struck by differences of quality than a degree." Somehow, sixty years after Slater's insight we are captivated by the ever expanding polychrome of mental disorders where just small *quantitative* differences matter.

medicine, either. The postmodern healthcare policy is to compartmentalize financial resources for '*multicultural counseling experts*' handling each ethnic or socio-economic groups, which Satel[22] branded as "indoctrinology."

Economically, there is a limit to such practices. After all, each village in a place like New Guinea is kept separate by an assortment in language, rituals, deities, and interests' differences. Their inhabitants seldom understand one another. The ultimate way of being accepted by them is, as William Graham Sumner[77] observed, joining them. Western cultural practices demand the minorities accept the dominant customs: "When I am at Rome I fast as the Romans do; when I am at Milan I do not fast. So likewise you, whatever church you come to, observe the custom of the place" (St. Ambrose 337–397 A.D.). There is no way a physician or a psychologist would be able to adjust to the whole spectrum of mores. Likewise, by adopting the principle of *hais cuaj txub kaum txub*, doctoring or science would inhibit any incentive to generate new data and exhibit, instead, as holism did, "sovereign disregard" for the obligation to provide verifications of adopted practices.[78] Clark Glymour and Douglass Stalker[79] uncompromisingly derided this gravitation of alternative medicine to holistic practices:

The reason why holism proved incapable of imposing any brakes on the progress of neurobiology is that the majority of practitioners in contemporary psychology and medicine are unable to get by without reductionism, even if implicitly. Therefore, psychologists pay an

> *"Holistic medicine is a pablum of common sense and nonsense offered by cranks and quacks and failed pedants who share an attachment to magic and an animosity toward reason. Too many people seem willing to swallow the rhetoric — even too many medical doctors — and the results are not benign."*

obligatory nod in the direction of *complexities and wholeness* and then go about their research by primarily scrutinizing each specific problem in *isolation*, in an effort to find wide-ranging rules to which complex phenomena may be reduced.

In conclusion, it is tempting to compare holism with monotheism. We owe to monotheism many wonderful things. Historically, the uniqueness of monotheism was in a dematerialization of God and conceiving of it as an omnipotent singular authority divorced from the separate forces of nature, as those of wind, rain, sea, or rivers, when each is presided over by various conflicting deities. But we also instinctively fear the absolutist demands of the intolerant nonconformist mindset. You do not have to believe in the Greek gods to realize that it was quite soothing to conceive of the world as controlled by numerous conflicting holy beings that ran routine day-to-day activities of the mortals. Although less formidable and occupying a small territory, these deities were possible to relate to, defy in anger, restrain by human artifacts, or mollify by specified rituals. Monotheism was a step forward in human history compared to the showing of adulation to a bunch of pagan gods. However, research is inescapably territorial and thus 'polytheistic.' Only by fragmenting a medical problem into specific steps governed by dissimilar mechanisms or genes can we ever hope to make it manageable and decipherable, and perhaps much later down the road cemented by a unified theory. Irrespective of whether one believes in vitalism or reductionism, according to Sir Alan Cottrell,[80]

> *"it remains a sound research tactic to proceed on the working assumption that all wholes are in principle understandable entirely in terms of their part, since this has been so consistently successful in the natural sciences and since it may be the means of bringing science right up to the edge of the supposed gap between the material and mental worlds, a gap which may then be seen to be either illusory or profound"* (p. 130).

SO WHAT?

Unlike the holism of experimental sciences that tends to overcome ignorance and numerous sources of uncertainty, clinical holism is quite certain of what sickness necessitates. It has become a license for the intuitive, a plea for a compassionate practice rather than an instrument for conducting rigorous (i.e. reductionistic) clinical research.

Clinical holism tells us that salvation will come with the adoption of new rationality. Operationally, that means using organic, biological, 'natural' agents and adhering to a diversity of complementary maneuvers and lifestyle changes. Its world view is counter to the search for the most proximal and biologically tractable component of disease, and hence cannot be a viable doctrine of health psychology. In human epidemiological studies, holism often appears as factorology, or as an engine buttressing peripheral paradigms (designated as Gresham's law or Goal Displacement strategies). It probably fits in the realm of the 'Why,' but proves useless in the analytical region of the 'How.'

Insofar as wholeness lies beyond the other rim of knowledge, holism by its own definition cannot take on the dimensions of full-scale theory for being much too amorphous and incomplete. It cannot hope to ever provide meaningful measurements at this grand scale when we have such difficulty testing more simple models.

Since a therapist's consciousness is also part — and an important part at that — of the treatment process, there is no boundary in holistic sense between patient and doctor. The latter ceases to operate as an independent agent and becomes a participant in a world that has to be comprehended after their mode of action is elucidated. When this insight is posted as a practical dictum of health practitioners, then what happens with patients whose stance is decidedly pragmatic?

Holism is a ploy to recruit public tolerance by demanding broadmindedness, to lessen the criticism of peers for imprecision as well as to avoid disregard of funding agencies, regardless of how cleverly its proponents argue otherwise.

8

---•---

If Health Psychology is the Answer, What was the Question?

Fathering Health Psychology

The opening lines of Chap. 1 asserted that health psychology was born to the parents of the 20th century. In truth, it is a brainchild of the Greek sage and physician Hippocrates (460–375 BC). Does this mean that health psychology and medicine are sister professions? Helen King[1] argues that the Western medical tradition deriving an origin of medicine from the 'twin fathers,' Hippocrates and Galen, follows the myth staged by Galen, a Roman physician who needed a solid father figure to legitimize his own methodological flaws and assuage his insecurity. On the model practiced by major religions, he nominated himself a prophet for Hippocrates. By adopting him as the Father, he purchased a respectable lineage traceable to no lesser a god than Apollo himself. Hippocrates' name is often called upon as a mythological patron saint of unrivaled purity and selflessness. He was an Asclepiad who received his training in medicine at the temple of Asclepios on the Island of Cos and battled illness by invoking the power of Asclepios. Therefore, the suggestion of tracing health psychology to Hippocrates is not intended to add prestige to the profession. Rather, by referring to antiquity I tend to join ranks with those who force a comparison of a limited increment of scholarship and success since "our intellectual ancestors, for all their fumbling, were asking precisely the same question we are asking today."[2] The paradox of a meager affinity between health psychology and 'orthodox medicine' is not in their differences, but in their resemblances, which goes back to the origin of both disciplines.

The handling of illness has been a central issue with medicine since its beginnings. The Coan School commanded by Hippocrates emphasized the importance of detailed clinical observations for determining the course and outcome of each disease. Presumably, Hippocrates was quite accepting, if not soberly opportunistic in the reliance on Asclepios for psychological insights and in the offering of healing. The ancient Greek city of Cnidus on the southwest coast of Anatolia was home to a different school of medicine. The Cnidians looked for essential internal or external causes of illness and strived to establish precise diagnoses before providing medications. They thus represented medicine in its contemporary sense. Ironically, the model of the father of medicine attributed disorders to psychosocial factors, family problems and nutrition, thus resembling the health psychology of today. The difference between the two schools boils down to the emphasis on organs, diseases, and the efforts of a physician in the city of Cnidus, as opposed to an accent on the sick, their environment, or diet, and what we today call 'doctor-patient' relations, on the island of Cos:

At the very early stages of the art of medicine, there was nothing unusual about instructing about life style and environmental influences along with fixing fractured bones, but the Cnidians insisted on much more: the need to establish the precise locations of the causes of illness, and treatment tactic. These demands could not be matched by their medical

"The Cnidians focus on the disease, while that of [the school] of Hippocrates was on the patient. The Cnidian physicians, like those of today, were reductionists, fine-tuners who directed their efforts to the classification of the processes of sickness and to exact diagnosis. They sought to know the specific local organ disturbances that caused the symptoms they so assiduously categorized"[3] (p. 9).

skills. Thus, the Cnidians were destined to disappoint their patients and vanish from the scene.* Still, the vestiges of their philosophy reverberated through medical history. Disguised as Paracelsian pharmacology, phlebotomies of medieval bloodsuckers, and Galenic rationalists, they acquired scientific respectability by bonding with science, and were finally acknowledged as

---

*We best know Cnidus today, perhaps, as a site of the famous statue of Aphrodite sculpted by Praxiteles in the fourth century BC because the open-minded people of Cnidus purchased the sculpture after the Coans had rejected it for its nudity.

professionals with the advent of the germ paradigm when the ancient aspiration of finding 'major cause' of illness became achievable.

It is uncertain whether these two 'schools' were as polarized as historians have it. If they were, they certainly prove that the scapegoats of one age became the scientists of another, since the Cnidians stand at the roots of the 20th century philosophy of medicine whereas the Coans gradually evolved into its Brahmins. The Coans did not overstate their ability. Their message was largely holistic and often as carefully phrased as an astrological forecast. Their popularity waxed and waned through several centuries of history. Some tricks and recommendations of the Coans were not articulated into a systematic toolkit for they did not derive their treatment from actual diagnosis, but tailored their efforts to the patients' needs:

One might concur with the assertion that "what we today call alternative medicines are really *remnants of* that classical paradigm, even though they started out claiming to be *alternatives to* it. ...."[4] The same century experienced a flashback of our remote history when the failures of medicine discussed in the opening chapter encouraged the practices of health psychology. The appeal of the latter was further enhanced with its emphasis on somatic ('physical') diseases.

"By making him [the patient] a member of his own therapeutic team, they achieved success that eluded their rivals; in this can be recognized the seeds of what has come to be called holistic medicine, *or at least holistic medicine divorced from some of the crackpot ideas which have encumbered it of late*"[3] (p. 10, ital. added).

Admittedly, physical illness is one of the most powerful stimulus situations determining psychological states. Historically, these 'stimuli' were understood and handled by the medical and paramedical professions, with only a few others who infrequently crossed the professional boundaries. That eagerness to help the somatically ill was noticed and much-admired inasmuch as the promise of health psychology to deal with somatic illness did not come with immoderate demands for a stake in the expenditures on healthcare that have risen in all industrial countries faster than the general rate of inflation. Inescapably though, these efforts exposed health psychology to the same perils that the rigid Cnidians had ignored in the early phase of gestation of medicine. Now, health psychology is challenged by input from the medical, academic, and regulatory communities: To what extent is the practice of health psychology expected to affect particular endpoints? How does health psychology's role intersect with the responsibilities of clinical social workers, marriage and family therapists, mental health counselors, nurse practitioners, nurse midwives, physical therapists, physician assistants and pharmacists, who work on a range of communal and family determinants of health? The latter professionals insist on the intimate links between health and the social, economic and political structure of society, and are also petitioning for independent status and the faith of their patients.[5] In short, were the objectives of health psychology stated in its Manifesto made with the intention of keeping them? Who, then, should foot the bill?

In Praise of the Slave-Physician

The quandary regarding the quality and virtue of 'mechanical,' physical-organic therapy as opposed to comprehensive, psychological healing, has an impressive pedigree. According to Plato, the differences between the physician-philosopher who treats 'noble and virtuous' free Athenian citizens, and the slave-physician who attends to the needs of slaves is in the fact that the latter never talks to patients separately, or lets them talk about their problems. He just prescribes the remedy. Why would he behave 'as if he had exact knowledge ...'? He is unable to learn from a better model since "the other doctor, who is a freeman," explains Plato,

> "carries his enquiries far back, and goes into the nature of the disorder; he enters into discourse with the patient and his friends, and is at once getting information from the sick and also instructing him as far as he is able, and he will not prescribe for him until he has first convinced him; at last, when he has brought the patient more and more under his persuasive influences and set him on the road to health, he attempts to effect the cure" (Law, 720; cited by Simon,[6] p. 227).

The point in citing this passage from Plato is not to indict the physician-philosopher but to suggest that in those cruel times the principle of *primum non noccere* was not attributable to slaves as they were costly but 'disposable.' Exhortations of the clever philosophers might have been more relevant for some worried aristocrats rather than slaves afflicted with serious disorders that were in need of being 'fixed' so as to enable them to continue to work and bring profits to their masters. The strategies employed by slave physicians were thus second-class therapies in appearance rather than in result.

Their pragmatic knowledge of what is required was derived from years of experience dealing with slave owners and slave dealers to ensure maximal work output at minimal charge. Unlike the itinerant physicians, as the majority of philosophers-physicians were at the time (even Galen wandered from city to city until he obtained his first appointment as physician of gladiators in Pergamum), slave-physicians were empiricists who stayed with their owners and were responsible for the mortality of their patients. To counterbalance the weakness of 'philosophical medicine,' Plato concedes:

> "If one of those empirical physicians [i.e. slaves] ... were to come upon the gentleman physician talking to his gentlemen patients, and using the language almost of philosophy, ... he would say, ... *'Foolish fellow, ... you are not healing the sick man, you are educating him; and he does not want to be made a doctor, but to get well'* " (Law, 875,; cited by Simon,[6] p. 227, ital. added).

There was another relevant feature of socially inferior slave-based medicine. Although less driven by the narrative of their patients and their subjective world (in many cases they did not share the same language to conjecture of that world) they were more objective and more 'tool-oriented.' The slave-doctors were apparently less bothered by the sensitivities of their patients, and when examining their naked bodies had a better understanding of their anatomy and pathology. In short, it was a *physician-dominant* kind of medicine.

By contrast, the physician-philosopher was more able academically, more inclined to explain the logic of their strategies, more controlled by their customers, and more dependent on their whims. It was a *patient-dominated* doctoring. In the 19th century Europe, the two kinds of medicine retained only very few of their features, such as an inferior status of the surgeons. In the practice of medicine a century ago, the two schools temporarily converged. Contemporary technology made them drift apart. The technological sophistication of medicine came with the realization of the fact that smart counsel, human touch, and refined conduct, however important and often needed, could hardly solve the problem of improving the state of health care.[4] Today, the 'slave-physician' and 'philosopher-physician' models are more and more polarized. The psychotherapist, holistic nurse, alternative practitioners and clinical psychologists take over the role played by the physician-philosopher, whereas contemporary orthodox practitioners are the present-day 'slave-physicians,' albeit much better equipped and wealthier. Correspondingly, the philosophy of treatment also differs in agreement with the so-called 'hidden decisions' or unwritten decisions, as they were designated by Meehl[7]:

In psychiatry, African American and Hispanic patients were often given drugs in the conviction that they were unlikely to benefit from psychotherapy as they were psychologically unsophisticated. Ironically, these

"Lower class patients are more likely to receive pills, shock, or supportive therapy than are middle and upper class patients, who are more likely to receive intensive, uncovering, long-term psychotherapy..." (p. 250).

patients benefited more in terms of reduced length of treatment, its efficacy and cost. The reason is that contemporary slave-physicians, very much like those of the antiquity *are* 'somatizers' since "they preferentially search for and diagnose somatic conditions to the exclusion of psychosocial problems."[8]

Is Health Psychology, Psychology of 'Health'?

What is Normalcy?

The question that has all but disappeared from our agenda is what does the word 'health' mean when yoked with psychology? Is health psychology a euphemistic disclaimer as opposed to the more demanding term 'medical psychology' (i.e. psychology of the sick) or is it psychology of sick behavior implicit in the term 'behavioral medicine' that are often used as synonyms? And how is the term 'health' defined in the context of health psychology? These questions are not simple. Samuel Johnson noticed that "definitions are hazardous," and a definition of health supports his warning. In the past, psychologists, anthropologists, physicians, and social philosophers have voluminously discussed the definitions of health and normalcy. It would be futile to provide more than a sketch of the debate. Health (i.e. functionally good health or 'wholeness') is one of those words that like normalcy defies definition, varies across cultures, and means different things to different people.

Science has not produced a single overwhelmingly persuasive definition of normalcy or health to which all psychologists adhere. Wrestling with the description of 'what is environmental health,' Sir Colin Berry answered with tongue in cheek that at the first glance it offers a trouble-free epistemological problem, much like the Polish dictionary definition of a horse ("what a horse is, is evident to everybody"). That designation may not be as laconic if the pragmatic meaning of a horse is considered. Likewise, the boundaries between the normal state and illness may also be drawn for different purposes and based on dissimilar assumptions. Consider the border between person an ordinarily shy and the social phobic, or a question of when excessive sensitivity to group approval becomes suggestive of the hysteroid dysphoric. It is normal to be charitable, but someone's generosity may be so extraordinarily different from other donors that an underlying brain dysfunction may be suggested. Easy acceptance of the assurance of normalcy is also unwise because each profession has a somewhat different perspective on *normal* performance, such that conflicts may easily arise in the absence of a consensual definition. In its sylleptic abuse, the word 'normal' is used when the data are normally distributed, when the state is conventional, innocuous, habitual, and common, or when deviations are so trivial as to be inconsequential.[9] In a cheerless academic tradition the same word may be used in different senses (consider, for example, the terms such as parity, derivative, or stock). In short, it is a label for some central tendency that may or may not have pathological connotations (e.g. normal does not mean ideal or trivially substandard) and thus abstains from value judgment. An asymmetry of breasts in a young woman is a sign of a mild cosmetic defect. It may thus indicate that health and norm are also esthetic categories.

The same sign might signal to a physician that she is likely to be scoliotic.[10] The key distinction between the two categorical options is that the first is a guess of 'clinical medicine' that deals with the *individual*, and thus it is a custom-made ('private') assumption whereas the second is a hypothesis about entire populations, or a hypothesis of scientific medicine, in Murphy's[11] terminology. Woven into this categorization is the view that cosmetic irregularity or *defect* is person-centered and thus health delivery is bounded by the perimeter of a patient's need and her belief system (e.g. cosmetic surgery or psychotherapy, if the woman in the above example is unhappy). The question of what health professionals should do when the probability of a benefit for group is not worth mentioning as much as it is convincing for a single individual? This is a general question pondered by health psychologists concerning the reliability of their measures.

The notion of health as synonymous to 'normal' — in the sense in which we use that term today as a statistical average with reference to a given population — was only introduced into clinical medicine in the 19th century. It contrasts with the ancient Greek tradition of normalcy as being 'natural,' or as nature intended it to be.[4] Since our knowledge is culturally determined, irregularity was synonymous with deviance, thus giving meaning to individualistic

Box 8.1   Top 20 non-diseases (voted by *www.bmj.com* readers), in descending order.[13]

1. Ageing	11. Childbirth
2. Work	12. Allergy to the 21st century
3. Boredom	13. Jet lag
4. Bags under eyes	14. Unhappiness
5. Ignorance	15. Cellulite
6. Baldness	16. Hangover
7. Freckles	17. Anxiety about penis size/penis envy
8. Big ears	18. Pregnancy
9. Grey or white hair	19. Road rage
10. Ugliness	20. Loneliness

agony. It is often difficult to distinguish deviance from disease. When observed unsystematically, "any human being is likely to emit at least a few behaviors which can be subsumed under almost any trait in the phenotypic or genotypic lexicon"[7] (p. 233). For Irving Maltzman,[12] disease must have two characteristics: "It must be a syndrome, and it must be judged a significant deviation from a standard of health." Admittedly, in making decisions on matters of health, Maltzman is at the mercy of expert judgments. Alas, the experts themselves either are not always sure, or are convinced that the meaning of disease is self-evident, much like the definition of the horse in the Polish dictionary. To show that the issue is not really settled one might refer to the *British Medical Journal*, which is often ready to expose professional ignorance. Its editor polled the readers on the definition of what is 'non-disease.' Responses came in all calibers of wit and vigor and was complete with a list of top 20 non-diseases (Box 8.1). This list might summarize the cases which doctors should not treat; it certainly does not reflect their patients' perspective since some of these conditions cause distress and might prompt people to look for medical assistance.

Health as Social Well-being

An alternative loose offshoot of the debate on health is revealed in the oft-cited, and stodgy definition by the World Health Organization of 1946 (reasserted in its declaration of 1978) that good health is "a state of complete physical, mental and social well-being, and not merely the absence of disease or infirmity." This definition confuses the physical state or mental health (presence of physical parameters or some objective testimony, which would at least add some objectivity) of an individual with the general sense of satisfaction with life, i.e. a judgmental decree. The requirement of public consonance for identifying good health is charged with the authoritarian intolerance of any discontent. What is complete satisfaction and to whom does it apply, an individual or society? This question, with a huge subjective charge, a philosopher might try to answer on behalf of society. It is not entirely surprising that a philosopher from a formerly Eastern European communist country suggested that the better a person is able to adapt "to *reasonable* social norms without pain and suffering," the longer and happier life such a social elasticity will guarantee a person.[14]

The word 'reasonable' emphasized the need to be predictable and sensible. Both the communists and Nazis insisted on faith in a doctrine that was aimed at delivering something *good* for people. But faith is not reasonable by definition and does not allow for logical debunking. Consequently, it may create a climate where normalcy is defined in ethical terms or introspectively as a shared expectation of what a person should do.[15] It will not elude the reader that health psychologists cannot promise a diagnosis of moral health or happiness since the word 'reasonable' would be strained when applied to some infamous dictatorial societies that stipulate that people should identify with their objectives. Psychologists can study these matters, but they are hardly equipped with special senses or novel instruments to diagnose health as currently defined. Regulators tend to answer the same question of satisfaction on behalf of an individual. Therefore, in order to cover both ends, the role of public health services as stipulated by the US Institute of Medicine is in "the fulfillment of society's interest in assuring conditions in which people can be healthy."[16]

For another view of psychological health along the same dimension, one can recall the notion of a *black norm* — a constant vigilance, suspicion, and edginess exhibited by Black Americans in response to the expected offence, public and cultural, emanating from their white colleagues and fellow citizens. This is a sensitive subject among psychologists since a state of mind bordering on *cultural paranoia*, may lead to a considerable scorn of laws that are *not* perceived as protecting an individual. Breaking such laws is understood to be unacceptable, particularly when one is caught and punished, but it does not have the same measure of moral condemnation as breaking *one's own* law.[17]

Almost forty years back, when reading James Baldwin's loaded prose, I came to realize that this manner of cushioning one's dignity against injustice, slander, hatred and humiliation is shared by any minority group living in similar conditions. Yet, its *understanding* does not make it normal. Paul E. Meehl[7] forcefully maintained that understanding aberrant behavior does not make that behavior ethically permissible or 'excusable.' He was facetious about the tendency of pronouncing 'normalcy' *as we are*, that is approving in others what is noticed in ourselves. He cautioned not to include ourselves in every judgment we pass on another person, or as Sperber[18] quipped, to "smuggle ourselves into every picture we paint of someone else."

Health and Asymptomatic Disease

One of Webster's definitions of health is that of "enjoying freedom from physical disease or pain." We can agree with the need to be free from pain, even if some might be compelled to discuss how to categorize pains and fatigue after work out or strenuous physical activity. But disease is not necessarily something that is felt immediately. Rather, it is a protracted state when a metabolic error or pathogens slowly bind an excessive share of organismal defenses for years or decades. Their assault is recognized, and diagnosed as such, when they overwhelm these defenses with advancing years such that no modification of our physiology is capable of preserving orderly function.*

An atherosclerotic plaque that is clearly a sign of metabolic disorder may not lead to an acute coronary syndrome and even the rupture of atherosclerotic plaques may not necessarily be symptomatic to be of 'actual interest' for a patient in Henri Bergson's language. Myocarditis may manifest no symptoms whatsoever or may debut with only vague symptoms, like irregular heartbeats. Parkinson's disease has a long presymptomatic phase, and someone who has at least 20–30% of functioning cells in the substantia nigra pars compacta may be considered normal for his age inasmuch as these individuals are unaware of their limitations. Yet it is very likely that such individuals might be proven to

---

*Such cases are often given the name of *dis-order*, which might be defined following Henri Bergson's (1859–1941) 1911 book, *Creative Evolution*, as a violation of a general way reality is *ordered*:

"The idea of disorder is then entirely practical. It corresponds to the disappointment of a certain expectation, and it does not denote the absence of all order, but only the presence of that order which does not offer us actual interest" (p. 274).

be cognitively inferior if formally tested. Other examples are osteoporosis, breast cancer, or diabetes that may exist for years without causing discomfort, let alone physical pain. That is why the ageless dictum coined by Armand Trousseau (1801–1867) that "there are no diseases, there are only sick people" is still in circulation.

A diagnosis of such illness as hypertension or diabetes rests on normative values established by science, i.e. a hypothesis of scientific medicine,[11] rather than personal insights or perceived symptoms. Thus, the statement that a man has hypertension requires that we have measured his blood pressure. By contrast, concluding that a man is fat might not mean that we know his body mass index or skin-fold thickness. It is an esthetic definition, i.e. a custom-made ('private') hypothesis. Ironically, many years back a fat child was perceived as a child resistant to infection. The antiquated medical doctrine for treating tuberculosis ('consumption' or 'burning up') has departed from the intuitive view that more food is better for boosting health and bodily resistance to infections. Each patient in the sanatoria for the treatment of pulmonary tuberculosis had to chomp through a gargantuan main meal three times a day, and then spend an hour in compulsory complete rest in order to gain weight so that they would *look* healthy.[19]

Still another example is the health of fetuses with evidence of genetic disease, which may not necessarily tell us whether a healthy fetus is at high risk for developing a disease in adolescence or adulthood. Taking into account this uncertainty, medical definitions include, however implicitly, the notion of the individual's propensity to manifest disease. It would be naïve to dismiss these factors as irrelevant for peoples' lives. Yet, the task of explaining when 'norm' evolves into 'disease' rests on specific health care professionals since the division between health and illness has become increasingly blurred, and with good reason (Chap. 2). Understandably, such clarification is a function of the resolution of our methodology. As the technology becomes more sophisticated and reliable, people can be tested for genetic traits long before they develop clinical evidence of the overt disease; one might ask whether someone with a gene defect linked to early-onset Alzheimer's disease is normal. What about some people who carry a 'recessive' gene, and may transfer a disease only if they get married to a person with the same recessive gene? Or some easy questions, such as, is someone with occasional labial herpes healthy? Is a man positive for HIV infection inevitably mortally sick? Given that contemporary preventive medicine is based on probabilities, and cannot predict with 100% certainty whether disease will ever appear, an invasion of someone's privacy with a good intention of disease impediment may be, on occasion, worse than waiting for the diagnosable signs or symptoms to emerge.

The capacity to generate symptoms is influenced by a host of factors, including 'state of mind' and personality, as much as the type of disorder. The absence of symptoms may be a sign of a high *iatrotropy* threshold. In normal persons, denial may serve the adaptive purpose of coping with adversity and sustaining an optimistic outlook in a hopeless situation. Illness is announced when a person experiences pain, fatigue, and fever or when pain is associated with fear, as happens in asthma and cardiovascular pathology. However, when the brain is impaired, the recognition of disease may be impaired, too. In such cases, the claim of wellness may be a sign of some neurological or neuropsychiatric disorder. This state, already mentioned above as anosognosia, is often associated with a right hemisphere lesion when a patient enjoys the feeling of 'well-being' and false freedom from illness. Patients with tardive dyskinesia may be completely oblivious to their abnormal involuntary movements.[20] Thus, a concept of normalcy is tightly coupled with that of insight and self-monitoring.

Health psychology does not focus on *pre*symptomatic disorders nor is it equipped to look for specific vulnerabilities and specific predictors of latent diseases. Despite the aura of historical respectability, the notion of 'vulnerability' has so often been abused that theorists now reach for their earplugs. In the past, a physician was seldom able to pinpoint acquired or inborn premorbid defects, or specify malfunctions in various stations in the chain of command of diverse functions. More frequently, therefore, the origin of illness was attributed to a plethora of environmental and host events, such that one's deterministic philosophy was not rewarded by an immediate gain in predictability and treatment success. (This style of theorizing was discussed in Chap. 7.) This does not mean that health psychologists do not have a say in matters of genetic counseling, the search for markers of somatic disease or psychopathology and/or their successful modeling, but largely, that remains the province of medicine and scientific psychology. Hence, by necessity, medicine tends to map its boundaries based on ills, either somatic or mental, rather than characterize the signs of health since many disorders are just exaggerated normal processes. Just consider a regular sneezing due to banal rhinitis as opposed to a burst of sneezing that occurs in about 25% of people when they look up at the sun, which is the photic sneeze reflex. Penile erection is a regular REM-sleep sign in healthy men yet it may evolve into painful sleep-disrupting episodes of priapism. Another example is a normal process that acquires a pathological character when misplaced in time. The temporary muscular paralysis during the REM period of sleep is normal, but when such an event breaks into the daytime, it is designated as narcolepsy. Narcolepsy is often disturbing to other people, but might otherwise be harmless. When one cannot resist the grip of sleep while sitting at an important meeting, it may contribute to the feeling of social *'dis-ease.'* At that end, the presence of *'disorder'* is not always possible to ascertain as it is determined by the sensitivity of our instruments. It is often a problem for both patients and physicians to wonder how many tests have to be passed before the case is pronounced as normal. To paraphrase a popular joke, a "healthy person is someone who has not been thoroughly examined in a university hospital." Were such examinations granted to everyone at a low cost and minimal inconvenience, some abnormalities would have easily been found in most of us, in full compliance with a popular cliché "the more you look, the more you find." The only access health psychologists have to these patients is through the medical staff provided by the hospital. To orient them to be ready to run every person by high-tech facilities is neither practical nor desirable. Nevertheless, we live in an age of rapid change, and it may not be impossible to envisage a solution for screening all within the present decade. Therefore, the strategy of health protection and with it, the role of the health psychologist, will ultimately depend on how we define ill health. If sickness is conceived of as the result of multifactorial 'physiological dysregulation' the door will be opened for all sorts of romantic declarations where dysfunction of the cardiovascular, pulmonary, gastro-intestinal, genitor-urinary, and renal systems will be seen together with cognitive and emotional upset to multiple stressors that will legitimize almost any remedy and delay an active treatment.

In sum, it is uncertain whether an exhaustive definition of the terms 'healthy' (health) or 'normalcy,' however imperative, will be readily met for they require answering the questions of diagnostic assessments and quantifications, reflecting on ethical and moral principles, social factors, esthetic judgment, self-monitoring and self-concept. In his inaugural lecture, Dieppe,[21] asked a rhetorical question, "What *is* health?" After defining health by what it is not (i.e. neither disease, illness or sickness) he concludes his probing with an elastic holistic statement: "Health literally means wholeness and can be interpreted as the ability of an individual to fulfill his or her potential." This circumlocution leads him to relinquish the definition of health altogether because it "seems to be the province of politicians, who just 'pontificate' about it"[21] (p. 611). There. Does all this clarify things?

Psychology versus Psychiatry

One may not be surprised that there is no consensus between psychological and medical means of guarding the patient's ("client's") health. By juxtaposing etymologies of the words we notice why. Psycho*logy* is the science of the mind whereas psych*iatry* is the science of doctoring the (unhealthy) mind. The message being that psychology holds science (research) in high regard. It does not cure in the way we expect in the medical environment, which presently derives its strength from the molecular biology paradigm.

Pies[22] suggested that professions have deep structures that make them unique. Table 8.1, which was borrowed from his paper, compares the deep structure of psychology and psychiatry and conveys a dose of bitterness in the dispute on the value of the two occupations as well as profound, old disagreements. The only function that is shared by the two professions is that of case *history taking* and, to a point, that of *differential diagnosis*. According to Pies, the similarity ends there. One might add, parenthetically, that a convincing argument in favor of the medical definition of health is '*diagnosis*

Table 8.1   Comparative approach of physicians and psychologists (after Pies[22]).

Components of 'deep structure' of medicine	Psychiatrist	Psychologist
Case history taking	✓	✓
Drug history taking	✓	—
Physical assessment	✓	—
Neurological assessment	✓	—
Referrals for laboratory diagnosis	✓	—
Considering ancillary tests	✓	—
Arriving at the right differential diagnosis	✓	✓ ?
Prescription of drugs	✓	—
Monitoring and interpreting drug plasma levels	✓	—
Monitoring therapeutic effects	✓	—
Monitoring potential untoward (central and somatic) effects	✓	—
Assuming responsibility for managing untoward effects	✓	—

ex-juvantibus,' i.e. diagnosis by medication when drugs (presumably specific) have healthful effects on those who are symptomatic whereas the same dose has little or no effect on normal individuals. Psychologists cannot continue the diagnostic procedure to the level of diagnosis "*ex-juvantibus*." In their differential diagnosis, they cannot deal with the spectrum of somatic disorders.

As physicians worked hard to make medicine more of a science, the boundary between mainstream medicine and health psychology has become increasingly more distinct. Referrals for laboratory diagnosis and the understanding of its results is another important divide that is difficult to bridge with the current curriculum of health psychology. Ever since Rudolf Virchow's era, laboratory analyses were driven by practical goals of defining the loss of normal order in terms of malfunctioning cells. The novelty of Virchow's claim came from the effort of 'fingerprinting' disease by the pattern of microscopic changes of the ailing tissue. All trappings to the latter approaches adopted by future generations of scientists were based on the progress of the methodology of cytological subtyping of tissues. It appears, however, that the same malignancy (e.g. prostate carcinoma) in two patients may look identical under the microscope, but may have different outcomes. These look-alike pathological tissues with dissimilar pathological behaviors suggest that the resolution of the histopathological profiling of tissues was not sufficiently sensitive. This explains the paradox of why one person reacts to a specific remedy whereas the same drug does not affect another person without attributing the effects to the role of past stressors, domineering mothers, and personality differences. Another example shows that adipocytes that are located perinodally participate in immune responses and have special properties allowing them to interact locally with lymphoid cells, whereas histologically similar adipose tissue of mesenteric or omental origin are devoid of this property.[23] Recently, the emphasis has shifted from a cell to a deficient enzyme, mediator, cytokine, or protein.

Table 8.1 further suggests that the diagnostic and therapeutic work-up starts with a patient presenting a symptom. It is a phased, orderly process starting with a relevant history taking, physical examination, followed by more invasive and costly tests, when needed. It continues into the differential and final diagnoses, treatment routine, monitoring its success and controlling untoward effects. Clearly, health psychology might avow to control the domain of mental involvement in deficient bodily functions, whereas the medical profession claims authority over all bodily functions as well as the sanity of mental functions themselves. Thus, the program of health psychology must be that of a discourse and consensus building with medicine that has its own explicit ways of reaching therapeutic goals. The definition of disease is so inextricably coupled with the medical profession and its institutions that health psychologists find it mandatory to define rather precisely their position vis-à-vis specific medical problems, show how to provide cost-effective help and reduce the incidence of disease endpoints. Such challenges require, according to Evans,[24] that health psychologists participate in a range of activities and research projects, such as:

* creation of physical pathology,
* responding to symptoms in the absence of true pathology and individuals' preoccupation with illness or disease,
* exploring increased or decreased susceptibility to infectious disease,
* explaining what intensifies, prolongs, or diminishes existing pathology,
* examining those who voluntarily engage in health-threatening behaviors,
* taking on health-enhancing life-style behaviors.

Given these ends, he declares, "Currently, research in health psychology is directed toward investigations that might add to an understanding of the disease process and that might prevent, diminish, or arrest this process."[24] To paraphrase British philosopher F.H. Bradley (1846–1924), this line looks like an effort to provide good reasons for things we believe on instinct. Less charitably, it is a suspect of occupational rhetoric intended to boost professional confidence. The 'understanding' depends, at a minimum, upon the ability to weigh evidence and explanations. That assumes knowledge of the tentative origin of disease, its course, and history of its control, prevention and rehabilitation. However, as time passes by, much of the current concepts of disease may disappear into oblivion whereas future therapies will rely less on painful and disabling general chemotherapy, radiology and surgery than they do today before new 'physical pathology' will be created. Agents targeting angiogenesis, growth factors, and toxic genes will terminate the major chronic suffering caused by 'existing pathology,' such as malignancies. The hopes are that new treatment strategies will reduce pain and toxicity; they will target disease on a molecular level, and will likely diminish common side effects as compared to present systemic remedies. Perhaps in its current state, health psychology could participate in implementing some of the goals listed by Evans. It can handle successfully though, only the last two of them, but they are part of our mothers' conviction that if you hear again and again about the need to adopt healthy habits, you eventually will. What do we do with those who do not wish to follow their mother's wisdom? And how much is it really up to us to stay healthy, if we do follow it?

Health Psychology as Salutogenesis

Health psychologists see themselves, at least in the US, as involved in the treatment and rehabilitation of the *physically* ill.[25] Among the goals of the *APA Division 38* are the "prevention, diagnosis, treatment and rehabilitation of physical and mental illness, the study of psychological, social, emotional, and behavioral factors in physical and mental illness, the improvement of the health care system, and formulation of health policy." Thus, this is a goal of dealing with *disease psychology*, or the *psychology of illness*. That would make sense, save for one proviso that there is no single health psychology for all diseases. 'The psychology of breast cancer' is dissimilar from psychological aberrations in infections, sudden loss of function after stroke, the rehabilitation process following fractured limbs, or psychological demands associated with the uncertainty of living with disease, pain and frailty of advanced age, terminal illness, and dying. However, due to limitations discussed above, the term 'health' in conjunction with psychology may be used rather euphemistically as the psychology of disease.

That compels some workers to uncouple health psychology from the problems of pathology. They highlighted a more viable alternative, that of preserving (good) health, or rather, helping to maintain a *normal* level of homeostatic processes. In his presidential address to the *APA Division of Health Psychology*, presented in 1979, Matarazzo[26] admitted the need to emphasize more vigorously the task of health maintenance. With this objective in mind, he proposed the term *behavioral health* "for a new interdisciplinary subspecialty within behavioral medicine specifically concerned with the maintenance of health and the prevention of illness and dysfunction in currently healthy persons." By contrast, the term *health psychology*, he set aside for a more discipline-specific psychology's role "as a science and profession in both of these domains" (p. 807).

For the new direction of dealing with health issues rather than illness, Aaron Antonovsky[27] coined the term 'salutogenesis' (*salus* = Latin for health). Salutogenesis is one of those successful words that are readily picked by many who wish to define themselves and their role. It is used to identify any system of actions or values that contribute to the promotion of *health of the healthy* even in potentially adverse situations. The insight came from Antonovsky's experiences with refugees who came to Israel from Nazi concentration camps after World War II, and who were relatively healthy regardless of years of unremitting brutality, humiliation, starvation, torture and hopelessness. The question of what was the protective shield that reduced psychopathological and somatic manifestations in some others has been often discussed in American and European psychiatry. Whereas for Antonovsky, salutogenesis is linked to his concept of 'sense of coherence' including (i) comprehensibility, (ii) manageability, and (iii) meaningfulness, numerous systems that sprang from it do not even pretend to be rational to be recommended as therapeutic. These are phenomena such as faith healing, pleas to religion, physiotherapeutically oriented procedures of naturotherapy, placebo, responding to love, messages of optimism, and the procedures of complementary medicine. More recently, a label of salutogenesis became popular even in the context of unorthodox birthing (Chap. 6).

Health psychology could certainly live more profitably with a narrow and more credible definition of professional goals rather than spread out into areas of somatic pathology where its competence is relatively marginal. In this regard, Antonovsky's views overcome the duality of Matarazzo's circumlocution between *behavioral health* and *health psychology*. However, it does not seem likely that the soundness of 'salutogenesis' is to be easily tested within the context of health care delivery of health psychology because of psychology's formal commitment to the spectrum of goals as defined in its Manifesto, and because salutogenesis is not user-friendly in its numerous attires. In addition, according to Merriam-Webster, *Medicine* is the science and art of dealing with the prevention, alleviation, and cure of disease, as well as the *maintenance of health* that is certainly a more mechanistic term for 'healing the health' using *health factors.*

Admittedly, public health benefits more from the dealings of prevention than deploying medicine for 'maintenance,' alleviation and cure of illness. Aldous Huxley explained why this is so in his immortal *Brave New World Revisited* of 1958:

"Penicillin, DDT and clean water are cheap commodities, whose effects on public health are out of proportion to their cost. Even the poorest government is rich enough to provide its subjects with a substantial measure of death control" (p. 7).

Lifestyle change is a different matter. To paraphrase Aldous Huxley, to achieve changes of lifestyle (the major end of salutogenesis) would take the cooperation of an entire people for it is like birth control, since it must be practiced by countless individuals, from whom the practitioner demands more intelligence and will power than the world's illiterate possess. One might argue though that 'normal' people may also need to be taken care of, inasmuch as there are disorders that are characterized by a lengthy presymptomatic phase and on occasion, clinical manifestations could be delayed following timely 'salutogenic' interventions into 'health.' It would be highly desirable to develop a toolkit for early detection of the late-onset decline of locomotion, emotional aberrations and cognition in healthy individuals with presymptomatic disorders (e.g. Alzheimer disease, various presentations of Frontotemporal Dementias, or Parkinson's disease), particularly among those who harbor susceptibility genes, and then work together with the medical profession to delay the arrival of a phase when clinical disease phenotype is obvious.

Bandwagons of Medicine and Health Psychology

To debate about what is right and what is undesirable in an area in which new policies are persistently going in and out of style is not a small problem for practicing health psychologists. With the current pace of validation of mainstream medical practices, the scientific analysis of health psychology recommendations, very much like those of integrative therapies, is still far away from determining their utility for health maintenance and clinical practice. That pace is partially imposed by a conservative trait of progress to move with the tide and to see things as everybody expects them to appear, even when they are "unproved, but popular ideas — the bandwagons of medicine."[28] The word 'bandwagon' is often used as a euphemism for the insecurity of those who are convinced that the leaders have more of a clue than they do as to what lies ahead. Bandwagons carry recommendations for dieting, weight-control, 'drinking plenty of fluids,' low-carb, exercise, statin treatment, discount drugs, primary care, vitamins, herbal remedies, biotechnology, and genome sequencing, among many other topics that require consensus building. There is no getting around the optimism with which some popular recommendations are doled out to the public. The key-word *bandwagon* submitted to *PubMed* yields over 200 commentaries and papers carrying the word in the title. Today, as before, some bandwagon travelers are regular hypotheses, and they might be making headway on the surf of forefront knowledge. Eagerly expected, these findings and ideas are misperceived by the public as something all set for practice before they were properly tested. Only several items of the bandwagon repertory are sampled here in alphabetical order, mostly by way of summary of what has been discussed in the preceding sections since they persist in classroom discussions.

Antioxidants

Antioxidants have joined the bandwagon family due to their alleged ability to serve as a 'rust-protector' for the body, putting a stop to a process called natural or pollutant related oxidation. Although there are many interesting pathophysiological leads, a list of herbs and agents that are advertised for allegedly 'good scientific agreement' regarding their antioxidants' benefits for health is exceedingly long. Among antioxidants there are some trace elements, endogenous agents (glutathione, melatonin, and estrogen), vitamin C, E, and β-carotene (a provitamin A) that share the shelves of drugstores with green tea, grapeseed extract, shiitake mushroom, aloe vera and many other agents. Shooting from the hip with antioxidant 'remedies' in normal individuals is plainly irrational.[29] It is uncertain whether or not over-the-counter antioxidants would produce a desirable tissue concentration for the promised therapeutic results when administered orally even in megadoses. Nor can one confidently advise patients with cancer to supplement their diet with large doses of antioxidants (e.g. vitamins C or E) for possible preventive or therapeutic anticancer effects. Reactive oxygen species play a pivotal role in many physiological reactions, and their excessive inhibition may be undesirable. In particular, they provide an important defensive barrier service by eliminating mutant cells. For example, radiation-induced apoptosis in cancer therapy is a needed effect and it is not clear whether high doses of vitamin C or other antioxidants would rather help malignancy to survive. In mice with brain tumors, at least, antioxidant-*depleted* diets have been observed to increase apoptosis rates in cancer cells and diminish tumor size.[30] It may be impossible or unethical to conduct such studies in humans. Still, it is best that we learn to wait until better methodological approaches have evolved to integrate evidence of what level of antioxidant treatment is desirable.

One of the recent U-turns of the antioxidant bandwagon regards estrogen. Although estrogen is known for its neuroprotective effect, it may be harmful when given in combination with progesterone. Such a combined drug given to postmenopausal women seems to heighten the risk of invasive breast cancer, ovarian cancer, heart disease, and thrombembolism (blood clots). These risks of comorbidity are so alarming as to trigger a panic among those who still take the drug, and might truly need it. The case taught the medical profession that the pharmacokinetic rationale of therapy may have been embarrassingly inadequate, inasmuch as it was revealed only after lengthy epidemiological studies. This is a tragic conclusion for several million postmenopausal women who, in the US alone, would have to live in a chronic hypoestrogenic state for over two decades after the menopause. The obstacles that remain for designing better estrogens as therapeutics are daunting. Estrogen is involved in so many molecular pathways that have multiple and often opposing actions in different bodily tissues that the problem for providing its more targeted delivery is high on the addenda. The future will show how soon hormone replacement therapy will reclaim the status of a safe 'lifestyle-improving' remedy, and at what cost. That leads to the next question.

"Brain Reserve" in Women: Estrogens by Any Other Name?

The rationale of the majority of studies on brain reserve is to investigate the molecular and neural mechanisms whereby estrogens maintain non-reproductive ('lifestyle improving') functions, arousal, memory, emotional reactivity, mood and locomotion. The hormone certainly does the job by altering neuronal excitability at the membrane level and in the genome. The direction of estrogen effects may be complex. On the cellular level, they show both calming and (more often) excitatory effects culminating in proconvulsant manifestations (apparently via NMDA and/or AMPA receptors in the hippocampus). A decade ago, Dr. P. Timiras of the University of California at Berkeley suggested that in women, estrogen is concerned with the processes needed for reducing wear and tear or what is defined as the brain reserve (see Chap. 3b). Her hypothesis poses a number of interesting questions: Is brain reserve a structural advantage that is best gained in early life? Is then intelligence a better predictor of brain reserve than the level of formal education? Is education undertaken postmenopausally effective in modifying the risk of cognitive decline or easing the severity of dementia? The answers to these questions are not available. They necessitate experimental analysis of experience-dependent synaptic plasticity. A number of groups mine the problem. An example is a program lead by Yu. Geinisman's group at Northwestern University School of Medicine (*www.cmb.northwestern.edu/faculty/yuri_geinisman.htm*). His laborious electron microscopy studies establish the presence of experience-dependent plasticity in the form of both new synapses and/or the remodeling of existing ones in the hippocampus that parallel learning. Among his models of learning were a trace eye blink conditioning and a synaptic model of memory, such as hippocampal long-term potentiation. Thus far, long-term changes have only been studied in *adult male* rats and rabbits (Geinisman, personal communication). A therapeutically relevant question has yet to be answered: Would estrogen protect the brain from being wiped out by dementia via facilitating the transformation of certain synaptic subtypes into more efficacious ones in his models and during which stages of ontogeny?

Compression of Morbidity

An influential principle of *compression of morbidity*,[31] i.e. an alternative word for 'successful aging' follows the recommendation by G. Bernard Shaw to use health to the point of wearing it all out: "Spend all you have before you die; and do not outlive yourself."[32] It posits that cumulative lifetime morbidity and disability which characterize the senior years could be shortened by squeezing morbidity into an increasingly brief period of time between the onset of disability and the age of death by better health habits (e.g. no smoking, lower body-mass index, exercise). Recent data seem to document the slowly improving age-specific health status for seniors, and the postponement of the onset of disability by more than five years in the low-risk group as compared with the high-risk group.[33] However, large, well-designed random controlled trials of 'successful aging' based on scoring systems which are of clinical significance in practice are still lacking.

Exercise and Fitness

The wholesome role of exercise ('gymnastics') for society, and physiological and psychological health has been recognized ever since Plato's *Republic*. A few decades of medico-biological research have confirmed that not only do healthy persons who engage in leisure-time physical activity become healthier and live longer; they also manifest adult vigor far into senescence near the end of life, improved mood, and sensation of being in control and thus benefit from lower health care costs. According to some authorities, an active life could have postponed 23% of all deaths (cited in Ref. 34). There is a strong relationship between reduced cardiovascular risk and increased fitness due to regular exercise. For community health professionals and laboratory researchers, the problem now is how to recruit at least 25% of individuals in the US, particularly women, who avoid lasting physical activities. Also, health psychology researchers have a lot to accomplish in order to elucidate the physiological mechanisms (vascular/endothelial, metabolic, neuronal, and endocrine) whereby exercise-related improvements are attained.

Muscle is the major source of protein needed for bodily defenses against illness, such as antibodies and white blood cell production. A gradual decline in lean body mass (sarcopenia) often begins in early middle age and is primarily due to the cumulative effects of oxidative damage, inflammation, insulin resistance, and other catabolic processes. There are also indications of an age-related decrease in the synthesis rate of myosin, the major anabolic protein. Muscle loss with aging may result from blunted response to nutrition, as well as reductions in appetite and food intake with advancing years, the so-called anorexia of aging. Loss of muscular protein means a far-reaching loss of function, which is exceptionally dangerous in the face of chronic disorders associated with aging. Sarcopenic obese (the 'fat frail') are at particular disadvantage as compared to those who are sarcopenic and non-obese. The best way to combat sarcopenia is by exercise along with adequate nutritional support, in order to maximize the response of muscle to anabolic stimuli, rather than by the use of anabolic agents, such as growth hormone or testosterone.

Surprisingly, the rule of thumb for a 'dose-response' relationship between exercise diversity, vigor, schedule and length, its mode (e.g. aerobic, muscular strength and endurance, walking, jogging, flexibility exercise, dancing and swimming) and specific outcome has yet to be established. Those who are recent exercise 'converts' after years of sedentary life may discover that although moderate activity is better than none, an excess of action may adversely affect health. The extent of cardiovascular stress during aerobic exercise may vary and be greatly increased by hyperthermia and dehydration (e.g. running long distances on a hot summer day). Both can reduce stroke volume during exercise thereby significantly reducing cardiac output. Thus, the most important cardiovascular adaptation to endurance training — an increased stroke volume during exercise — is violated. The increased plasma norepinephrine response to dehydration-induced hyperthermia further adds to stress thereby potentially unmasking previously unrecognized cardiovascular insufficiency. One should bear in mind that a rigorous profiling of activity programs based on an accurate monitoring of its effects (e.g. cardio-respiratory endurance, muscular endurance and strength, flexibility, bone density, steroid hormones levels, lipid profile and fibrinolytic capacity, etc.) is still lacking to allow firm advice for all the needs and circumstances of the individual.

Exercise and Imagery

Experimentally, the role of locomotion in sensory-motor rehabilitation was demonstrated twenty years ago when Joe P. Huston and associates took advantage of an interesting marker, a vigorous rotation that sets in following unilateral lesions of the substantia nigra in rodents. In their study, some animals that received unilateral 6-hydroxydopamine-induced damage were suspended in a hammock for the next seven postoperative days. It appeared that by forestalling their locomotion, they also precluded morphological recovery of the crossed nigro-thalamic projections. By contrast, such projections were proven to be re-established in control animals who were allowed to stay active immediately after the lesion. Thus, lesion-induced locomotion, though a part of a neurological syndrome, proved essential for a successful mending of aberrant cerebral asymmetry.

These findings seemed difficult to implement for motor or cognitive rehabilitation of the elderly and individuals with brain lesions. It was uncertain to what extent exercise training would affect health parameters of the hospitalized population and improve their lifestyle. In the majority of studies, the benefit of exercise may emerge as robust as it does because their participants were being selected for limited comorbidity (the 'healthy user effect'). They also had a high degree of compliance with established standards for patients' inclusion. The staff and doctors running such tightly controlled studies are also more carefully selected for their interest and skills. The staff quality certainly motivates their patients. Therefore, the benefits of the same interventions for a population larger than that taking part in small, though randomized controlled studies, may be different.[35]

Is there a way to circumvent, even if partially, the need for obligatory locomotion in disabled patients by using mental imagery? Possibly. In his book, *Mental Imagery in the Motor Context* (Blackwell, Oxford, 1997), Marc Jeannerod showed that actions are represented when their sequence was only mentally prepared for execution; a simulated movement seems to activate the same neural circuitry, including motor pathways as well as the autonomic system, as though an individual was actually performing it. It would be desirable to verify whether merely imagining, or watching an act carried out by someone else and rehearsing it mentally, would add to maintaining an adequate level of nervous functioning and its rehabilitation in hospitalized populations. Movements are intimately tied to emotional responses (from Latin *emoveo, exmovere* — to move, lift, shake) in environmental approach-withdrawal inventories. Expanding on this, clinical health psychologists might find it interesting to follow up these studies by examining to what extent by simply forming an idea of various movements, a patient could alter CNS homeostasis (e.g. by augmenting GABAergic inhibition or offsetting stress-induced activation of some neurotransmitter systems).

Fats of Life

Consumers tend to capture something that is important to them as either 'good' or 'bad,' rather than as a dynamic and complex gamut or as the ratio between fats and other nutrients. Which fats are 'healthy' and which are 'wrong' is a question of time. There was a period in nutritional science when all fats were a component of 'wellness' on par with vitamins (*vitamin F*). It was considered desirable to consume ω-6 fatty acids, which are now recognized as 'snake oil.' The reason is that humans need ω-3 fatty acids and they are deficient in enzymes needed to convert ω-6 fatty acids into ω-3 fatty acids. The latter must be obtained from dietary sources. Today, foods high in ω-3 fatty acids are considered a desirable addition to diet. The fascination with ω-3 fatty acids as a possible salubrious dietary agent began with the observation that the Greenland Inuit had low mortality from coronary heart disease on a diet rich in fat. But the Inuit also move more actively to obtain and then process the seal and whale that provide them with ω-3 fatty acids than a typical sedentary dieter, or a patient with cardiovascular disease.

In the aftermath of World War II, Eastern European children and millions of children in Russia were given fish oil (high in ω-3 fatty acids, as well as a high concentration of vitamin A) on a regular basis. Such an oil supplement was as mandatory as vaccination, and given to provide the starving children with fat-soluble vitamins. In 1996, a conference on the role of highly unsaturated fatty acids in nutrition and disease prevention hosted by Barcelona worked under the motto 'Fats of Life.' Perhaps, fish oil was indeed, a real 'fat of life.' Curiously, this WW II generation had a very low rate of allergies, much as do the Inuit.[36] That is not to suggest that people with asthma need to modify their dietary intake, unless it fits their taste and wallets. The nature of protective ω-3 fatty acid action on the cardiovascular system is not fully understood nor is the daily amount of oil needed to grant their benefits known. Therefore, the recommended 'two-three servings' a week may not provide the dose ingested by the Greenland Inuit. (See *www.nal.usda.gov/ fnic/foodcomp* and *www.omega-3info.com* for more information on ω-3 fatty acids.)

Not everybody is convinced that the data at hand are sufficiently convincing of the merit of oily fish to make a firm dietary recommendation for normal individuals, let alone coronary patients, without further studies. However, the majority believe that it would not hurt and be worth a try. It is reminiscent of a story George Gamow (*Thirty Years That Shook Physics*, Heinemann, 1966) related about Niels Bohr, who had a horseshoe hanging over the front door of his country cottage for luck. Asked if he believed in this superstition, he firmly answered, "Absolutely not," and then added, "But you know, they say it does bring luck even if you don't believe in it!"

High-Fiber Breakfast

As in many other areas of modern life, selecting what to eat is not a question of choosing between competing cures. Why then have recommendations to eat cereals with breakfast suddenly acquired the authority of a healthy lifestyle? The answer is in the practice of temperance and vegetarianism of Grahamites (after American clergyman Sylvester Graham) that was almost exclusively directed at unrefined foods, such as wheat and rice — the royalties of the cereals, and these prized items of diet were behind the bloom of the modern breakfast-cereal industry. The reliance on a high-fiber diet has become a cheap way to 'divine' over health improvement, a kind of nutritional 'magic bullet' against cardiovascular diseases, high blood cholesterol, hypertension, central obesity and diabetes. It may not be useless to increase the intake of high-fiber foods since there are indications that the ingestion of fiber protects against adenomatous polyps and colorectal cancers. Yet, it took some time to find out that the consumption of fruit and vegetables or daily wheat-bran supplements had no effect on the development of new colorectal adenomas, which are considered the precursors of most large-bowel cancers. "Credibility is a terrible thing to lose," summarizes Stephan D. Zucker in his commentary of some of these studies for *Gastroenterology* in 2000.

Hygiene

The choice of a belief that we follow is an action codifying which laws and values we will not hesitate to violate. Among the principles we comply with is that of our mothers' admonitions to stay away from anything unclean, such as feces, vomit, unclean people, spittle, pus, blood, sexual fluid, and rubbish, some animals, cockroaches, stray pets, and decayed or spoiled food. An unclean environment is sickening to the majority of people. Disgust is considered a biologically beneficial emotion, since it keeps us away from 'contagions' attributed to filth.[37] However, diverse bacterial strains that colonize (but not infect) the host in infancy and early childhood due to lax control over habitat purity may conceivably avert atopic sensitization and the development of allergic diseases with advancing years.

Children living on a farm appear to develop asthma and allergic sensitization less frequently than children in an urban environment. These kids are likely to have regular contact with pets and livestock, which is a typical feature of life on a small European farm. They breathe the same air as the animals do, inhale the dust, touch animals' skin and waste, play with them, and fetch home fresh milk and freshly laid eggs. As it turns out, exposure to farm animals has been found to be major factor protecting individuals from allergy. By contrast, breast feeding, dietary habits, frequency of respiratory infections, passive smoking, and housing conditions have been unable to explain the heightened immune tolerance among farm children.[38] The transition from an agrarian to an industrialized society in Finland during the last decade, along with more rigorous hygienic standards was accompanied by a striking increase in allergies. The *'farm factor,'* which is a euphemism for a primitive lifestyle, is now a prevalent unifying hypothesis explaining the promotion of immune tolerance in the developing world.[39] The notion that early-life exposure to domestic animals, a farming environment or passive exposure to other sources of endotoxins or pollutants may modulate the development of atopy and allergic manifestations has evolved as the most important insight in the prevention of allergic disorder. It shows that the common recommendations to avoid allergen exposures and triggering factors, 'whenever possible' are inadequate and impractical. With this, the prerequisite of hygiene shrank to the status of a recommendation that has a particular probability of being true (e.g. alcohol-based rubs that have been used in Europe for as long as 30 years may be useful in epidemics of influenza or SARS).

Is there any specific farm bacterial infection that is responsible for the protection against allergy? *Lactobacilli* and *Eubacteria* were found in the intestinal flora of non-atopic Estonian infants.[40] By contrast, *Clostridia*, were relatively more prevalent in allergy-prone Swedish infants of the same age. Paolo Matricardi[41] and colleagues compared serology tests (IgE antibodies) for six pathogens in 240 allergic male Italian air force cadets with a similar number of non-atopic controls. The result was straightforward. All non-atopic cadets had higher markers for pathogens transmitted by the oral route, with statistical significance for *T. gondii*, hepatitis A virus, and *H. pylori*. In the entire sample, the frequency of high atopy was almost three times higher among participants with no antibodies to these pathogens (20% vs. about 8%). There were no other socioeconomic or demographic differences between the two groups.*

Regardless of some inconsistencies, the beauty of the hygienic hypothesis is that it illustrates the validity of the ancient admonition, '*First Understand, Then Advise*.' It does not imply that hand washing should be banned or that children should now be encouraged to camp near farm animals. All we need to learn is how microbial turnover provides 'immune-massages' in early life, so as to inhibit Th2 responsiveness. The risk of allergy is reduced with increased exposure to infections through contact with older siblings or attendance at a day-care facility during the first six months of life (see Ref. 42 for a review). Therefore, learning about the factors that shape the immune profile of a child would ultimately let us mimic the response of our immune system without relaxing the standards of our hygienic lifestyle.[41†]

---

*It is well recognized that normal (nonpathogenic) luminal flora is an effective barrier against pathogenic microorganisms. Therefore, antibiotics decrease the susceptibility of animals to infection; and germ-free animals are more vulnerable to infection than their non-treated counterparts are. The famous Russian immunologist, Elie Metchnikoff (1845–1916), recommended ingesting some bacterial culture (e.g. *Lactobacilli*) in order to populate the intestinal tract with those useful bacteria. Lactobacillus species are the same agents that turn milk into yogurt. They are present in the vagina and in the human mouth, and help protect against urinary and oral infections, as well as other chronic ailments. Lactobacilli are known to be potent inducers of IL-12, which is a key cytokine in Th1 immunity profile.

†An amusing and informative 'encyclopedia of feces' by Ralph Lewin (*Merde: Excursions in scientific cultural, and sociohistorical coprology, 1999*), tells us that in the animal kingdom, ingesting samples of parental feces is an essential biological act that serves to inoculate offspring with useful complement of gut flora. Hippos (*Hippopotamus amphibius*) spend most of their time in a pond of their own feces along with that of their family. That attracts lots of fish eager to feed on the offerings. Such baths do not cause any morbidity because the animals' skin and mucous evolved antibacterial factors to protect them against their bacterial environment. The harmony within the flora that inhabits the healthy gut can protect against infections and gut disturbances; it can reduce susceptibility to both infections and allergies.

Mediterranean Diet

How do we reconcile the longevity of some health recommendations and theories with the low fidelity of scientific facts on which they are based? An interesting example of how little verification is essential for trust is the following: In the early 1950s, while in Naples, Ancel Keys[43] was impressed with the very low incidences of coronary heart disease among the locals. He attributed the health of Italians to their food, which was later dubbed the 'Mediterranean diet.' That diet differed from traditional American cuisine emphasizing eggs, bacon and meat in that it was low in meat and dairy products, and used more bread, cereals, legumes, beans, vegetables, and fruit. Even today we still know very little about the nutritional composition of the salubrious diet beyond carbohydrates, proteins and fats. With so little known about its biochemistry, Mediterranean diet(s) have become a part of the Green Revolution and a standard for the promotion of 'optimal health' and well-being, as well as nutritional defense against the diseases of affluence in the Western world. Its benefits could have been associated with the smaller size of meals in Italy, the pace of food ingestion, legumes/fruit ratio, meat/fish ratio, olive oil, amount of fruit, salt, some spices, 'wine in moderation,' or perhaps an absence of alcoholic wine or wine vinegar altogether due to Islamic sensibilities, freshness of the produce, edible wild plants, reduced ingestion of caffeine beverages during meal, an absence of food-preservatives, cooking techniques, good air, mild winter and a lack of pollutants, genes and a cheerful disposition of the diners, and the physical effort needed to pay for the meal. Perhaps, it was just a slice of pizza that reportedly confers benefits because of the tomato sauce loaded with the antioxidant carotenoid lycopene, and so on. All these variables differ in different Mediterranean countries; they change as a function of season and thus are hardly applicable as a model all over the world. Mesmerized by the novel fad, the American public never asked whether the absence of some victuals commonly ingested by the population of Crete or Cyprus would disqualify the domestic emulations of the cuisine served in various parts of the Mediterranean Basin.

Public concerns over the role of diet have prompted the US Surgeon General to embark on a special investigation led by a group from the Department of Medicine, Veterans Affairs Medical Center in San Francisco. Following a study, Warner Browner and his group[44] arrived at the conclusion that if the relationship between dietary fat and cancer were as strong as has been reported in some studies, about 42,000 (2%) deaths of adults each year in the

US could have been postponed by three to four months. Finally, there was a study armed with predictive power. In essence, it posited a question: what is the point of organizing a state campaign to reduce fat intake for such a meager incentive to increase longevity? It is therefore not astonishing that the funding office protested the result of the Browner's group to the extent that the Surgeon General considered the study flawed and tried to preclude its publication. The JAMA, however, published the paper and followed it up with a lively debate on the topic. The hypothesis that the consumption of fat, especially from animal sources, increases the risk for colon cancer has been repeatedly tested in numerous case-control and cohort studies, but no study has shown an association between dietary patterns and colorectal cancer risk. Recently, an authoritative review in *Current Opinion in Lipidology*[45] indicated again that the hypothesis of an increased cancer risk with a high-fat diet should be considered weak. Not only does this reassure doctors and their patients, it also identifies a major field that still needs careful research to disprove erroneous theories.

Mothers' Wisdom

Inescapably, we are all on the same cross-cultural wavelength. Amy Tan, a best-selling novelist of Chinese extraction recalled being taken to the funeral of one of her playmates. She was shocked by the image of the lifeless little girl she used to have fun with. "This is what happens", she suddenly took notice of her mother leaning over and whispering in her ear, "when you don't listen to your mother." An American, Stefanie Weiss of the *Washington Post* (August 5, 2003) began a campaign of contesting some amusing pieces of mothers' wisdom (e.g. don't sit with legs crossed; you'll get varicose veins, don't go swimming within a half-hour of eating; you'll get cramps and drown, don't drink ice water when eating cheese fondue; you'll get a knot in your stomach and die, don't go out in the cold with wet hair; you'll get pneumonia). There are countless other bits and pieces that have become the favorite mantra for the generations of overanxious mothers who prod their children to follow their wisdom of health maintenance:

This line from Aaron Wildavsky,[46] was meant to protest the ubiquity and subtlety of sanctions and regulations based on tenuous norms or shared expectations that were

"Our neurosis consists of knowing what is required for good health (Mother was right: Eat good breakfast! Sleep eight hours a day! Don't drink! Don't smoke! Keep clean! And don't worry!)"[46] (p. 122).

taken over by health psychology. Bound by its own declarations, the latter persisted in historical imbalance by investing in the spiritual and physical health of the sick while taking little notice of the mounting evidence that one's nosological destiny could be 'programmed' before birth. Whereas bandwagons are byproducts of applied science, whose popularity to a degree is an artifact of scholarship and clever propaganda, the lines of mother's wisdom are part of the folklore that once created, tends to self-reproduce and propagate. Why do these law-like beliefs persist in different reincarnations as health recommendations? Their mysterious longevity is often seen in a peculiar overprotective trait, such as the lust for governing, 'tyranny of the weak over the strong,' 'the Emotional Incest Syndrome,' and others. Another explanation might be that these maxims are simply rooted in the deeply held convictions that our health is contingent upon our good behavior and in avoidance of temptations. Historically, that was a reliable low-budget health care for dearth of a better one. The amusing thing about loving instructions is that they are counter to Jean Piaget's (1896–1980) recommendation to prod, contemplating "What would happen if...," such as to provide (a developing child) with a chance to imagine the future without harming himself or herself. Mother knows how to save from harm. Therefore, her instructions are coined with Biblical assertiveness: "Thou shalt not do..." or "Thou shalt fear ...." Some of them look like generational curses endowed with the vitality of 'meme' that help them spread through generations.* A number of barely camouflaged memes of mother's wisdom are so influential that — to paraphrase Dave Gross (*http://www.lycaeum.org/drugs/other/tattoo/meme.html*) — some people refuse to abandon complying with them even when the dubious validity of the suggestions is pointed out to them.

We are easily seduced even past adolescence when government agencies and committees, or even some well-meaning individuals, aim at emotional persuasion in the conviction that otherwise people would choose to act differently; or when governments emulate our mother's voice in order to prescribe safety standards of what commissars of health prematurely endorsed as a 'healthy' stuff. The difference between concerns and instructions are many, an important one is that of a distinction between a relative and an absolute risk.

---

*The word was coined by Richard Dawkins as the counterpart of 'gene' for replicating, non-biological, conceptual entities (e.g. ideas, catch-phrases, opinions, cultural artifacts, customs, etc.) (*The Selfish Gene*, Oxford University Press, New York, 1978; 2nd edition, 1989).

Whereas the first might be used to caution about the hazards facing a person who carelessly submits to the allegedly contaminated environment, the second mandates restrictions based on weak evidence (e.g. labored epidemiological findings, public demands, theoretical convictions, premature publications on the topics of pressing health needs, and poorly quantifiable risk factors).

Nicotine Bashing

There are many reasons to give up cigarettes. Among them, wrinkled skin, gray hair and balding, gum disease, cardiovascular disease, decline in lung function and emphysema, acute myeloid leukemia, damage to abdominal blood vessels, cataracts, cervical cancer, impotence, fertility problems, enhanced risk of getting cancer of the throat, mouth, esophagus, kidneys, pancreas, or the bladder and just about every organ in the body. Finally, over 80% of all cases of lung cancer are related to smoking. That is a convincing list, which grows ever longer (*http://www.cdc.gov/tobacco/sgr/sgr_2004/index.htm*). In *The Lancet* message on *Medicine and Health Policy* of April 12, 2003, Rafael Bengoa, the WHO's director of management of non-communicable disease maintains: "Global cancer-prevention activities should be focused on two main factors — tobacco smoking and diet." He also added the need to curb infections of various kinds. But health psychologists are more likely to focus on the first paragraph, leaving the germs to other health professionals since smoking claims more deaths in the US than suicide, homicide and car crashes combined.

The weight of epidemiological evidence is significant. Nonetheless, there are some limitations. A number of studies have been criticized as confounded by other variables, including the socioeconomic status of smokers, or a confusion of the term 'tobacco smoking' and 'nicotine-seeking behavior,' and others.[47] From scores of studies and recommendations, it is clear that many smokers *will* develop cancer, but it is not as clear that some will *not*, and in many cases scientists currently do not have the ability to identify and classify those persons except in retrospect. In fact, the truth is that *most* smokers will never develop the disease. Those in danger are a minority. Nicotine is metabolized by the enzyme, cytochrome P450 2A6 (CYP2A6), which is predominantly expressed in the liver. It is the most important enzyme in nicotine metabolism. Polymorphisms in the CYP2A6 gene were

hypothesized to impact on both smoking behavior and lung cancer susceptibility.[48] It has been suggested that the CYP2A6 genotype modulates the rate
of smoking: an absence of the CYP2A6 enzyme reduces the risk of lung cancer, because individuals lacking this enzyme will either refrain from smoking,
or at least will not become ardent smokers. They would hardly enjoy smoking
because a standard nicotine dose in a cigarette would yield a significantly prolonged half-life. The same enzyme is responsible for the clearance of many
environmental pollutants, including structurally unrelated pre-carcinogens. As
CYP2A6 metabolically activates a number of pre-carcinogens that are inhaled
with tobacco smoke, the lack of this enzyme may also reduce susceptibility to
lung cancer. This provocative hypothesis has many inconsistencies and has yet
to be confirmed. It is uncertain, though, if individuals would be willing to
undergo genetic testing as part of their assessment as to whether or not it is
safe to inhale. It thus seems more easy to recommend abstaining form smoking altogether and for all.

Exposure to cigarette smoke is said to have been associated with prenatal morbidity by causing perinatal death, placental infarctions, congenital
malformation, growth retardation, attention deficit disorder, spontaneous
abortions, sudden infant death syndrome, and allergy. How could women not
give up smoking in the face of all the medical evidence that defines tobacco
as a mass killer? The point is that with the exception of small but consistent
growth retardation in the offspring of smoking mothers, tobacco smoke has
yet to be proven to cause the foregoing conditions. This is not to say that the
declared relations are not present, but that the problem is that of judgment or
rather, acting on interpretation of the same data, something that the anti-
smoking lobby has not seriously considered. More importantly, however,
those babies become addicted to nicotine before they are born, and then initiate smoking as high-school students and then sustain an interest in tobacco.
The harmful effects of passive smoking for pregnant mothers, as well as that
of the secondary smoking of children could conceivably be associated with
CYP2A6 induction. One might wonder whether the (paradoxically) greater
rate of lung cancer among adult African American men who smoke less than
adult whites (e.g. *http://mdhealthdisparities.org/html/data.html*) is not 'programmed,' even if partially, by the prenatal/infantile CYP2A6 induction or
enzymatic induction due to their casual inhaling of tobacco smoke at an earlier age. The advantage of exploring this hunch is that if correct, it would provide a better way of reducing racial disparities in lung cancer mortality and

morbidity in general. It will shift the priorities of health care to the hygiene of pregnancy and early infancy, and deemphasize the socioeconomic and lifestyle factors of adults who have a hard time sacrificing their habits. This suggests that juvenile smoking requires primarily long term, sustainable changes that focus on the need of *mothers* to alter their lifestyle rather than emphasizing interventions such as taxation, banning tobacco advertising or restricting places where smokers can light up, none of which are of significant concern to minors (see *Prevention*, below).

Nicotine is the chief reason why people continue smoking. Yet, any chemical substance is associated with more than a single outcome. Nicotine is no exception. It is a psychomotor stimulant that has diverse effects. It is known to have neurorestorative, antianxiety, antipsychotic, and antidepressant actions. The nicotinic receptor family is widely distributed in the mammalian nervous system. Its various subtypes are located in many regions of the brain, including areas that are important for cognitive functions (attention, learning and memory), such as the hippocampus and the frontal cortex. Enhancing nicotinic cholinergic transmission is allegedly neuroprotective, and thus might be therapeutically beneficial for Alzheimer's and Parkinson's patients.[49] In neuroleptic-induced Parkinson's disease, acute nicotine application reportedly induces positive changes of symptomatology.[50]

Given current concerns about the increasing incidence of smoking among children and adolescents, one might wonder whether nicotine is a marker of self-treatment efforts. One study that followed the life histories of 492 children up into adulthood showed that a third of them were hyperactive. Their symptoms and medical histories were used in establishing the revised (3rd edition) Diagnostic and Statistical Manual of Mental Disorders (DSM-III-R) ADHD diagnoses. The study demonstrated that by age 17, 46% of ADHD children began smoking on a daily basis as opposed to 24% of the controls. That disparity was retained in adulthood. There were significantly different lifetime tobacco dependency rates — 40% for the ADHD children as compared to 19% for the age-matched controls. There was a significant difference in rates of daily smoking and tobacco dependency between those with ADHD who had used stimulant medication in childhood and the controls.[51] It is uncertain whether or not nicotine helps treat ADHD symptoms. But a placebo-controlled double-blind experiment provided at least a tentative answer to that possibility.[52] The study was based on a small sample of six smokers and 11 nonsmokers who were outpatient referrals for ADHD as diagnosed by DSM-IV criteria. The smokers underwent overnight deprivation from smoking, and were administered a 21 mg/day nicotine skin patch for 4.5 hours during a morning session. The nonsmokers were similarly administered a 7 mg/day nicotine skin patch. Active and placebo patches were given in a counterbalanced order, approximately a week apart. Nicotine caused a significant overall improvement, as assessed using the Clinical Global Impressions Scale, although only among the nonsmokers. All participants in that study showed improvement in time estimation, reduction in reaction time and inattention, and increased vigor, as determined by the Profile of Mood States test. However, more research is needed to ascertain that tolerance to these effects would not develop over time.*

Prevention

When it comes to health, people often deviate from the beliefs of market management. They place a premium on real or imagined present benefits rather than on some profit to be gained in the future. Prevention becomes a province of token charity. Being able to pursue distant health goals requires special foresight motivations. We all rely on the unmitigated optimism that we will survive to harvest future rewards regardless of present unhealthy behaviors. It is difficult in our culture to institutionalize concerns about insurance and mortality statistics in the young in preparation for their own deaths before they become adults. What we call the 'generation gap' is, in fact, openness to diverse inputs and a dissimilar perspective on points in time and mortality. Thus, the question is how to enlighten the young and healthy, who are not preoccupied with their morbidity nor feel it imperative to invest into preventing illness before they reach their fifth or sixth decade of life.

---

*The book on nicotine is not closed. It has potential benefits in obesity and ulcerative colitis. The latter is predominantly a disease of nonsmokers, and formulations of nicotine, which permit its slow release in the colon may be of therapeutic value in ulcerative colitis.[53] Thus, scaring those who smoke may deprive one of some of its potential benefit. It would be wise to calm down wholesale nicotine bashing until, at least, a different nicotine formulation is available to provide the needs of inexpensive nicotine-replacement therapy for its recreational use. As a cigarette burns, temperature at its tip reaches 700°C. This heat breaks down the tobacco to produce various poisons. There are over 4,000 chemical compounds and over 300 toxic substances that the smoker is inhaling. Tobacco smoking is thus a dangerous habit; a gamble with health, particularly if a smoker is already unhealthy, but chiefly when burning tobacco leafs is used as a vehicle for nicotine is delivery.

The choice between treating a symptomatic sickness (an individual's position regarding risk) and the modifying risk factor attributable to the future problem in people with bad habits (populational risk) is of a crucial and age-dependent merit for a person. Not surprisingly, there may be a justified resistance to instructions that promote a policy for offsetting risks in the future by investing into something while we are young (see *Mother's Wisdom* above). Efforts to convince a young person that food restriction has sound neuroprotective effects and prolongs lifespan; that obesity has deleterious effects on bone density and decreases resistance to stress, is hardly able to win a child to a less pleasurable (and calorie-restricted) diet by the sheer force of rhetoric. Much has been written on the topic of such resistance to the ways of intercepting diseases and reducing their potential consequences. The spirit of the debate is splendidly captured by the familiar joke of John Allen Paulos about a young boy who was quietly masturbating in his room when his mother walked in:

"Don't do that, son, you'll go blind."

"Mom, couldn't I do it just until I need glasses?"

The mother explains (correctly) that the aim of preventive measures is to *modify risk*, rather than to treat an illness. The son sees it differently, as the public commonly does. The moral of the joke is that the boy was reluctant to delay gratification on the conviction that optometrists would save his failing sight in due time. His present fantasies were perhaps also more compelling than his mother's concerns of a remote future. More generally, mother seems unable to dispel the trend of her child to be optimistically biased regarding his susceptibility to harm since, according to Weinstein's[54] seminal idea, people have a tendency to claim that one is less at risk than one's peers. After all, he might have intuitively grasped (also correctly) that managing risk factors is about dealing with probabilities applied to populations. The boy must have got the picture that uncertainties persist regardless of the frequencies of outcomes. Weinstein[55] did not limit optimistic bias to any particular age, it must be the privilege of youth since he established that it was inversely related to perceived frequency of occurrence and personal experience. Although our mothers have the advantage of age, as well as the advantage of familiarity with the current winds of science or an overconfidence in current scientific knowledge[56] may be associated with the same error that is based on common sense.

Red Wines: The French Paradox Revisited

The amendments to an itemized list of lifestyle changes are like corrections to the front-page headlines in a newspaper. Eventually, they may catch-up with the news, but even if noticed, they might be overtaken by other news or may themselves require some revisions. Alcohol has escaped the rule of obscurity of exonerated sins. Moderate alcohol consumption ("one to three drinks daily") is no longer posted as a marker of unhealthy behavior together with poor diet, smoking, or a sedentary lifestyle. It is advertised for its ability to reduce the risk for cardiovascular events and even diabetes. That seemingly protective effect may result from a number of factors (e.g. decreased platelet aggregation, increase in fibrinolytic activity, or increased high-density lipoprotein level). With the recognition of the salubrious effect of red wines that contain chemopreventive agents known as polyphenols, wine has become somewhat more respectable, almost on par with aspirin. These molecules are reportedly responsible for the French paradox, i.e. the puzzle of an unusually low rate of cardiovascular mortality among the smoking and fat-eating French, who in addition are not so eager to exercise. Of all polyphenolic compounds, the stilbene *resveratrol* was recently singled out as the most interesting agent.

Resveratrol is known as one of a family of chemical defense agents synthesized in several plants (peanut, grapevine, and pine) in response to pathogen attack, UV irradiation or exposure to ozone. As a 'stress chemical' it is accumulated in plants growing in harsher conditions. Therefore, wines produced in Spain, Australia or Latin America are reputed to contain more resveratrol than those produced in milder climates. In 1993, *Nature* published a study by scientists of Bayer AG in Germany who succeeded in transferring stilbene synthase genes from grapevine into tobacco, thereby making these transgenic plants more disease resistant.

Resveratrol is alleged to have numerous pharmacological properties which include inhibition of arachidonate metabolism in leukocytes and platelets, modulation of lipid metabolism, inhibition of platelet aggregation and lipid peroxidation, reduction of expression and activity of cyclooxygenase-2, inhibition of angiogenesis, antimutagenic effects, and induction of apoptosis in tumor cells. This impressive list promises to help in a range of diseases (infectious, ocular, respiratory, endocrine, vascular, geriatric, and malignant as well as neurodegenerative). Resveratrol seems also to possess an antiepileptic potential, mimic the effect of calorie restriction, and increase cell survival. The excitement with resveratrol has recently swept the media with the announcement that the 'red wine molecule extends life.' A number of websites (e.g. *www.youngagain.com*) promote this new panacea as a relatively inexpensive food supplement. In a word, if resveratrol turns out to be a major constituent of the *Fountain of Youth* then Ponce de Leon could have found in 1513 a better wine in his native land rather than in Florida.

Those miraculous effects have elevated resveratrol to a heavyweight of the dietary movement for the prevention or reversal of morbidity and increase of longevity even though the underlying biological mechanisms through which these beneficial effects are mediated have yet to be elucidated. Therefore, despite the enthusiasm of many believers, a critical attitude towards the application of these compounds is warranted. As a nontoxic agent, it would be an exciting cancer chemopreventive drug. However, well-designed pre-clinical studies in mammals and human clinical trials remain mandatory. Polyphenols are certain to make wine deeper in color and taste better. They confer astringency and structure to the beverage and predict its response to preservation. But whatever wine's real benefits, "It wouldn't be around since pre-biblical times," as Irving Maltzman[12] quipped, "if it did not lubricate social interactions and provide a feeling of gemütlichkeit" (i.e. joviality, relaxation). Besides, wine is not an obligatory vehicle for resveratrol. Peanuts, blueberries, or cranberries and alcohol-free wine could be ingested by those who trust the efficacy of this longevity agent but have ideological or health objections to imbibing alcohol. Thus, one should not recommend moderate alcohol consumption to persons who do not currently drink.

Science by Committee

US Senator McGovern's committee was founded in 1968 with a mandate to eradicate malnutrition in America (see Ref. 57 for an excellent account). Political offices have a tendency to perpetuate their assignments and outlast their terms. There is nothing so permanent, observed the Nobel Prize winning economist Milton Friedman, as a temporary government program. Eager for a new health target, the committee set a goal to fight the 'hidden hunger' or 'malnutrition of fat.' McGovern was sympathetic to the conviction voiced by Professor Mark Hegsted of the Harvard School of Public Health that restricting fat intake would ultimately benefit Americans' health. Indeed, the Rand Institute have reported that obesity is more strongly linked to chronic diseases than living in poverty, smoking, or drinking.[58] Yet, that is not the same as stating that adiposity is consequent to dietary fat.*

Ironically, the committee's report acknowledged the existence of the controversy, but was based on the assumption that Americans had nothing to lose by following the committee's advice. That was a lightheaded decision protested by the American Medical Association. Fighting cholesterol is not necessarily associated with health benefits. Reporting on their findings on fat and cholesterol concentrations in 3,572 Japanese American men aged 71–93 years in *The Lancet*, Dr. Irwin Schatz and colleagues partially address this issue. They tell us that high death rates among elderly people may be associated with *low* cholesterol levels. These findings will certainly give pause to the zealous efforts of lowering cholesterol in elderly people to concentrations below the advised limit. Men with very low cholesterol levels (below 160 milligrams per deciliter (mg/dl)) seem prone to premature death. In a word, tinkering with fats could disrupt the repair machinery of the membranes in stress and aging, it might lead to alterations of membrane permeability to hormones, peptides, and pathogens. But this admonition cannot be written in black and white. Hemorrhagic stroke risk does appear to be inversely related to total cholesterol, whereas nonhemorrhagic stroke risk was positively related to total cholesterol. Cancers of the lung and the liver, lymphatic as well as hematopoietic cancers are seemingly more common at low total cholesterol levels.[61] Low-level cholesterol might be potentially dangerous since it is used in regeneration and for synaptic plasticity in neurons. Cholesterol deficiency was shown to encourage tau phosphorylation, reduce synapse

---

*Although Hegsted maintained at the time that dietary standards are mandatory, he also appreciated that an optimal design of diets requires a consideration of numerous factors such as food supplies, food habits, the individual profiling of people and their specific needs as well as better profiling of different lipids for different needs and hazards. In order to reduce the headache of decision-making, the standards were based on 'nutrient density,' which seemed most useful for designing a rational diet.[59] This kind of 'science by committee' was in effect a death sentence for dietary fat before an optimal diet was defined. Inexplicably, Hegsted himself was rather disdainful of 'science by committee.' When discussing the protein portion of the FAO/WHO Report on Energy and Protein Requirements of 1973, he maintained that by the time people on the committee found an issue they could agree upon, that issue represented nobody's opinion and was likely to be misleading or useless. But his repudiation came much too late. "If we knew what an optimal diet was," conceded Hegsted[60] in retrospect, "additional research in nutrition would not be necessary." One might be amused to note that his misgivings follow the script of the famous *Mitchell's Law of Committology*, "After the solution screws up the project, all those who initially endorsed it will say, 'I wish I had voiced my reservation at the time.'" Alas, the damage was done. McGovern's recommendations were in the public domain and supported by many who were eager to obtain grant money.

formation and thus could possibly fuel neurodegeneration in Alzheimer's disease[62] rather than protect from it. Reduced HDL cholesterol appears to be a marker of depression and suicidality. Assessing, by semistructured interview, the lifetime history of 650 patients, aged 18–59 years, who were consecutively admitted to a psychiatric hospital for attempted suicide, Golier and associates[63] found that psychiatric patients with low cholesterol levels are twice as likely to make a fatal suicide attempt. That association was obtained only in men; no association between cholesterol level and attempted suicide was obtained in women. These observations have prompted the speculation that lipid deprivation, and a decreased consumption of polyunsaturated fatty acids, especially ω-3 fatty acids, might lead to behavioral or emotional disturbances, depression and suicide. Engelberg[64] proposed that cholesterol could determine the availability of the serotonin receptor and its transporter. A reduction in serum cholesterol levels may lead to a reduction of membrane fluidity, with a consequent decline in 5-HT uptake from the blood. Thus, from what is known about the role that serotonin neurotransmission plays, low cholesterol levels might contribute to antisocial personality disorder and impulsivity. Juvenile cynomolgus monkeys who were kept on a low-cholesterol diet were more aggressive, less affiliative, and had lower cerebrospinal fluid concentrations of 5-hydroxyindoleacetic acid than did their higher-cholesterol level counterparts.[65]

The role of dietary fat in cardiovascular morbidity and dementia has polarized the community of scientists engaged in nutrition research into 'low-fat' and 'unrestricted diet' advocates. This recovery of the pro-fat claims may have to survive the test of scrutiny, inasmuch as the public is increasingly more edgy and skeptical. Although some of the cholesterol evidence was compelling, results of other findings were mixed. Moreover, recent epidemiological studies based on samples with greater statistical power and longer follow-up periods, and after controlling for potential confounding variables showed a positive correlation between cholesterol concentrations and suicidality.[66] John-A. Skolbekken[67] disheartened by inconclusiveness of the studies predicted in 1995:

Admittedly, the jury is still out on the issue of cholesterol benefits and dangers, but it also

"New chapters in this controversy will obviously be written and it should not come as a big surprise if the pendulum swings back and forth for some time still" (p. 302).

out on the issue of a recommending a

cholesterol restriction regimen for all. That caution is also roused by the possibility that cholesterol lowering drugs, such as statins will soon be available over the counter in the UK.

Self-knowledge as Salvation

The Paris doctor Philbert Guybert, a member of the rationalist movement of 17th century France, produced in 1623 one of the most successful self-help manuals. Once unique, such guidebooks are now common in bookstores. Numerous editorial, opinion-forming publications and books for the lay public are calling for a disciplinary generalization under the labels of 'self-management,' 'self-regulation,' 'self-efficacy,' 'coping,' and 'self-improvement.' A recent sample of self-help hardcover books on The New York Times bestseller list dole out instructions on how to reclaim one's 'authentic identity', how improve one's body and one's life, counsel on "breaking through the blessed life", and provide lovemaking tips. Their doctrines of self-help overlap with instructing on the changes in the patients' self-concepts, perception of health and disease, habits, behavior, and readiness to exercise self-enforcement, not only in somatic disorders but also in psychotherapy.[68] They promise to deliver every conceivable benefit, such as how to practice self-talk, self-love, and self-efficiency in achieving self-therapeutic goals. They go as far as to assure their consumers that they will learn to think as Albert Einstein did. Although there are a few interesting models of self-help strategies, they are relevant for the 'worried well.' Enabling patients to make informed choices about their treatment may reduce the risk of litigation, but it is doubtful if public education would increase satisfaction with the process of care if it is unsuccessful. One well-meaning book divulges the following insight: "the most important tool is one I can't give you — selfknowledge. In the final analysis, it isn't me, or your doctor, or anyone else, who knows what's best for you. For that knowledge, you and you alone are the expert."[69]

The reader might have had a quiet chuckle, apparently recalling that the shrine of Apollo's oracle is said to be adorned with a similar recommendation to emphasize something almost unreachable. Karl Jaspers (1883–1969) wrestled with the predicament of the Socratic "Know thyself" and expressed doubts that one can ever approach the limits of self-understanding. For those who miraculously prevailed over the difficulty, it makes but little practical difference whether or not they have additional therapeutic sessions to realize that a search for medical solutions to health problems could be more painful that the sickness itself. Regardless of such understanding, such a decision is better made together with a medical practitioner: if an ailing patient can be more profitably treated with physical therapy, pharmacological means or surgery, ministering self-knowledge, understanding, wellness, and Panglossian optimism would be a waste of time and a prescription for trouble.

As an idea, self-help seems a wonderful response to health care fiscal problems. Physicians or therapists would also like to know how much personal reserve a patient can call upon. But the final cost/benefit analysis of the 'self-help index' or 'toughness index' has yet to be provided. And what is the *cost* to a nation in an age of laissez-faire, of perpetual reliance on self-help when medicine has found some vital answers to curtail the impact of disorders that originate in prenatal programming? What is the *benefit* to the people of dependence ('self-reliance') on a network of nutritional stores when there is a need to localize and eradicate chronic inflammatory processes in the body? Is 'self-help' part of the wisdom of assigning the responsibilities? Knowles[70] fittingly argued that people do not worry about health until they lose it. That is why the idea of health rights, as he felt, should be replaced by health duty, so to speak, or 'an individual moral obligation to preserve one's own health.' Matarazzo's[26] proposition follows rather closely that of Knowles by defining behavioral health as

Does that mean that our clients should know something about biomedical science and techniques of which their therapists may not know much, or is it that when it comes to self-help, everything is different? Well, no. These declarations are only possible in the absence of precise standards and tested methodology.

"an interdisciplinary field that stresses *individual responsibility* in the application of biomedical science knowledge and techniques to the maintenance of health and the prevention of illness and dysfunction by a variety of self-initiated individual or shared activities" (p. 813, ital. added).

What the advocates of self-healing imply, but stop short of explaining, is that self-help is a ploy to buy time before a better solution is on hand. People may conceivably benefit from self-help when it is deployed before their health was already sabotaged to the point when disease becomes symptomatic. However, as was mentioned already, it is difficult for somatically healthy and psychologically competent human beings to 'self-force' themselves into the role of patients obeying unsolicited instructions and invasive explorations. Still more on the negative side, self-help can cause unnecessary treatment delays and create a chronicity gap when health care would ultimately be provided too late and in too small a dose to influence the outcome.

The American celebration of a single-minded subscription to the social ethic that declares all persons responsible for themselves ("self-made") has added more appeal to the idea of self-help and has become part of the health psychology message. This neo-Freudian or, perhaps, neo-Buddhist insight implies that we have no one to help us, and thus, if help is required, salvation must come from within. It also teaches us that whatever happens to a person here and now, requires a great deal of personal reserve, rather than deflecting the blame onto the family, the working environment, economic circumstances, linguistic barriers, the wicked forces of racism, or sexism, an unsympathetic family, or bad friends. Just the same, when lecturing on helplessness, and providing advice on how to do better, we are driven by something deeper than selfless therapeutic impulses. We express moral indignation at someone displaying social, cognitive, physical and emotional incompetence. Much as with psychological over-treatment, one might expect some problems with an 'overdose' in promoting 'self-help' since it is every bit self-indulging in loading onto anxious, often disoriented, powerless, and lonely patients the responsibility for their own somatic or psychopathological destiny. A tentative definition of 'self-help' is any self-directed activity that *has the effect of benefiting the state of health.* However, in 1954, Abraham M. Maslow, cautioned in *Motivation and Personality* that the free-choice situation works best for *healthy* people:

> *"Sick, neurotic people make wrong choices; they do not know what they want, and even when they do, have not courage enough to choose correctly"* (p. 350).

Vegetables as Anticancer Foods

By now you know that your mother's warning that "you'll never grow up if you won't eat your vegetables" is not about your height, it is the 'morbidity and mortality reduction claim.' But her metaphor is still in vogue. Bernard Stewart, an adviser to the International Agency for Research on Cancer, was cited by the *Lancet* of April 12, 2003 (p. 1278) as saying that "With our low intake of fresh fruit and vegetables and our high intake of fatty foods, together with a lack of exercise, we have managed to pull down on our heads [sic] a spectrum of disease, of which colorectal and breast cancer are only a couple." He points out that the World Health Organization already has on its short list 15–20 agents that provide the basic anticancer armamentarium. In the meantime, not to fear: "It is a relatively simple message — everyone should be eating about 500 g of fresh fruit and vegetables a day. And that's enough," he assured. There … Few sane people would quarrel with the need for roughage. But standardized methods for computing fiber consumption (its frequency, amount, type and solubility, preparation methods, source and associated diet) are lacking, a fact which leads to inconsistencies and scarcity of good-quality studies. Therefore, imputing protection from cancer to that 'one-size-fits-all' dose of vegetables strikes one as daring to the point of being irrelevant. It can be assailed on many grounds — the public health view point, ecological prospects, and disease prevention.

Ecologically, in view of the shrinking land and water resources in the world, it makes better sense to orient students beyond the needs of providing an individual lunch bag. Such perspective means overcoming the fear of and resistance to genetic technology that could ultimately result in food crops resistant to salinity, drought and disease, and produce safety-controlled foods with superior nutrient quality, enriched with desirable phytonutrients, and adequate culinary properties. In the future genetically altered foods would hopefully permit us to provide nutrition-tailored therapies based on the genetic makeup of individual patients. None of us can pretend to be aware of the amount of phytonutrients in a 500 g dose of vegetables presumably needed to avert the Armageddon "we have managed to pull down on our heads." It takes decades to make a lasting dent on our inherited susceptibility genes. Given the enormous variability of micronutrient composition in food crops it is hardly possible to tell when a desirable dose is achieved on our plate, let alone in our tissues, since the bioavailability of each nutrient or its cocktail is not under our control. More to the point, many of nutrients we wish to ingest to get better or protect ourselves from probable ailments are largely *non-bioavailable*. Since the food-based approach is only optional rather than prescribed, a caveat is that hypotheses (or longevity-increase claims) for any across-the-board recommendations must ultimately lead to testable consequences — a process that may take years, even decades — if science is to advance. An underlying principle of epidemiological analysis of nutrient effects, much as in drug studies, is that of their homogeneity and the uniformity of the samples. Given the heterogeneity of diet, as well as that of the dieters, is colossal, it is not surprising that a clear answer to the level of intake of plants and fruits as well as their type has yet to emerge. What's more, there are indications that a population subsisting on vegetables would not benefit from all salubrious micronutrients in the presence of subclinical inflammatory processes and infections. Thus, to recommend improving infected populations through diet would be an oversimplification. Eradicating perinatal infections and their control in adults might prove a simpler and a more successful health care policy for the next generations (e.g. Chapter 2). This leads to the next point.

War on Obesity

We all must have taken for granted the need to 'fight obesity.' The declaration of war is a legal avowal of hostilities between forces or countries when low-level hostilities do not secure a desired victory. It is not quite certain though, who is the enemy in the war on obesity and how the enemy is to be defeated: by identifying all those with genetic a liability, targeting the food industry, asking celebrities (presumably anorexic) to encourage children to eat healthier foods, promote exercise, introduce a tax on high-fat foods items, limit the amount of calories ingested (reduce meal size, dietary fat, carbohydrates, etc.) or mandate all of the above and also reduce the impact of economic disparities? To have the upper hand, potential combatants have to follow the rules determined by a formal decision-making process. The latter requires that a goal be unambiguously identified beforehand (e.g. reaching a specified body mass index, or increasing the longevity of the population) in order to know when the 'war' is won. Kevin R. Fontaine and his colleagues report (*http://www.mindfully.org/Health/2003/Obesity-Life-Lost8jan03.htm*) that weight beyond a body mass index of 23–25 is capable of lessening life expectancy, regardless of age. For argument's sake, let us assume that *Pax Romana* is to be declared when an average body mass index for the US population drops to around an acceptable 25. Alas, excessive precision in stating what is 'norm' can be more trouble than it is worth. By computing a more realistic index, that of 'years of life lost' due to obesity for adults aged 18 to 85 years, Fontaine found that the danger of exceeding the index appears to be maximal for white individuals in younger age groups. Given that overweight people are more likely to be black and of low socioeconomic status, it was surprising to discover that among blacks, excess weight may *not* decrease life expectancy until body mass index reaches 32 to 33 for men and 37 to 38 for women (substantial excess weight!).

Although these differences have yet to be explained, Fontaine's dissenting findings tell us that the risk of morbidity cannot be characterized by the same populational 'corpulence digit.' Including a wider group of people at risk (including such racial/ethnic groups as Mexican-Americans and Pacific-Islander Americans, who are known to have high prevalence of obesity) and a larger sample size are likely to be more accurate. Still, it is possible to wonder now, if adiposity increases susceptibility to disease, why would presumably more vulnerable groups not show reduction in longevity? How likely it is that investing money to merely reduce population weight to an accepted criterion would *not* make people healthier? Food ingestion is said to act like secondary smoking. Therefore, *the Surgeon General's Call to Action to Prevent and Decrease Overweight and Obesity* (*www.surgeongeneral.gov/ topics/obesity/default.htm*, last updated May 27, 2004) guides parents:

> "Be a good role model for your child. If your child sees you enjoying healthy foods and physical activity, he or she is more likely to do the same now and for the rest of his or her life."

This is reminiscent of mothers' incentive to enforce 'what everybody knows is true.' Nonetheless, biological research of possible underlying causes has not been made superfluous since the Surgeon General's recommendation had been received. One might wonder if the obesity pandemic is attributable, even if only in some measure, to an adverse embryonic (fetal) environment, such as utero-placental insufficiency, maternal undernutrition, preterm births, and teen pregnancies.

Yahoos Arrival?

On its first page the *Washington Post* of August 14, 2003 ran a sensational report titled *EU's Ailing Arrivals from the East*. Its gist was that Hungary's cancer rate highlights the 'health gap' between the low-income, former communist East and the affluent West. So, where is the beef? There is certainly plenty to think about. The paper mentions mishandled chemicals, pesticides and other pollutants during that county's race toward industrialization. Yet,

Dr. Otto Szabolcs, deputy director of the National Institute of Oncology in Hungary cited in that article is on the side of prudence. In the spirit of common lore he acknowledges primarily "lifestyle and diet" — "very tasty, but high in fat and also poor in fruits and vegetables." There are many things Hungary does *not* have or is deprived of — much as people in Croatia, Poland or Russia, for that matter — contaminated water supplies, crowded housing, and poor sanitation after decades of wretched management. There was not a word in the report devoted to the inadequate handling of infection as a possible risk for malignancies in Hungary. There is some evidence, however, about *Chlamydial* infections of the genital tract that often lead to preterm birth (Chap. 2), and which, according to Dr. T. Nyari of Szeged University Department of Medical Informatics, are the most imperative perinatal problem in Hungary. *C. trachomatis* infection is suspected to lead to ovarian and uterine cancer. As a urogenital infection it may be implicated in asymptomatic prostatitis. *C. pneumoniae* infection may also be an independent risk factor for lung cancer. Both are implicated in other kinds of cancer, including non-Hodgkin's lymphoma (*www.herkules.oulu.fi/isbn951425533X/html/x1636.html*). The presence of past infections or the presence of inflammation markers such as homocysteine or C-reactive protein are hardly ever flagged in nutritional studies. Their identification is costly and unreliable, but we cannot afford to ignore them. By using Koch's postulates it is almost impossible to show *Chlamydia* as a causative agent in malignancies. Regardless of the outcome of the future studies it is wise never to attribute to other causes that which could be accounted for by infection.

'Yo-yo' Syndromes and Laparophobia: Biology or Culture?

'Yo-yo' has become a symbol of the constant and often futile struggle of patients trying to quit smoking, bulimics fighting with "ugly fat" or slimming, and gaining obesity patients on all sorts of diets. Like Sisyphus, the 'absurd hero' of Albert Camus (1913–1960) they are always at the foot of the mountain, always find their burden again. Very few overweight individuals escape the Sisyphean curse, and those who do and stay longer than a year or two with their weight loss would have to be subjected to an analysis of their psychologic profiles.

A recent survey of schoolgirls between 1993 and 2003 in southern Ontario (Canada) showed that nearly a third of girls aged 10 to 14 felt they were 'too fat' and were trying to shed pounds (*www.pulse24.com/News/ Top_Story/20040511-005/page.asp*). One might be curious why anorexia is never mentioned as an epidemic on par with obesity. As of this writing, the search engine Google gives 27,000 hits on 'yo-yo dieting.' Anorectics are ardent exercisers, driving the rest of the population into the 'frenzy of fitness.' Between 1987 and 2001, the number of Americans who exercised 100+ days a year increased from 9 million to over 18 million. From 1990 to 2001, there was a 63% increase in membership of health clubs. Is this not a sign of a pandemic in the making? The pendulum seems to be swinging far in that direction, and society has now an immoderate fear of adiposity. Hundreds of young women in the US starve themselves to death or binge and purge and exercise in their efforts to stay slim because of the insatiable craving for companionship they fear to be unable to find otherwise.

Why is an effort to get brighter in order to fit into the college norm highly commendable while the trend of slimming to measure up to the standards of society preposterous? An important part of the answer to this question belongs to the way we reflect, talk and represent ourselves. It is commonly suggested that only some genetically vulnerable phenotypes ('behavioral anorexia phenotypes') respond with pathological hypophagia in the presence of sociocultural pressures (e.g. those who are said to manifest perfectionism, rigidity and obsessiveness; have enhanced sensitivity to social approval, prone to body dissatisfaction culminating in dysmorphic delusions, anxiety, irritability, and shame). However, normal 'self-monitors,' who may be obsessed with countless distressing preoccupations and feel embarrassed by their sagging skin, balding scalps, unshapely feet, and unimpressive pectoral muscles, also engage in a continuous checking of what their peers presumably think of their appearance. Such individuals are neither dysfunctional nor delusional to the extent of being labeled as having body dysmorphic disorder. Although many of them tend to read (implicitly) too much of interest in their persona into the minds of others, that is not a schizotypic feature, and they cope handsomely as self-help customers who keep pushing dumb bells, jog on treadmills, and support an army of practitioners for body fixing who represent a novel subdivision of discretionary health care — 'vanity-maintenance.'

Why are anorexics different? That is often not so clear since like many other things, anorexics may differ in degree more than they do in kind. Susceptible individuals, mostly adolescents (although cases of 'tardive anorexia' are known) develop severe and persistent fears of their body weight that are commonly unreasonable as they are relatively independent of body mass index. Operationally, their 'patienthood' is established when their weight declines to the level when malnutrition could cause mortal complications. Do then these individuals develop what can be defined as culturally (socially) acquired phobia? The role of fear in anorexia is always compelling since it implies the presence of a specialized neural circuitry, a sort of innate 'fear module' and a central focus for fear-related memories that are likely to be activated at critical periods of development. Once operational, that circuitry is difficult to disable by extinction (in terms of learning theory). In the past, even 'heroic' efforts such as lobotomy, once reserved for treating schizophrenia, were tried in anorexia. However, for some reason, phobias are defined in the *DSM-IV* as fears of environmental (i.e. extrinsic, 'extracorporeal') prompts, which phobic individuals commonly tend to escape. In anorexia, the only way out of a distressing situation is away from the presumably 'fat' body. Consequently, the label of anorexia is a term defining (somewhat) a coping strategy rather than the character of disease. The latter is triggered by specific phobia such as fear of stoutness, and thus *laparophobia* (a term derived from the Greek word '*lapar*' for belly). This term is a small improvement on anorexia. Practically though, it may be as peculiar as diagnosing agoraphobia when we guess it to be a façade for autonomic distress. So, what should be treated, how and when?

The puzzle of chronic self-starvation is that, unlike obesity, it seems so counterintuitive biologically. From an evolutionary point of view, it might be thought of as a vestige of a submissive response of individuals of the lower social ranking that are threatened in a stressful competition for scarce resources. Laparophobia might thus share its neurochemical territory with that of harm avoidance, anxiety, depression and suicidality. Consequently, disturbances in monoaminergic and lately serotonergic pathways have received much attention in the search for the neurobiological underpinning of self-starvation. Serotonin receptor and transporter genes have remained the major focus for efforts to identify genetic liability of the disorder, albeit thus far with positive and negative results. However, anorexia is a centrally reinforced self-starvation that is achieved in times of plenty rather than imposed during food scarcity. Also, self-starvation is often an attempt of lean individuals that wish to get trimmer. It is likely to be pathophysiologically different from that in binging anorexics, who are commonly those who cannot terminate the 'yo-yo' sequences.

One might also ponder a view (that does not rule out the role of anxiety and phobia) that anorexia is a remnant of some rewarding circuits that were once needed for curbing parents' appetite when they were supporting young and when a stronger self-preservation instinct would have conflicted with the preservation of the species. This notion follows that of Peter Kropotkin (1842–1921), who is better known as an anarchist than as an inspired social ecologist. That idea diminishes the role of the 'bottom-up' metabolic signals. Instead, it calls attention to the authority of 'top-down' mechanisms that produce an abstemious Spartan when, for some reason, these adaptations go wrong and such devices are unnecessarily overactivated. If, in obesity, the prefrontal cortex were assumed to be deficient in restraining an impulse to overindulge (Chap. 4) then some subcategories of laparophobia might be conceived of as caused by a (prematurely?) overactive prefrontal cortex that causes some individuals to channel their lives into an irrational pursuit of thinness. The paradox of this environmental 'autonomy' is that it is coincident with conformist personality and an augmented craving for social acceptance.

It is desirable to find ways of disrupting an established circuitry of self-representation as compared to that of representing others, and learning more as to how such prefrontal hyperexcitability is fine-tuned by serotonin input during the early stages of pre- and postnatal development. This also includes understanding the ways serotonin interacts with a burgeoning list of orexigenic and anorexic neuropeptides, GABAergic receptors, as well as NMDA/ AMPA receptors. If the only admonition were psychopharmacological, then it could be hoped that a 'serotonergic mindset' of anorexia pathophysiology would be minimized. At the very least, serotonergic modulating therapy ought to show success, more definite than reducing the rate of relapse of the disorder. That calls for exploring the virtues of other putative pharmacotherapy candidates. The well-established aberrations of glutamatergic neurotransmission in neuronal development in anxiety disorders and anorexia suggest that drugs that potentiate GABAergic neurotransmission, as well as non-competitive NMDA antagonists, such as memantine (mentioned in Chap. 4), are thought to be helpful.

Health Delivery Map

What Can Be Done?

The success of health psychology will be determined by the understanding of mutual needs and collaboration between laboratory scientists and clinicians representing both psychology and medicine. The history of merging with medicine occupations such as dentistry, nursing, midwifery, osteopathy, pharmacy, optometry, and podiatry, was thorny and instructive as to what such mergers entail. As they joined medicine, all have become subordinate to the medical profession and have essentially adopted its philosophy. It is not certain whether health psychology is ready to make that choice. The osteopathic system put forth an alternative conception of health care and treatment that promoted *wellness* rather than illness and emphasized prevention rather than treatment. It would have been a well-forgotten episode in the history of healing if not for its leaders' ability to redefine goals, and abandon the ideological wars of identity.[71] In short, osteopathy accepted medicine wholeheartedly, and attempted to draw on its strength in order to enhance its own professional standing. Rather than fighting the medical profession as its founder was inclined to do, osteopathy joined it. The same can be said about dentistry, which never challenged medicine's claims to knowledge or expertise.[72]

Why have physicians acquired so much influence and power despite the fact that, in times gone by, health psychology seems to have branched from the same tree? A likely answer is that medicine evolved into a highly standardized occupation with a number of restricting provisions that it cared to enforce (Box 8.2). The most that can be said in favor of contemporary medicine, regardless of its shortcomings, is that the scientific potential that it amasses generates the longer-term promise for population health improvements. There are no distinct signs that medicine has already turned a corner. Pathological insights have yet to be matched by equal progress in the management of many conditions. Yet, the historical record clearly shows that the promises of medicine have ultimately been brought to fruition. Health psychology is infinitely more syncretic and inclusive than medicine and other paramedical professions. It thus relaxes barriers to membership in dealing with the sick who are expected to be complex, and having unique features. Psychologists and cultural anthropologists did help to galvanize a resurgence of interest in the personalized approach to patients. Such efforts are relevant when dealing with minorities, migrant and immigrant populations, as well as children. Yet, 'individualized' handling, however acceptable to patients, may not necessarily help their condition, actually aggravating sickness in those with multiple complaints and persistent pain. By comparison, the current trend in medicine is that the more *cure* is needed, the more an outcome is viewed as the property of *disease*. That trend prompts the list of tentative

Box 8.2   How a 'new order' in medicine has been achieved (adapted after Ref. 73).

- By defining objectives. Showing that the management of diseases will be determined by five major means: *Preventive, Etiologic, Pathophysiological, Symptomatic* and *Restorative*
- By controlling educational standards and curriculum on a national scale. Setting a high threshold for obtaining professional education and training
- By unifying the services and procedures, setting the limits and legislation for novel practices
- By imposing a rigorous control over the content of practitioners work
- By waging a battle with illegal and unethical practitioners. Regulating standards of behavior of professionals
- By encouraging high standards of professional courtesy
- By demanding a clear division of labor within the profession and between health care occupations
- By drawing upon a strong bond with science to further the legitimacy of claims to exclusive professional expertise
- By confronting occupations that conflicted in philosophy, expertise, and practice with those of mainstream professionals

goals (in a 'womb-to-tomb' logic) in Box 8.3, which seems desirable in the context of a more disease-oriented health psychology curriculum. Thus far, the accomplishments of health psychology, measured against these tasks have been uninspiring since the focus of the profession was on the gamut of 'unhealthful' behaviors. Now what?

The Skill Mix?

Doctors are no longer lonely players who used to spend over 60% of their time visiting the sick in the family setting prior to the early 30s. Now they visit the sick at home in less than 1% of cases. They work in a complex system of health delivery that rests on team efforts comprised of different participants, and based on the notion of *skill mix*. The presence of a psychologist helps identifying problematic patients who are prone to impulsive behavior, rudeness, verbal abuse, outbursts of anger, and noncompliance. Another category in need of psychological assistance consists of patients with sleep disorders, mild cognitive impairment, eating disorders and obesity. All of them require the assessment of mental disorder, its severity, personal and cultural history, drug history, family

Box 8.3   The 'womb-to-tomb' goals of health psychology.

- Work with health professionals at various levels in order to improve the quality of health delivery to women of childbearing age and 'difficult mothers' so as to improve their lifestyle in order to advance the viability of their progeny in middle to later life.
- Support investments into new vaccination programs, so as to reduce the incidence of cardiovascular morbidity and to improve the utilization of phytonutrients by the body.
- Counsel families with problematic children (e.g. those with hyperactivity, eating disorders, bullying and violent behaviors) as well as people at risk for a wide range of genetic disorders (neurodegenerative, psychopathological, or malignant) to plan their lives.
- Identify strategies directed at improving the health status of underserved groups (e.g. minorities, inner city residents, populations in remote communities or those released from prison).
- Prioritize research for early detection and an enhanced accuracy of diagnosis of cognitive decline, heralding dementias.
- Educate the public in the need for moderation in self-treatment with alternative remedies and vitamins.
- Input medical and psychological information that might temper the contemporary tide of publicity surrounding medical or pharmacological discoveries causing 'bandwagon effects.'
- Prioritize individual health in the atmosphere of confusing messages and mass anxiety.
- Encourage bonds with physicians to aid in the management of patients *after* they are discharged from the hospital as recovered and 'healthy.'
- Bring skills to the management of end-stage diseases and geriatric patients, including nursing home residents.

difficulties or substance abuse. They need time for counseling, problem solving, or cognitive-behavioral therapies that are best handled by health psychologists alone or together with general practitioners.

Skill mix was advocated for quite some time in psychiatry as an inevitable adjustment to the fact that psychiatrists, consultation-liaison psychiatrists, psychologists and social workers had to discuss their respective roles in managing the same patient. One of the skill mix versions is a split treatment concept. The concept debuted in an effort to change the style of management of psychotic patients when a physician (or a nurse) conducts pharmacotherapy whereas a 'psychotherapist,' most commonly a non-physician, handles all non-pharmacological therapy. This multi-professional team-work concept in primary health care moved it a certain distance from the classical hierarchical 'doctorcentric' model.[74] However, changes in policy do not automatically translate into changes in practice. The question regarding this model is: would the increased roles of non-physician personnel result in service development/ enhancement rather than labor substitution? No less important is the question: would patients object to the decentralization model, which emphasizes the substitution of health psychologists or nurses for doctors whenever feasible? Indeed, the ability of non-physician personnel to substitute rather than to complement doctors will depend not only on their qualifications as seen by the administration but also, and perhaps largely, on their acceptance by the public that traditionally expects to see a doctor. Thus, teamwork does not *ipso facto* guarantee that it would be easy to overcome initial apprehension of the patients and win their confidence. Patient satisfaction is the major outcome measure of any medical system, a gauge contributed by the 'philosopher-physician' model and marketing considerations.

Given that consultation-liaison psychiatry specializes in physical/ psychiatric comorbidity, somatization, and issues involved in management of these disorders,[75] the presence of health psychologists would require a model operationalizing their services vis-à-vis those of other professionals. Until this happens, health psychologists are likely to hear what despirited but determined Eliza Doolittle in "My Fair Lady" demanded from her suitor: "Don't talk of fall! Don't talk at all! Show me!"

A Glance Back for a Fleeting Look Ahead

Since the dawn of medicine, physical touch has primarily been a diagnostic tool. Leopold Auenbrugg (1722–1809), a famous librettist for Salieri, and the court composer of Joseph II improved the touch by proposing to 'tap' on the chest to obtain information about the physical events inside. Such a technique, familiar to all wine producers who check on the level of wine in the barrels, was a significant improvement in corroborating the story of the sick patient and finding its locus.

In 1816, Renè Théophile Hyacinthe Laënnec (1781–1826), an amateur flutist and illustrious physician, invented the stethoscope as the method of eavesdropping on the sounds emanating from the chest. Not only did the stethoscope begin to direct the study of disease and recovery, it also cemented medicine as a profession by augmenting some of its syndromes with the patterns of noises of the heart, lungs, and gut. The stethoscope enriched the ritual of physical examination practically to the state we are familiar with today. Unwittingly though, by establishing a 'flute-length' distance from the patient's sensibilities and contagion, Laënnec's invention was the first in the list of medical technologies distancing the physician from the patient. It was the first step on the road to reducing the dose of touching.

In 1868, the German physician Carl Wunderlich introduced a mercury thermometer for examining axillary temperature,[76] which further increased the space between doctors and patients. Physicians, or should we say 'slave-physicians,' have become still better artisans. 'Hot' and 'cold' did not require a story or a doctor with sensitive tactile functions. With it, it became clear that although "the hand is the instrument of instruments" (*Aristotle, De Anima, 3.8*), it is also a tool for its own demise. In this day and age, the armoury of diagnostic tests is so impressive that an elaborate physical examination and touching is no longer in vogue. Since the clinical diagnosis is obtained by means of diverse laboratory tests or after consultation with specialists[77] it seems uncertain whether there is a need to spend time on such antiquated techniques of physical examination as palpation, percussion, and auscultation. Not surprisingly, young physicians tend to recoil from the physical examination if they have access to the more decisive laboratory results or brain imaging information. Consequently, training at the bedside in the US has declined from an incidence of 75% in the 1960s to less than 16% today. Scrutinizing this development before the age of imaging modalities, Robert Wartenberg[78] pointed out that what is needed for neurological diagnosis is often so simple that it is imprudent to refuse carefully studying the craft. Yet, almost fifty years later, Phoon[79] more assertively questioned, "Must doctors still examine patients?" His reasoning primarily doubts the function of the physical examination since diagnostic procedures are based on precise 'high-resolution' assessments of different organs and tissues. An antiquated tactile 'physical examination,' he believes is hopelessly outgunned, and "a diagnostician, using only his senses and wits, would virtually disappear, since reliance on technology would be nearly complete." The days of Hippocratic 'bedside healing' are apparently over. Medicine solved the caring/expertise dilemma by asserting that professional worth is measured by what one is able to get done rather than by one's wishful thinking:

One might feel sad over the increased distance of patients and a reduced ability to understand their viewpoint through dialogue. But it looks as though in the struggle for genuinely democratic medicine, machines win over the groomed senses. They are an extension of the no-

"While there is obviously much that can and should be done to improve modern medicine's friendliness, there ultimately may be an inherent limit to what it can do in this regard, a limit that will force modern medicine to chose, on occasion, between being more humanitarian and being more effective"[4] (p. 516).

nonsense 'slave medicine' of antiquity. So far, the trend appers to be irreversible. In part, because doctors, like all other human beings, as Nietzsche famously warned in *The Gay Science*, released from their 'slave morality,' would now behave like gods. They are in charge, indeed. Phoon[79] believes that, "physical examination *will* become largely obsolete as a *diagnostic* tool" (*ital.* in the orig.). Is the decline of 'touch medicine' a problem for health care delivery? The answer is 'Yes.' The real issue for this discussion is how much it is a problem for health psychology. It seems uncertain whether health psychologists would experience the void of 'personal touch' to the same extent as the rest of the medical community. Undeniably, they would need to find out how their virtues could be articulated in a different media when health care assumes a variety of different forms.

Since there will never be enough qualified doctors to meet patient needs, the health care of the future may well reduce its dependence on the doctor-patient dyad by turning to 'e-medicine.' Indeed, the physical bonds between patients and their half-listening doctors cannot be restored to their archaic form. Therefore, the 'humanistic-touch' health care will have to yield to an electronic one of virtual reality or 'teletouch' that would not require an obligatory course for doctors on bed-side manners, popular psychology and spirituality. As a decision-making tool, the Internet will acquire a special role. Is there a hope for e-medicine in our health care future? Perhaps. The Internet does not have to display doctors' and patients' ethnic or racial identity, thereby removing the issue of 'doctor-patient race concordance' from the agenda of achieving greater satisfaction with care.[80] In the age of the Internet, it is meaningless to ask a Western doctor to master multicultural knowledge for managing immigrant patients. In addition, a skilled dermatologist, say in Bombay, would scrutinize skin images submitted by a patient from Maryland for a fraction of the cost charged by a doctor in the US for similar work. That is how some jobs will go abroad. In the longer run, to be truly competitive, US-based physicians should always be a notch better or they will have to reduce their fees.

For the majority of remote populations, the Internet has provided a cradle for a new form of telemarketing of health that now includes all medical activities from diagnosis to therapeutics. Telemedicine is not a new word (for early telemedicine, see *www.hesca.org/history/early-telemeds.jpg*). Its benefits were convincing already in the 60s. From those modest beginnings, it has become an inevitable substitute for the proximal care in emergencies in the rural environment, in countries with low population density or difficult topography when doctors cannot be personally present at a requested consultation at the specified time. Telecare will provide an immediate answer to the problem of the second opinion and 'physician-shopping'; it will bring care to patients who cannot travel; it will make health care infinitely more satisfying when the public appreciates that this new medium is genuinely egalitarian; it will give a remote rural community the ability to reach top health professionals. Without the advent of the Internet, assistance to these populations would never have gotten off the ground. For the same reason, telemedicine and information technology have the potential to make working in rural areas more attractive to young health care professionals.

The contemporary generation might settle for meaningful impersonal relations with a health professional via TV monitors and a virtual medical environment. Those who today are beginning to type on the keyboard almost together with their toilet training represent the future patients whose choices and commands will determine the future face of public health. Michael H. Brooke[81] cautioned us that the members of the 'television generation' will probably be more peculiar and solitary, and yet more networked rather than personally interactive. They grow into the consumers of health care, seeking impersonal answers from their computers. Many of these kids will soon graduate from medical schools and become residents; then some of them will be professors who would not force-feed their students to memorize the fact of diseases or laboratory normative values. Instead, they will demand the understanding of the general concepts and a rapid access to appropriate sources of information.[81] We already see this happening as a new generation of patients is less concerned with obtaining 'respect' and 'touch' as compared to their parents.

Admittedly, at this stage, the Internet is still larval and a long way before it addresses all the needs of any electronic customer. Surfing the Web may be a laborious process given that some sites migrate, become outdated or require a password. Efforts to achieve easy drug access may lead to potentially disagreeable consequences. There is no doubt, however, that practical and professional issues will be learned 'on the job' as *Hospitals Without Walls* continue to evolve.[82] These hospitals have countless doors open for health psychology. It seems that by developing virtual help, health psychology power would flourish to the point where its expansion might match that of medicine.*

Epilogue

As a profession, health psychology has been sustained by the needs of those unhappy patients with multiple complaints who were disenchanted with the quality of health care (Chap. 3). Physicians suspect such complexities to be contributed by comorbidity, and manage the cases accordingly (say, pondering over urological problems emerging in a depressed and obese elderly cardiac patient) without bickering over the model. Psychologists are more tempted to view such difficult patients as necessitating a 'holistic' approach based on a biopsychosocial concept. The initial excitement with the health psychology approach and the enthusiasm of its practitioners was not translated into viable health paradigms. Why not? There many answers.

One answer is that many aspects of health care were interpreted as dependent on or requiring an inspiration from the social theory of disease. It is perfectly acceptable that being aware of their social commitment, some health psychologists value their contribution to a broad social agenda and continue to struggle within the model of reliance on traditions, investment in hopes, social bonds, proper counseling, and belief in the world of positive expectations. However, social psychologists have a quite limited experience in matters of health. Nor could they spearhead the fight for many valid causes, such as food quality control and a wider use of solar energy, or a campaign against toxic pollutants and contaminants, the population explosion, radioactivity or non-ionizing radiation (electromagnetic fields),

---

*The "Journal of Medical Internet Research" (Medline-abbreviation: *J Med Internet Res*) provides information in the healthcare field defined as 'eHealth' or 'consumer health informatics' (e.g. *www.jmir.org/2003/4/index.htm*).

the effects of noise, climate changes, and global warming. All these issues can surely affect our health. But health psychology is not a new brand of social activism. Its professors cannot prepare pundits for goals remote from the roles of their students as clinicians; they cannot produce zealots in health promotion activities. In Evans'[83] view, health psychology departments can ill afford to train intruders or mini-experts in the areas where specific professional groups are involved.

An added reason is that health psychology cannot reshape the style of medical care in the territory where it is technically inferior, underpaid, and ideologically marginal. In order to prepare a new generation of health professionals for a credible partnership with general practitioners in helping patients with Q syndromes, psychology needs to attract clinician-educators from diverse fields of medicine to work together with psychologists in supplementing their curriculum. Such a curriculum would help to understand how and when adjusting environmental manipulations would make sense as compared to waiting until medicine learns how to engineer the genome to fit its environment better. Unless that mission is accomplished, a potential practitioner would unavoidably drift to either the area of classical clinical psychology or to that of alternative practices. Drawing as it does upon a number of eccentric therapies that make steady inroads as acceptable ways of managing illness in the US (e.g. Chap. 6), health psychology may only repel some of the stock of more hardheaded young students who will not join the ranks in fear of risking their scientific respectability.

But, perhaps a different excuse is that while medicine is in dire need of reinvention, health psychology is not a key to the solution as a viable profession and has been in tacit crisis ever since its emergence. Its leaders mistook their honest goals and mission statements for achievements. Medicine prompts any allied occupation to prove that it has a sufficient range of tools, rather than a credible philosophy, since medicine in its contemporary state has ascended clinging by the fingernails to the rope of technical progress. The centuries-long struggle within the medical profession helped to establish some normative guidelines that elevated professional standards. An old but telling example is the struggle between barbers (many of whom doubled as military medics, treating on battlefield) and physician-surgeons, which ended by the first decade of the sixteenth century. Barbers were skilled artisans and they won the battle for recognition based on their surgical skills. Yet, they had to pay the price for being elevated to the level of barber-surgeons by attending lectures in anatomy and pass rigorous master's examinations to achieve the degree. Only then were they accepted into the 'brotherhood' (professional guild) in order to continue training in surgery and achieve the status of doctors.[84]

With its growing technological arsenal, medicine treats psychology as a high-profile research occupation but rather low-status treatment craft, and a job with minor community influence at that. Thus, any desire to attain professional status and a share of management of the somatically ill would necessitate a significant change of the face of health psychology. Specifically, if health psychology were to be associated with medicine it would have to model itself after the medical profession in terms of its curriculum, matriculation, and toolkits. The term 'toolkit,' as used here, refers indiscriminately to the entire range of devices potentially available to a profession, whether linguistic, mechanical, bioelectric, chemical, or nutritional. Biofeedback, psychotherapy, drugs, approval of drinking or sanctioning abstinence from wine, curbing smoking or unprotected sex, and even ingestion of breakfast cereals might be considered as legitimate items of the toolkit assuming that, consequently to their use, health is decidedly promoted or that adaptation of the sick to their environment is enhanced. This point has a broad, 'anthropological' meaning, so to speak, since the *Hominidae* have long been defined as the 'toolmakers.' If the above toolkit is taken as an index of a professional status, health psychology may be in danger of having a rather limited level of professional adaptation unless it acquires the tools and such major components of the professional glue as autonomy, authority (the body of knowledge based on formal training), and legitimacy of membership.

The hopes of adopting pharmacotherapy did *not* prove to be a realistic venture acceptable to all. An acquisition of healthy behaviors thus has remained the most prevalent theme in health psychology. In the scholarly literature, this type of healing is labeled 'popular health reform' because its gurus are frequently untrained laypersons.[85] They have adopted the stance that a physical condition is harmed by stressors, such as those introduced by social inequality, shame, loss of trust and cohesion, low self-esteem, income disparity, psychological tension, and racial hatred. These are significant factors, but their remedy will not significantly change mortality and morbidity of the population.[80] Collectively, they are the familiar scarecrow, similar to the bad air and carnal irregularities of the 19th century health thinkers. More significantly, patients cannot afford to wait for society to inch its way forward and even less so to create an impression of advancement in the minds of those who feel demoralized. It is demonstrably obvious that lifestyle modifications alone as well as the management of psychological stressors cannot defeat the current epidemic of disorders of civilization. Such theorizing would be a terrible mistake, a kind of Thomas Moor psychology, because implicit within it is Moor's celebrated worldview that everything in Utopia was perfect and even chamber pots in it were made of gold. He was apparently convinced that his constipated elderly would voluntarily open their anal sphincters when seated on golden toilets. Only much later has it become known that changes in lifestyle factors may not necessarily produce a corresponding change in risk.

Discussing the fact that the principles of health psychology were not matched by the tools required for responsible functioning in the health delivery system, one of the founding members of the profession, Cynthia Belar held that health psychology gave away too much of what it has developed.[25] She had it right. It is important to add, though, that health psychology failed to capitalize on those conquests of knowledge in psychology that it was capable of developing. Some of this modern methodology was shifted to cognitive neurosciences, neuropsychiatry and molecular psychiatry, thereby leaving a new profession outside of research work that has been the basis of scientific modernity. The field was overtaken by rigorous research and was unable to keep in step with the scholarship needed for practical public health work. Some new programs and tools may yet be discovered — in which case health psychology would have a fresh chance to justify its health care ambitions. Without such a find the alternative arguments or excuses will struggle to stay alive since it has to compare itself in the bountiful harvest of scientific results that have metamorphosed the community of health practitioners. The problems of health psychology appear to be even more profound. The founding principals of the occupation were much too archaic to nurture its own set of unique concepts as expected and were unable to borrow from other disciplines; it did not devote some of its resources to long-term exploratory research. In addition, from its creation, health psychology has inherited some of the weakness experienced by professional psychology in the past. As Donald R. Peterson prophetically warned:

Peterson's recent summary on the quality of education of professional psychologists is a

"Psychology had more trouble than most disciplines in defining itself as a profession. By the lofty ideals of its academic tradition, professional work has often seemed more of an embarrassment that an achievement"[86] (p. 572).

painful admission of someone who for decades was an astute leader of the movement.[87]

The word 'profession' (from Latin, *profiteor fessus sum*) has several connotations: as a public declaration of a mission, a claim of belief, faith or opinion, and as an ability to declare and teach, pontificate, in short, 'to profess.' Other definitions emphasize the presence of specific skills or practices that rest on a period of apprenticeship ('a calling requiring expert knowledge and often long and intense academic preparation'). Students entering the field wish to be reassured that their investment in the future of a new profession is wise and that they will provide relevant answers to the old and new question of health care crises. This synopsis was unable to back-up this hope with faith and passion, and give a helpful career counsel. For students aspiring to a health care calling, there comes a point at which they must chose between creating the vibes of 'care' and generating knowledge. Both choices are important, but only one is science. During their undergraduate years, these students also learned that rules for academic psychology and for health psychologists are dissimilar. The main reason for supporting health psychology — according to a *Division 38 Mission Statement* — might be its projected practical use as "*vital members of multidisciplinary clinical and research teams in rehabilitation, cardiology, pediatrics, oncology, anesthesiology, family practice, dentistry, and other medical fields.*" Such emphasis on vocational training was not supported thus far by an effort to enrich the repertoire of problem-solving tools and overlooks the major tool of the expert evolution, that of acquiring relevant medical knowledge. Given the rate of proliferation of specialized journals in all aspects of medicine, it has become impossible to keep up with the new winds of science by an occasional flick through the main journals. The only way to foster that knowledge is to participate in the research endeavor that would make these incoming students fit into a health care 'marketplace.'

With these points in mind, the questions of where health psychologists enmesh with medical professionals, and to what extent their aid can be buttressed by current reimbursement schemes seem quite premature. Admittedly, health psychology is capable of developing a number of tentative solutions for health improvement along the lines of the goals in Box 8.3, but the way they are phrased will very much depend upon our programmes. What are the questions to answer first, and what assumptions can we accept? Will health psychology share common assumptions with medicine as it makes an effort to design its foothold in the medical territory? Is there a territory between them? Is there a home for a new practitioner in that territory to carry on producing health psychologists? In the diplomatic answer of the Cat, to *Alice in Wonderland*, the way we ought to go depends a good deal, on where we would want to get to. If we wish to go to the frightening somberness of the same bedside where medical practitioners are supposed to spend most of their time, a more acute question is: Will medicine recognize health psychologists' relevance and adequacy of their skills? More passionately, is health psychology possible?

The past two decades have been kind to health psychology regardless of the fact that it has not met its goals. Although health psychology is not necessarily in a crisis and can still draw on an outstanding scientific tradition of psychology it does not have unlimited time. In our dynamic era, a profession that is not in the health marketplace with its ideas and services fast enough and that cannot be improved and reinvented over and over is bound to rapidly lose its value. Many occupations operate within certain time-windows, some of which are very narrow. The threat is that as the public enchantment with alternative/complementary therapies wanes, the discipline of health psychology, too, will remain a footnote in the glorious history of scientific psychology and medicine, relegated to an obsolete field of placebogenic procedures with a decreased income and curbed power. One health care practice cannot be 'truer' than another can; it can only be more efficacious, potent, inexpensive and convenient in order to survive. Museums of medicine are full of the proposed innovative techniques and treatments that failed to progress from blueprints to reality, or worse still, never worked as expected.

SO WHAT?

For people living two millennia ago, being near damp and fetid places was frightful. They worried about malaria, one the most dreaded and prevalent infections in tropical areas throughout the world. The sound of the term malaria (*mal-aria*) is a reminder of its hypothesized cause — bad air — emanating from marshes and waste disposal sites. Acting on this fear, Roman engineers drained the marshes around Tiber. Much to the public joy, malaria was gone together with the offensive haze. The solace of sanatoria as cures of tuberculosis was also attributed to healthy air and improved living conditions.

The futile efforts of many noble scientists to trail flawed doctrines, however successful at times, remind us of a parable of the man who ran into a lion. Shouting "bang-bang," the man held up his umbrella and took aim. The lion sank to the ground, mortally wounded. A miracle? Well, unlikely. As the man with the umbrella uttered his cry, a hunter posted behind him fired his real gun. Manes Sperber,[18] acquainted us with this parable when wrestling with his own doubts: "Did psychology produce this revolutionary century by changing human beings in a totally unexpected fashion?" His answer is relevant to the present theme: "If there had been no man with an umbrella, the result would have been the same. But the bang-bangers, of whom there are many, stare in fascination at the miracle-working umbrella and have no eyes for the hunter and his rifle" (p. 197).

Bibliography

Chapter 1
The Point of Departure: The Pillars of the Health Psychology Edifice

1. Critchley M. The citadel of the senses and other essays. New York: Raven Press, 1986.
2. Shorter E. From paralysis to fatigue. A history of psychosomatic illness in modern era. New York: The Free Press, 1993.
3. Schofield W. The role of psychology in the delivery of health services. *Am Psychol* 1969: 565–584.
4. Margulis L, Sagan D. What is life? Berkeley: University of California Press, 1995.
5. Riley J. Sickness, recovery and death: A history and forecast of ill health. Iowa City: University of Iowa Press, 1989.
6. Freidson E. Profession of Medicine. A study of the sociology of applied knowledge. Chicago: The University of Chicago Press, 1988.
7. Lundberg G. Severed trust: Why American medicine hasn't been fixed. New York: Basic Books, 2000.
8. Cochran G, Ewald P, Cochran K. Infectious causation of disease: An evolutionary perspective. *Persp Biol Med* 2000; **43**: 406–448.
9. Evans AS. Causation and disease: A chronological journey. New York: Plenum Medical Book Co., 1993.
10. Veen J. Drug resistant tuberculosis: Back to sanatoria, surgery and cod-liver oil? *Eur Respiratory J* 1995; **8**: 1073–1075.
11. Tomes N. The making of a germ panic: Then and now. *Am J Public Health,* 2000; **90**: 91–198.
12. Uwins PJR, Webb RI, Taylor AP. Novel nano-organisms from Australian sandstones. *Am Miner* 1998; **83**: 1541–1550.
13. Belongia E, Goodman J, Holland E, *et al.* An outbreak of *herpes-gladiatorum* at a high-school wrestling camp. *NE J Med* 1991; **325**: 906–910.

14. Mack T. A different view of smallpox and vaccination. *NE J Med* 2003; **348**: 460–463.

15. Webster R. Enhanced: A molecular whodunit. *Science* 2001; **293**: 1773–1775.

16. Calabrese LH. Thalidomide's tightly controlled "comeback". *Cleveland Clin J Med* 1999; **66**: 136–138.

17. U'Ren R. Psychiatric diagnosis and the market. *Persp Biol Med* 1992; **35**: 612–616.

18. Van Praag HM. Past expectations, present disappointments, future hopes or psychopathology as the rate-limiting step of progress in psychopharmacology. *Hum Psychopharmacol-Clin Exp* 2001; **16**: 3–7.

19. Harte J. Toward a synthesis of the Newtonian and Darwinian worldviews. *Physics Today* 2002; **October**: 29–34.

20. Valenstein E. Blaming the brain. The truth about drugs and mental health. New York: The Free Press, 1998.

21. Walsh V. Turning points — Learning to face facts. *Curr Biol* 1997; **7**: R335–R336.

22. Carmichael A, Ratzan RE. Medicine: A treasure of art and literature. New York: Hugh Lauter Levin Assoc., Inc., 1991.

23. Porter R. The rise of physical examination. In: Bynum WF, Porter R, eds. Medicine and five senses. Cambridge: Cambridge University Press, 1993: 179–197.

24. King S, Weaver A. Lives in many hands: The medical landscape in Lancashire, 1700–1820. *Med Hist* 2000; **44**: 173–200.

25. Haggard H. Devils, drugs, and doctors. New York: Pocket Book, Inc., 1946.

26. Schiedermayer D, McCarty DJ. Altruism, professional decorum, and greed — Perspectives on physician compensation. *Persp Biol Med* 1995; **38**: 238–253.

27. Jutte R. The historiography of nonconventional medicine in Germany: A concise overview. *Med Hist* 1999; **43**: 342–358.

28. Lipsitt DR. The challenge of the "difficult patient" (*Deja vu* all over again — only more so). *Gen Hosp Psych* 1997; **19**: 313–314.

29. Nahm FKD. Neurology, technology, and the diagnostic imperative. *Persp Biol Med* 2001; **44**: 99–107.

30. Lyons J. The American medical doctor in the current milieu — A matter of trust. *Persp Biol Med* 1994; **37**: 442–459.

31. Wildawsky A. Doing better and feeling worse: The political pathology of health policy. *Daedalus* 1977; **106**: 105–123.

32. Friedenberg RM. Health care rationing: Every physician's dilemma. *Radiology* 2000; **217**: 626–628.

33. Dormandy T. The white death. New York: New York University Press, 2000.

34. Ader R. On the development of psychoneuroimmunology. *Eur J Pharmacol* 2000; **405**: 167–176.

35. Temoshok L. Biopsychosocial studies on cutaneous malignant melanoma: Psychosocial factors associated with prognostic indicators, progression, psychophysiology and tumor-host response. *Soc Sci Med* 1985; **20**: 833–840.

36. Ogawa K, Hirai M, Katsube T, *et al.* Suppression of cellular immunity by surgical stress. *Surgery* 2000; **127**: 329–336.

37. Siegel BS. Love, medicine and miracles. New York: Harper & Row Publisher, 1986.

38. Bovbjerg D, Valdimarsdottir H, Zahariae R. Psychoneuroimmunology in oncology. In: Schedlowski M, Tewes U, eds. Psychoneuroimmunology. New York: Kluwer Academic, 1999: 473–489.

39. Edelman S, Craig A, Kidman AD. Can psychotherapy increase the survival time of cancer patients? *J Psychosomat Res* 2000; **49**: 149–156.

40. Schapiro IR, Ross-Petersen L, Saelan H, *et al.* Extroversion and neuroticism and the associated risk of cancer: A Danish cohort study. *Am J Epidemiol* 2001; **153**: 757–763.

41. Goodwin P, Leszcz M, Ennis M, *et al.* The effect of group psychosocial support on survival in metastatic breast cancer. *N Engl J Med* 2001; **345**: 1719–1726.

42. Segerstrom S. Optimism, goal conflict, and stressor-related immune change. *J Behav Med* 2001; **24**: 441–467.

43. Petticrew M, Bell R, Hunter D. Influence of psychological coping on survival and recurrence in people with cancer: Systematic review. *Br Med J* 2002; **325**: 1066.

44. Ader R, Cohen N, Felten D. Psychoneuroimmunology: Interactions between the nervous system and the immune system. *Lancet* 1995; **345**: 99–103.

45. Penninx B, Guralnik JM, Pahor M, *et al.* Chronically depressed mood and cancer risk in older persons. *J Natl Cancer Inst* 1998; **90**: 1888–1893.

46. Penninx BWJH, Guralnik JM. Chronically depressed mood and cancer risk in older persons — Response. *J Natl Cancer Inst* 1999; **91**: 1080–1081.

47. Cummings J. Depression and Parkinson's disease — A review. *Am J Psychiat* 1992; **149**: 443–454.

48. Myslobodsky M, Mintz M, Ben-Mayer V, *et al.* Unilateral dopamine deficit and lateral EEG asymmetry: Sleep abnormalities in hemi-Parkinson patients. *Electroenceph Clin Neurophysiol* 1982; **54**: 227–231.

49. Myslobodsky M, Lalonde F, Hicks L. Are patients with Parkinson's disease suicidal? *J Geriatr Psychiatry Neurol* 2001; **14**: 120–124.

50. Lalonde F, Myslobodsky M. Are dopamine antagonists a risk factor for breast cancer? An answer from Parkinson's disease. *The Breast* 2003; **12**: 280–282.

51. Zubenko G, Zubenko W, Spiker D, *et al.* Malignancy of recurrent, early-onset major depression: A family study. *Am J Med Genet* 2001; **105**: 690–699.

52. O'Donnell MC, Fisher R, Irvine K, *et al.* Emotional suppression: Can it predict cancer outcome in women with suspicious screening mammograms? *Psychol Med* 2000; **30**: 1079–1088.

53. Forlenza MJ, Baum A. Psychosocial influences on cancer progression: Alternative cellular and molecular mechanisms. *Curr Opin Psychiatr* 2000; **13**: 639–645.

54. Gunn J, Taylor PJ. Introduction. In: Gunn J, Taylor PJ, eds. Forensic psychiatry: Clinical, legal and ethical issues. Heinemann: Bitterworth, 1993: 1–20.

55. Sutter MC. Assigning causation in disease: Beyond Koch's postulates. *Persp Biol Med* 1996; **39**: 581–592.

56. Burnet M. Changing patterns. An atypical autobiography. William Heinemann: Melbourne. Melbourne: William Heinemann, 1968.

57. Slovic P, Fischhoff B, Lichtenstein S. Facts versus fears: Understanding perceived risk. In: Kahneman D, *et al.*, eds. Judgments under uncertainty: Heuristics and biases. Cambridge: Cambridge University Press, 1982: 463–492.

58. Ewald PW. Evolution of infectious disease. Oxford: Oxford University Press, 1994.

59. Timmer E, Voorn WJ, Tjiptadi, *et al.* Variability of the duration of life of living creatures. Amsterdam: IOS Press, 2000.

60. Solomon G. Psychoneuroimmunology: Interactions between central nervous system and immune system. *J Neurosci Research* 1987; **18**: 1–9.

61. Medawar PB. Advice to a young scientist. Reading, MA: Basic Books, 1979.

62. Thomas L. The youngest science. Notes of medicine-watcher. New York: The Viking Press, 1983.

63. Meehl P. Law and fireside inductions: Some reflections of a clinical psychologist. *The J Soc Issues* 1971; **27**: 65–100.

Chapter 2
'Bad Boys' and Prenatal Programming

1. Durfee K. Crooked ears and the bad boy syndrome: Asymmetry as an indicator of minimal brain dysfunction. *Bull Menninger Clin* 1974; **38**: 305–316.

2. Yule W, Taylor E. Classification of soft signs. In: Tupper D, ed. Soft neurological signs. Orlando, Florida: Grune & Stratton, Inc., 1987: pp. 19–43.

3. Venes J. Surgery of craniosynostosis. Symposium on development of the basicranium. Bethesda, MD: US Department of Health, Education, and Welfare, 1976: 443–454.

4. Pruzansky S. Radiocephalometric studies of the basicranium in craniofacial malformations. Symposium on development of the basicranium. Bethesda, MD: US Department of Health, Education, and Welfare, 1976: 278–298.

5. Robson P. Persistent head turning in the early months: Some effects in the early years. *Dev Med Child Neurol* 1968; **10**: 82–92.

6. Wender P. Minimal brain dysfunction in children. New York: Wiley International, 1971.

7. Towbin A. Neuropathologic correlates. In: Tupper D, ed. Soft neurological signs. Orlando, Florida: Grune & Stratton, Inc., 1987: pp. 157–178.

8. Barker DJP. Mothers, babies and disease in later life. London: BMJ Publishing, 1994.

9. Rasmussen KM. The "fetal origins" hypothesis: Challenges and opportunities for maternal and child nutrition. *Annu Rev Nutr* 2001; **21**: 73–95.

10. Ingraham LJ, Myslobodsky M. Coping with uncertainty: What would an animal model of Schizophrenia look like? In: Myslobodsky M, Weiner I, eds. Contemporary issues in modeling psychopathology. Boston: Kluwer Academic, 2000.

11. Mintz M, Myslobodsky MS. Emergence of PTSD-type reactivity in Sprague-Dawley rats following prenatal gamma-irradiation. In: Myslobodsky M, Weiner I, eds. Contemporary issues in modeling psychopathology. Boston: Kluwer Academic, 2000.

12. Kramer M, McLean F, Olivier M, *et al.* Body proportionality and head and length "sparing" in growth-retarded neonates: A critical reappraisal. *Pediatrics* 1989; **84**: 717–723.

13. Hogan DP, Park JM. Family factors and social support in the developmental outcomes of very low-birth weight children. *Clin Perinatol* 2000; **27**: 433–459.

14. Matte T, Bresnahan M, Begg M, *et al.* Influence of variation in birth weight within normal range and within sibships on IQ at age 7 years: Cohort study. *Br Med J* 2001; **310–314**: 684.

15. Lorenz JM, Wooliever DE, Jetton JR, *et al.* A quantitative review of mortality and developmental disability in extremely premature newborns. *Arch Pediatr Adolesc Med* 1998; **152**: 425–435.

16. Menninger WC. Emotional factors in pregnancy. *Bull Menninger Clin* 1943; **7**: 15–24.

17. Meehl PE. Why I do not attend case conferences. Psychodiagnosis. Selected papers. New York: Norton & Co., 1977: 225–302.

18. Murrell NL, Scherzer T, Ryan M, *et al.* The AfterCare project: An intervenion for homeless childbearing families. *Fam Community Health* 2000; **23**: 17–27.

19. Malamitsi-Puchner A, Tzala L, Minaretzis D, *et al.* Preterm delivery and low birthweight among refugees in Greece. *Paediatr Perinat Epidemiol* 1994; **8**: 384–390.

20. Misra D, O'Campo P, Strobino D. Testing sociomedical model for preterm delivery. *Paediatr Perinat Epidemiol* 2001; **15**: 110–122.

21. McWhorter JH. Losing the race: Self-sabotage in black America. New York: Free Press, 2000.

22. Leigh WA, Lindquist MA. Women of color health data book: Adolescents to seniors. Washington, DC: NIH. Office of the Director, 2001.

23. Myslobodsky M. Preterm delivery: On proxies and proximal factors. *Paediatr Perinat Epidemiol* 2001; **15**: 381–383.

24. Busse WW, Lemanske RF. Advances in immunology — Asthma. *N Engl J Med* 2001; **344**: 350–362.

25. Paul WE, Seder RA. Lymphocyte-responses and cytokines. *Cell* 1994; **76**: 241–251.

26. Hospers J, Rijcken P, Schouten J, *et al.* Eosinophilia and positive skin tests predict cardiovascular mortality in a general population sample followed for 30 years. *Am J Epidemiol* 1999; **150**: 482–491.

27. Wilder RL. Hormones, pregnancy, and autoimmune diseases. *Neuroimmunomodulation* 1998; **840**: 45–50.

28. Warner JA. Primary sensitization in infants. *Ann Allergy Asthma Immunol* 1999; **83**: 426–430.

29. Bjorksten B. Environment and infant immunity. *Proc Nutrition Soc* 1999; **58**: 729–732.

30. Ray NF, Thamer M, Fadillioglu B, *et al.* Race, income, urbanicity, and asthma hospitalization in California — A small area analysis. *Chest* 1998; **113**: 1277–1284.

31. Miller JE. The effects of race/ethnicity and income on early childhood asthma prevalence and health care use. *Am J Public Health* 2000; **90**: 428–430.

32. Le Souef PN, Goldblatt J, Lynch NR. Evolutionary adaptation of inflammatory immune responses in human beings. *Lancet* 2000; **356**: 242–244.

33. Lesouef PN, Goldblatt J, Lynch NR. Genome screen and candidate gene studies in parasitized populations. *Clin Exp Allergy* 1999; **29**: 31–34.

34. Strannergård O, Strannergård I-L. The causes of the increasing prevalence of allergy: Is atopy a microbial deprivation disorder? *Allergy* 2001; **56**: 91–102.

35. Yazdanbakhsh M, van den Biggelaar A, Maizels RM. Th2 responses without atopy: Immunoregulation in chronic helminth infections and reduced allergic disease. *Trends Immunol* 2001; **22**: 372–377.

36. Riedler J, Eder W, Oberfeld G, *et al.* Austrian children living on a farm have less hay fever, asthma and allergic sensitization. *Clin Exp Allergy* 2000; **30**: 194–200.

37. Reichrtova E, Ciznar P, Prachar V, *et al.* Cord serum immunoglobulin E related to the environmental contamination of human placentas with organochlorine compounds. *Environ Health Perspect* 1999; **107**: 895–899.

38. Schildkraut JM, Demark-Wahnefried W, DeVoto E, *et al.* Environmental contaminants and body fat distribution. *Cancer Epidemiol Biomarkers Prev* 1999; **8**: 179–183.

39. Savoy LB, Lim JD, Sarnaik SA, *et al.* Prevalence of atopy in a sickle-cell-anemia population. *Ann Allergy* 1988; **61**: 129–132.

40. Gilstrap III LC, Ramin SM. Urinary tract infections during pregnancy. *Obstetrics and Gynecology Clinics of North America* 2001; **28**: 581–591.

41. Blattner P, Dar H, Nitowsky H. Pregnancy outcome in women with sickle cell trait. *JAMA* 1977; **238**: 1392–1394.

42. Goldenberg RL, Hauth JC, Andrews WW. Mechanisms of disease — Intrauterine infection and preterm delivery. *N Engl J Med* 2000; **342**: 1500–1507.

43. Goncalves L, Chaiworapongsa T, Romero R. Intrauterine infection and prematurity. *Ment Retard Dev Disabil Res Rev* 2002; **8**: 3–13.

44. Mardh P. Influence of infection with *Chlamydia trachomatis* on pregnancy outcome, infant health and life-long sequelae in infected offspring. *Best Pract Res Clin Obstet Gynaecol* 2002; **16**: 847–864.

45. Read JS, Klebanoff MA. Sexual intercourse during pregnancy and preterm delivery — Effects of vaginal microorganisms. *Am Obstet Gynecol* 1993; **168**: 514–519.

46. Dudley DJ. Pre-term labor: An intra-uterine inflammatory response syndrome? *J Reprod Immunol* 1997; **36**: 93–109.

47. Hill JA, Choi BC. Maternal immunological aspects of pregnancy success and failure. *J Reprod Fertil* 2000; **55**: 91–97.

48. Greig J. Enzootic abortion in ewes: A preliminary note. *Vet Rec* 1936; **42**: 1225–1227.

49. Entrican G, Buxton D, Longbottom D. Chlamydial infection in sheep: Immune control versus fetal pathology. *J R Soc Med* 2001; **94**: 273–277.

50. Hillier SL, Nugent RP, Eschenbach DA, *et al.* Association between bacterial vaginosis and preterm delivery of a low-birth-weight infant. *NE J Med* 1995; **333**: 1737–1742.

51. Sobel JD. Vaginitis. *NE J Med* 1997; **337**: 1896–1903.

52. Peacock JL, Bland JM, Anderson HR. Preterm delivery — Effects of socioeconomic factors, psychological stress, smoking, alcohol, and caffeine. *Br Med J* 1995; **311**: 531–535.

53. Eng T, Butler W. The neglected health and economic impact of STDs. In: Eng T, Butler W, eds. The hidden epidemic: Confronting sexually transmitted diseases. Wahsington, DC: National Academy Press, 1997: 28–68.

54. Sorlie P, Rogot E, Anderson R, *et al.* Black-white mortality differences by family income. *Lancet* 1992; **340**: 346–350.

55. Smith GD, Neaton JD, Wentworth D, *et al.* Mortality differences between black and white men in the USA: Contribution of income and other risk factors among men screened for the Multiple Risk Factor Intervention Trial. *Lancet* 1998; **351**: 934–939.

56. Kuehr J, Frischer T, Karmaus W, *et al.* Early-childhood risk-factors for sensitization at school age. *J Allergy Clin Immunol* 1992; **90**: 358–363.

57. Arshad SH, Stevens M, Hide DW. The effect of genetic and environmental-factors on the prevalence of allergic disorders at the age of 2 years. *Clin Exp Allergy* 1993; **23**: 504–511.

58. Frischer T, Kuehr J, Meinert R, *et al.* Risk-factors for childhood asthma and recurrent wheezy bronchitis. *Eur J Pediatr* 1993; **152**: 771–775.

59. Evans M, Palta M, Sadek M, *et al.* Associations between family history of asthma, bronchopulmonary dysplasia, and childhood asthma in very low birth weight children. *Am J Epidemiol* 1998; **148**: 460–466.

60. Brooks AM, Byrd RS, Weitzman M, *et al.* Impact of low birth weight on early childhood asthma in the United States. *Arch Pediatr Adolesc Med* 2001; **155**: 401–406.

61. Oliveti JF, Kercsmar CM, Redline S. Pre- and perinatal risk factors for asthma in inner city African-American children. *Am J Epidemiol* 1996; **143**: 570–577.

62. Cheung Y, Low L, Osmond C, *et al.* Fetal growth and early postnatal growth are related to blood pressure in adults. *Hypertension* 2000; **36**: 795–800.

63. Eriksson J, Forsen T, Tuomilehto J, *et al.* Fetal and childhood growth and hypertension in adult life. *Hypertension* 2000; **36**: 790–794.

64. Fuentes-Afflick E, Hessol NA, Perez-Stable EJ. Testing the epidemiologic paradox of low birth weight in Latinos. *Arch Pediatr Adolesc Med* 1999; **153**: 147–153.

65. Markides K, Coreil J. The health of Hispanics in the southwestern United States: An epidemiologic paradox. *Public Health Rep* 1986; **101**: 253–265.

66. Cotch MF, Pastorek JG, Nugent RP, *et al. Trichomonas vaginalis* associated with low birth weight and preterm delivery. *Sex Transm Dis* 1997; **24**: 353–360.

67. Levitt NS, Lambert EV, Woods D, *et al.* Impaired glucose tolerance and elevated blood pressure in low birth weight, nonobese, young South African adults: Early programming of cortisol axis. *J Clin Endocrinol Metab* 2000; **85**: 4611–4618.

68. Kistner A, Celsi G, Vanpee M, *et al.* Increased blood pressure but normal renal function in adult women born preterm. *Pediatr Nephrol* 2000; **15**: 215–220.

69. Kelly YJ, Nazroo JY, McMunn A, *et al.* Birthweight and behavioural problems in children: A modifiable effect? *Int J Epidemiol* 2001; **30**: 88–94.

70. Knowles J. Introduction: Doing better and feeling worse: Health in the United States. *Daedalus* 1977; **Winter**: 1–7.

71. Li XM, Stanton B, Cottrell L, *et al.* Patterns of initiation of sex and drug-related activities among urban low-income African-American adolescents. *J Adolesc Health* 2001; **28**: 46–54.

72. Blum RW, Beuhring T, Shew ML, *et al.* The effects of race/ethnicity, income, and family structure on adolescent risk behaviors. *Am J Public Health* 2000; **90**: 1879–1884.

73. Upchurch DM, Levy-Storms L, Sucoff CA, *et al.* Gender and ethnic differences in the timing of first sexual intercourse. *Fam Plann Perspect* 1998; **30**: 121–127.

74. Norris AE, Ford K, Shyr T, *et al.* Heterosexual experiences and partnerships of urban, low-income African-American and Hispanic youth. *J Acquir Immune Defic Syndr Hum Retrovirol* 1996; **11**: 288–300.

75. Stanton B, Li XM, Black MM, *et al.* Anal intercourse among preadolescent and early adolescent low-income urban African-Americans. *Arch Pediatr Adolesc Med* 1994; **148**: 1201–1204.

76. Stanton B, Li XM, Black M, *et al.* Sexual practices and intentions among preadolescent and early adolescent low-income urban African-Americans. *Pediatrics* 1994; **93**: 966–973.

77. Persson I, Ahlsson F, Ewald U, *et al.* Influence of perinatal factors on the onset of puberty in boys and girls: Implications for interpretation of link with risk of long term diseases American. *Journal of Epidemiology* 1999; **150**: 747–755.

78. Matsuhashi Y, Felice M, Shragg P, *et al.* Is repeat teenage pregnancy in adolescents a "planned" affair? *J Adolesc Health Care* 1989; **10**: 409–412.

79. Slater E. The neurotic constitution. A statistical study of two thousand neurotic soldiers. *J Neurology and Psychiatry* 1943; **6**: 1–16.

80. Critchley M. The citadel of the senses and other essays. New York: Raven Press, 1986.

81. Silverman W. "Fixing" human reproduction. In where's the evidence? Oxford, England: Oxford University Press, 1998.

82. Chadwick R, ten Have H, Husted J, *et al.* Genetic screening and ethics: European perspectives. *J Med Philos* 1998; **23**: 255–273.

83. Nelkin D, Tankredi L. Dangerous diagnostics: The social power of biological information. New York: Basic Books, 1989.

84. Watson J. Good gene, bad gene. What is the right way to fight the tragedy of genetic disease? Time, 1997–1998: 86.

85. Streiner DL, Saigal S, Burrows E, *et al.* Attitudes of parents and health care professionals toward active treatment of extremely premature infants. *Pediatrics* 2001; **108**: 152–157.

86. Montello M, Lantos J. The Karamazov complex. *Persp Biol Med* 2002; **45**: 190–199.

87. Nelson J. Microchimerism: Incidental byproduct of pregnancy or active participant in human health? *Trends Mol Med* 2002; **8**: 109–113.

Chapter 3
Between Psychiatry and Medicine: Illness in Search of a Place

1. Symonds C. The assessment of symptoms following head injury. *Guys Hospital Gazette* 1937; **51**: 461–468.

2. Engel G. A unified concept of health and disease. *Persp Biol Med* 1960; **3**: 459–485.

3. Lipsitt DR. The challenge of the "difficult patient" (*Deja vu* all over again — only more so). *Gen Hosp Psych* 1997; **19**: 313–314.

4. Hughes R. Culture of complaint: The fraying of America. New York: Oxford University Press, 1993.

5. McWhinney I. Beyond diagnosis. *N Engl J Med* 1972; **287**: 384–387.

6. May R. The meaning of anxiety. New York: W.W. Norton & Co., Inc., 1979.

7. Goldstein JH. Darwin, Chagas', mind, and body. *Persp Biol Med* 1989; **32**: 586–600.

8. Hadler NM. If you have to prove you are ill, you can't get well — The object lesson of fibromyalgia. *Spine* 1996; **21**: 2397–2400.

9. Sharpe M, Mayou R, Bass C. Concepts, theory and terminology. In: Mayou R, *et al.*, eds. Treatment of functional somatic symptoms. Oxford: Oxford University Press, 1995: 3–16.

10. Nimnuan C, Hotopf M, Wessely S. Medically unexplained symptoms: How often and why are they missed? *QJM-Mon J Assoc Physicians* 2000; **93**: 21–28.

11. Reitsma B, Meijler W. Pain and patienthood. *Clin J Pain* 1997; **13**: 9–21.

12. Katon W. Panic disorder and somatization. Review of 55 cases. *Am J Med* 1984; **77**: 101–106.

13. Kroenke K, Mangelsdorff AD. Common symptoms in ambulatory care — Incidence, evaluation, therapy, and outcome. *Am J Med* 1989; **86**: 262–266.

14. Carson AJ, Ringbauer B, Stone J, *et al.* Do medically unexplained symptoms matter? A prospective cohort study of 300 new referrals to neurology outpatient clinics. *J Neurol Neurosurg Psychiatry* 2000; **68**: 207–210.

15. Noyes R, Holt CS, Happel RL, *et al.* A family study of hypochondriasis. *J Nerv Ment Dis* 1997; **185**: 223–232.

16. Barsky AJ, Borus JF. Functional somatic syndromes — In response. *Ann Intern Med* 2000; **132**: 329–330.

17. Reiger D, Goldberg I, Taube C. The de facto US mental health services system: A public health perspective. *Arch Gen Psychiat* 1978; **35**: 685–693.

18. Fadiman A. The spirit catches you and you fall down. New York: Farrar Straus & Giroux, 1998.

19. Lewis A. The survival of hysteria. *Psychol Med* 1975; **5**: 9–12.

20. Micale MS. Charcot and the idea of hysteria in the male: Gender, mental science, and medical diagnosis in late nineteenth century France. *Medical History* 1990; **34**: 363–411.

21. Beitzer J. Ventriloquized bodies. Narratives of hysteria in nineteenth-century France. Ithaca: Cornell University Press, 1993.

22. Goering L. "Russian nervousness": Neurasthenia and national identity in nineteenth-century Russia. *Med History* 2003; **47**: 23–46.

23. Dupre E. Les cenestopathies. *Mouvement Medical* 1913: 3–12 (Translated by M. Rohde).

24. Sperber M. Masks of loneliness. Alfred Adler in perspective. New York: Macmillan Publishing Co., Inc., 1974.

25. Christensen J. Defining the irritable bowel syndrome. *Persp Biol Med* 1991; **38**: 21–35.

26. Read N W. Functional dyspepsia: A case of indecision. *Gastroenterology* 1999; **116**: 761–762.

27. Lambert J, Talley N. The role of Helicobacter pylori in non-ulcer dyspepsia: A debate. *Gastroenterol Clin North Am* 1993; **22**: 141–167.

28. Pitari G, Zingman L, Hodgson D, *et al.* Bacterial enterotoxins are associated with resistance to colon cancer. *Proc Natl Acad Sci USA* 2003; **100**: 2695–2699.

29. Bermond P. Therapy of side effects of oral contraceptive agents with vitamin B6. *Acta Vitaminol Enzymol* 1982; **4**: 45–54.

30. Viniker DA. Hypothesis on the role of sub-clinical bacteria of the endometrium (bacteria endometrialis) in gynaecological and obstetric enigmas. *Hum Reprod Update* 1999; **5**: 373–385.

31. Morrell MJ. Epilepsy in women: The science of why it is special. *Neurology* 1999; **53**: S42–S48.

32. Slotkoff AT, Radulovic DA, Clauw DJ. The relationship between fibromyalgia and the multiple chemical sensitivity syndrome. *Scand J Rheumatol* 1997; **26**: 364–367.

33. Cathebras P, Lauwers A, Rousset H. Fibromyalgia. A critical review. *Ann Med Interne* 1998; **149**: 406–414.

34.   Goshorn RK. Chronic fatigue syndrome: A review for clinicians. *Semin Neurol* 1998; **18**: 237–242.

35.   Wilson RB, Gluck OS, Tesser JRP, *et al.* Antipolymer antibody reactivity in a subset of patients with fibromyalgia correlates with severity. *J Rheumatol* 1999; **26**: 402–407.

36.   Wartenberg R. Neuritis, sensory neuritis, neuralgia. New York: Oxford University Press, 1958.

37.   Dalakas M. Discussion in NIH Conference: The stiff-person syndrome: An autoimmune disorder affecting neurotransmission of γ-Aminobutyric acid. *Ann Intern Med* 1999; **131**: 522–530.

38.   Levy L, Dalakas M, MK F. The stiff-person syndrome: An autoimmune disorder affecting neurotransmission of γ-Aminobutyric acid. *Ann Intern Med* 1999; **131**: 522–530.

39.   Lee P. The economic impact of musculoskeletal disorders. *Quality of Life Research* 1994; **3**: S85–S91.

40.   Robson P. Persistent head turning in the early months: Some effects in the early years. *Dev Med Child Neurol* 1968; **10**: 82–92.

41.   Friedenberg RM. Health care rationing: Every physician's dilemma. *Radiology* 2000; **217**: 626–628.

42.   Stirling A, Worthington T, Rafiq M, *et al.* Association between sciatica and propionibacterium acnes. *Lancet* 2001; **357**: 2024–2025.

43.   Donnay A. On the recognition of multiple chemical sensitivity in medical literature and government policy. *Internat J Toxicol* 1999; **18**.

44.   Ashford NA, Miller CS. Chemical exposures: Low levels and high stakes. 2nd edn. New York: Van Nostrand Reinold, 1998.

45.   Bynum W, Porter R. Medicine and the five senses. Cambridge: Cambridge University Press, 1993.

46.   Shorter E. Multiple chemical sensitivity: Pseudodisease in historical perspective. *Scand J Work Environ Health,* 1997; **23**: 35–42.

47.   Jamal GA. Gulf War Syndrome — A model for the complexity of biological and environmental interaction with human health. *Adverse Drug React Toxicol Rev* 1998; **17**: 1–17.

48.   Haley R. Is Gulf War Syndrome due to stress? The evidence reexamined. *Am J Epidemiol* 1997; **146**: 695–703.

49.   Rook G, Zumla A. Gulf War Syndrome: Is it due to a systemic shift in cytokine balance towards a Th2 profile? *Lancet* 1997; **349**: 1831–1833.

50.   Soetekouw P, de Vries M, Preijers F, *et al.* Persistent symptoms in former UNTAC soldiers are not associated with shifted cytokine balance. *Eur J Clin Invest* 1999; **29**: 960–963.

51.   Hotopf M, David A, Hull L, *et al.* Role of vaccinations as risk factors for ill health in veterans of the Gulf War: Cross sectional study. *Br Med J* 2000; **320**: 1363–1367.

52.   Haley RW, Billecke S, La Du BN. Association of low PON1 type Q (type A) arylesterase activity with neurologic symptom complexes in Gulf War veterans. *Toxicol Appl Pharmacol* 1999; **157**: 227–233.

53.   Haley RW, Marshall WW, McDonald GG, *et al.* Brain abnormalities in Gulf War Syndrome: Evaluation with H-1 MR spectroscopy. *Radiology* 2000; **215**: 807–817.

54. Levin HS, Eisenberg HM, Benton ALE. Mild head injury. New York: Oxford University Press, 1989.

55. Goldstein M. Traumatic brain injury: A silent epidemic. *Ann Neurol* 1990; **27**: 327–327.

56. McKinlay WW, Brooks DN. Methodological problems in assessing psychosocial recovery following severe head injury. *J Clin Exp Neuropsychol* 1984; **6**: 87–99.

57. Oddy M, Humphrey M. Social recovery during the year following severe head injury. *J Neurol Neurosurg Psychiat* 1980; **43**: 798–802.

58. Symonds CP. Observations on the differential diagnosis and treatment of cerebral states consequent upon head injuries. *Br Med J* 1928; **2**: 828–832.

59. Myslobodsky MS, Glicksohn J, Singer J, *et al.* Changes of brain anatomy in patients with posttraumatic stress disorder: A pilot magnetic resonance imaging study. *Psychiatry Res/ Imaging* 1995; **58**: 259–264.

60. Reiser SJ. Technology and the use of the senses in twentieth century medicine. In: Bynum W, Porter R, eds. Medicine and the five senses. Cambridge: Cambridge University Press, 1993.

61. Wessely S, Nimnuan C, Sharpe M. Functional somatic syndromes: One or many? *Lancet* 1999; **354**: 936–939.

62. Derrick E. "Q" fever, new fever entity: Clinical features, diagnosis, and laboratory investigation. *Med J Australia [reprinted in Rev Infect Dis, 5:790–800, 1983]* 1937; **2**: 281–299.

63. Katon WJ, Walker EA. Medically unexplained symptoms in primary care. *J Clin Psychiat* 1998; **59**: 15–21.

64. Abel LCJ, Rizzo LV, Ianni B, *et al.* Chronic Chagas' disease cardiomyopathy patients display an increased IFN-gamma response to *Trypanosoma cruzi* infection. *J Autoimmun* 2001; **17**: 99–107.

65. Hunter P. The English sweating sickness, with particular reference to the 1551 outbreak in Chester. *Rev Infect Dis* 1991; **13**: 303–306.

66. Rose G. The strategy of preventive medicine. Oxford, England: Oxford University Press. Oxford, England: Oxford University Press, 1992.

67. Taviner M, Thwaites G, Gant V. The English sweating sickness, 1485–1551: A viral pulmonary disease? Comment. *Medical History* 1998; **42**: 96–98.

68. Lee H. Haemorrhagic fever with renal syndrome: An emerging disease. *Nephrology* 1996; **2**: **Suppl. 1**: S88–S93.

69. Ewald PW. Evolution of infectious disease. 2 edn. Oxford: Oxford University Press, 1995.

70. Hotopf M, Mayou R, Wadsworth M, *et al.* Childhood risk factors for adults with medically unexplained symptoms: Results from a national birth cohort study. *Am J Psychiat* 1999; **156**: 1796–1800.

71. Dantzer R, Bluthe RM, Laye S, *et al.* Cytokines and sickness behavior. Neuroimmunomodulation, 1998: 586–590.

72. Kronfol Z. Cytokines and mental health. Boston: Kluwer Academic, 2003.

73. Johnson RW. The concept of sickness behavior: A brief chronological account of four key discoveries. *Vet Immunol Immunopathol* 2002; **87**: 443–450.

74. Raison CL, Marcin M, Miller AH. Antidepressant treatment of cytokine-induced mood disorders. *Acta Neuropsychiatr* 2002; **14**: 336–343.

75. Rief W, Pilger F, Ihle D, *et al.* Immunological differences between patients with major depression and somatization syndrome. *Psychiatry Research* 2001; **105**: 165–174.

76. Neveu PJ, Bluthe RM, Liege S, *et al.* Interleukin-1-induced sickness behavior depends on behavioral lateralization in mice. *Physiol Behav* 1998; **63**: 587–590.

77. Neveu PJ, Liege S. Mechanisms of behavioral and neuroendocrine effects of interleukin-1 in mice. *Neuroimmunomodulation* 2000; **917**: 175–185.

78. Stein DB. Psychogenic somatic symptoms of the left side. Review and interpretation. In: Myslobodsky M, ed. Hemisyndromes: Psychobiology, neurology, psychiatry. New York: Academic Press, 1983: 415–445.

79. Vuilleumier P, Chicherio C, Assal F, *et al.* Functional neuroanatomical correlates of hysterical sensorimotor loss. *Brain* 2001; **124**: 1077–1090.

80. Mintz M, Myslobodsky M. Two types of hemisphere imbalance in hemi-Parkinsonism coded by brain electrical activity and electrodermal activity. In: Myslobodsky M, ed. Hemisyndromes: Psychobiology, neurology, psychiatry. New York: Academic Press, 1983: 213–238.

81. Mailis-Gagnon A, Giannoylis I, Downar J, *et al.* Altered central somatosensory processing in chronic pain patients with "hysterical" anesthesia. *Neurology* 2003; **60**: 1501–1507.

82. Ptacek LJ. Ligand-gated ion channelopathies — Mutations in different genes causing one disease. *Neurology* 2000; **55**: 1429–1430.

83. Gates JR. Epidemiology and classification of non-epileptic events. In: Gates J R, Rowan A J, eds. Non-epileptic seizures. 2nd edn. Boston: Butterworth/Heinemann, 2000: 3–14.

84. Penfield W. Epilepsy, the great teacher. *Acta Neurol Scand* 1967; **43**: 1–10.

85. Anttila P, Metsahonkala L, Mikkelsson M, *et al.* Comorbidity of other pains in school-children with migraine or nonmigrainous headache. *J Pediatr* 2001; **138**: 176–180.

86. Perquin CW, Hazebroek-Kampschreur A, Hunfeld JAM, *et al.* Pain in children and adolescents: A common experience. *Pain* 2000; **87**: 51–58.

87. Wu H, Guidetti P, Goodman J, *et al.* Kynurenergic manipulations influence excitatory synaptic function and excitotoxic vulnerability in the rat hippocampus in vivo. *Neuroscience* 2000; **97**: 243–251.

Chapter 4
The Deadly Trio

a) The Obesity Epidemic

1. Pine D, Wasserman G, Coplan J, *et al.* Cardiac profile and disruptive behavior in boys at risk for delinquency. *Psychosom Medicine* 1996; **58**: 342–353.

2. Rose G. Sick individuals and sick populations. *Int J Epidemiol* 1985; **14**: 32–33.

3. Sorensen T, Stunkard A. Does obesity run in families because of genes? An adoption study using silhouettes as a measure of obesity. *Acta Psychiatr Scand, Suppl* 1993; **370**: 67–72.

4. Blundell J, King N. Overconsumption as a cause of weight gain: Behavioural-physiological interactions in the control of food intake (appetite). *Ciba Found Symp* 1996; **201**: 138–154.

5. Kral J. Morbidity of severe obesity. *Surg Clin North Am* 2001; **81**: 1039–1061.

6. Hill J, Peters J. Environmental contributions to the obesity epidemic. *Science* 1998; **280**: 1371–1374.

7. Nestle M. Food Politics: How the food industry influences nutrition and health. Berkeley: University of California Press, 2002.

8. Murphy G. Personality: A biosocial approach to origins and structure. New York: Harper, 1947.

9. Bengmark S. Ecoimmunonutrition: A challenge for the third millennium. *Nutrition* 1998; **14**: 563–572.

10. Levitsky DA. Putting behavior back into feeding behavior: A tribute to George Collier. *Appetite* 2002; **38**: 143–148.

11. Blum K, Cull J, Braverman E, *et al.* Reward deficiency syndrome. *Am Scientist* 1996; **84**: 132–145.

12. Rosenberg P, Herishanu Y, Beilin B. Increased appetite (bulimia) in Parkinson's disease. *J Am Geriatr Soc* 1977; **25**: 277–278.

13. Wang G, Volkow N, Logan J, *et al.* Brain dopamine and obesity. *Lancet* 2001; **357**: 354–357.

14. Schultz W. Getting formal with dopamine and reward. *Neuron* 2002; **36**: 241–263.

15. Robinson T, Berridge K. Addiction. *Annu Rev Psychol* 2002; **54**: 101–129.

16. Blundell JE. What food do people habitually eat? A dilemma for nutrition, an enigma of psychology. *Am J Clin Nutr* 2000; **71**: 3–5.

17. Duncan J, Emslie H, Williams P, *et al.* Intelligence and the frontal lobe: The organization of goal-directed behavior. *Cognitive Psychology* 1996; **30**: 257–303.

18. Shoda Y, Mischel W, Peake P. Predicting adolescent cognitive and self regulatory competencies from preschool delay of gratification. *Dev Psychol* 1990; **26**: 978–986.

19. Wegner D. White bears and other unwanted thoughts. New York: Penguin, 1989.

20. Somerset Maugham W. The complete short stories of W. Somerset Maugham. Garden City, New York: Doubleday & Company, Inc.

21. McReynolds WT. Toward a psychology of obesity — Review of research on the role of personality and level of adjustment. *Int J Eating Disord* 1982; **2**: 37–57.

22. Goldman R, Jaffa M, Schachter S. Yom Kippur, Air France, dormitory food, and eating behavior of obese and normal persons. *J Personal Soc Psychol* 1968; **10**: 117–123.

23. Boutelle K, Kirschenbaum D, Baker R, *et al.* How can obese weight controllers minimize weight gain during the high risk holiday season? By self-monitoring very consistently. *Health Psychol* 1999; **18**: 364–368.

24. Luria AR. Higher cortical functions in man. London: Tavistock, 1966.

25. Lhermitte F, Pillon B, Serdaru M. Human autonomy and the frontal lobes. I. Imitation and utilization behavior: A neuropsychological study of 75 patients. *Ann Neurol* 1986; **19**: 326–334.

26. Lhermitte F. Human autonomy and the frontal lobes. II. Patient behavior in complex and social situations. The "environmental dependency syndrome". *Ann Neurol* 1986; **19**: 335–343.

27. De Renzi E, Cavalleri F, Facchini S. Imitation and utilization behaviour. *J Neurol Neurosur Psychiat* 1996; **61**: 396–400.

28. Graff-Radford N, Russell J, Rezai K. Frontal degenerative dementia and neuroimaging. *Adv Neurol* 1995; **66**: 37–47.

29. Janssen JC, Warrington EK, Morris HR, *et al.* Clinical features of frontotemporal dementia due to the intronic tau 10(+16) mutation. *Neurology* 2002; **58**: 1161–1168.

30. Murad A. Orbitofrontal syndrome in psychiatry. *Enceph-Rev Psychiatr Clin Biol Ther* 1999; **25**: 634–637.

31. Gautier J-F, Chen K, Uecker A, *et al.* Regions of the human brain affected during a liquid-meal taste perception in the fasting state: A positron emission tomography study. *Am J Clin Nutr* 1999; **70**: 806–810.

32. Braun C, Chouinard M. Is anorexia nervosa a neuropsychological disease? *Neuropsychol Rev* 1992; **3**: 171–212.

33. Fuster J. The prefrontal cortex. New York: Raven Press, 1989.

34. Diamond A. Developmental time course in human infants and infant monkeys, and the neural basis of inhibitory control in reaching. In: Diamond A, ed. The development and neural basis of higher cognitive functions. New York: Academy of Sciences, 1990: 637–676.

35. Valenstein ES. Channelling of responses elicited by hypothalamic stimulation. *J Psychiatr Res* 1971; **8**: 335–344.

36. Macht M, Simons G. Emotions and eating in everyday life. *Appetite* 2000; **35**: 65–71.

37. Epel E, Lapidus R, McEwen B, *et al.* Stress may add bite to appetite in women: A laboratory study of stress-induced cortisol and eating behavior. *Psychoneuroendocrinol* 2001; **26**: 37–49.

38. Campfield LA, Smith FJ. Transient declines in blood-glucose signal meal initiation. *Intern J Obesity* 1990; **14**: 15–33.

39. Tuomisto T, Tuomisto M, Hetherington M, *et al.* Reasons for initiation and cessation of eating in obese men and women and the affective consequences of eating in everyday situations. *Appetite* 1998; **30**: 211–222.

40. Hou C, Miller B, Cummings J, *et al.* Artistic savants. *Neuropsychiat Neuropsychol Behav Neurol* 2000; **13**: 29–38.

41. Miller B, Cummings J, Mishkin F, *et al.* Emergence of artistic talent in frontotemporal dementia. *Neurology* 1998; **51**: 978–982.

42. Regard M, Landis T. "Gourmand syndrome": Eating passion associated with right anterior lesions. *Neurology* 1997; **48**: 1185–1190.

43. Williamson DF. Pharmacotherapy for obesity. *JAMA* 1999; **281**: 278–280.

44. Harrison AA, Everitt BJ, Robbins TW. Central 5-HT depletion enhances impulsive responding without affecting the accuracy of attentional performance: Interactions with dopaminergic mechanisms. *Psychopharmacol* 1997; **133**: 329–342.

45. Cummings D, Weigle D, Frayo R, *et al.* Plasma ghrelin levels after diet-induced weight loss or gastric bypass surgery. *NE J Med* 2002; **346**: 1623–1630.

46. Muurahainen N, Kissileff H, Lachaussee J, *et al.* Effect of a soup preload on reduction of food intake by cholecystokinin in humans. *Am J Physiol* 1991; **260**: R672–R680.

47. Korotkova T, Sergeeva O, Eriksson K, *et al.* Excitation of ventral tegmental area dopaminergic and nondopaminergic neurons by orexins/hypocretins. *J Neurosci* 2003; **23**: 7–11.

48. Ciriello J, Rosas-Arellano M, Solano-Flores L, *et al.* Identification of neurons containing orexin-B (hypocretin-2) immunoreactivity in limbic structures. *Brain Res* 2003; **967**: 123–131.

49. Agarwal M, Hughes P, Haliga A, *et al.* Relevance of cholesterol screening in the United Arab Emirates. A preliminary study. *Eur J Epidemiol* 1995; **11**: 581–585.

50. van den Pol AN. Narcolepsy: A neurodegenerative disease of the hypocretin system? *Neuron* 2000; **27**: 415–418.

51. Blass EM, Hoffmayer LB. Sucrose as an analgesic for newborn infants. *Pediatrics* 1991; **87**: 215–218.

52. Myslobodsky M. Petit Mal Epilepsy. A search for precursors of petit mal activity. New York: Academic Press, 1976.

53. Banks W. Is obesity a disease of the blood-brain barrier? Physiological, pathological, and evolutionary considerations. *Current Phamaceut Design* 2003; **9**: 801–809.

54. Henson M, Castracane V. Leptin in pregnancy. *Biol Reprod* 2000; **63**: 1219–1228.

55. Chehab F, Mounzih K, Lu R, *et al.* Early onset of reproductive function in normal female mice treated with leptin. *Science* 1997; **275**: 88–90.

56. Schwartz M, Woods S, Porte DJ, *et al.* Central nervous system control of food intake. *Nature* 2000; **404**: 661–671.

57. Schuman M, Gitlin M, Fairbanks L. Sweets, chocolate, and atypical depressive traits. *J Nerv Ment Dis* 1987; **175**: 491–495.

58. Lakatos I. Proofs and refutations. The logic of mathematical discovery. Cambridge: Cambridge University Press, 1994.

59. Patel K, Schlundt D. Impact of moods and social context on eating behavior. *Appetite* 2001; **36**: 111–118.

60. Stettler N, Zemel B, Kumanyika S, *et al.* Infant weight gain and childhood overweight status in a multicenter, cohort study. *Pediatrics* 2002; **109**: 194–199.

61. Weingarten H. Cytokines and food intake: The relevance of the immune system to the student of ingestive behavior. *Neurosci Biobehav Rev* 1996; **20**: 163–170.

b) Cognitive Decline: Factors and Targets

1. Clarke CA, Mittwoch U. Puzzles of longevity. *Perspect Biol Med* 1994; **37**: 327–336.

2. Kalache A, Keller I. The graying world: A challenge for the twenty-first century. *Science Progress* 2000; **83**: 33–54.

3. Fuchs V. Health care for the elderly: How much? Who will pay for it? *Health Aff (Millwood)* 1999; **18**: 11–21.

4. Critchley M. The citadel of the senses and other essays. New York: Raven Press, 1986.

5. Rojas-Fernandez CCM. Dementia with Lewy bodies: Review and pharmacotherapeutic implications. *Pharmacotherapy* 1999; **19**: 795–803.

6. Berthier ML, Leiguarda R, Starkstein SE, *et al.* Alzheimer's disease in a patient with posterior cortical atrophy. *J Neurol Neurosurg Psychiatry* 1991; **54**: 1110–1111.

7. Levy MH, Hart WM, Sonstein FM, *et al.* The incredible shrinking brain. *Surv Ophthalmol* 1995; **39**: 315–322.

8. Gainotti G, Marra C, Villa G. A double dissociation between accuracy and time of execution on attentional tasks in Alzheimer's disease and multi-infarct dementia. *Brain* 2001; **124**: 731–738.

9. Martin A, Brouwers P, Lalonde F, *et al.* Towards a behavioral typology of Alzheimer's patients. *J Clin Exp Neuropsychol* 1986; **8**: 594–610.

10. Parasuraman R, Greenwood P, Sunderland T. The apolipoprotein E gene, attention, and brain function. *Neuropsychology* 2002; **16**: 254–274.

11. Rabinowicz A, Starkstein S, Leiguarda R, *et al.* Transient epileptic amnesia in dementia: A treatable unrecognized cause of episodic amnestic wandering. *Alzheimer Dis Assoc Disord* 2000; **14**: 231–233.

12. Slater E. The neurotic constitution. A statistical study of two thousand neurotic soldiers. *J Neurology and Psychiatry* 1943; **6**: 1–16.

13. Cummings JL. Clinical neuropsychiatry. Orlando: Grune & Stratton, Inc., 1985.

14. Jabourian A. Vascular dementia and heart rhythm's disorders. *Ann Medico-Psychologiques,* 1996; **154**: 642–646.

15. Liao DP, Cooper L, Cai JW, *et al.* The prevalence and severity of white matter lesions, their relationship with age, ethnicity, gender, and cardiovascular disease risk factors: The ARIC study. *Neuroepidemiology* 1997; **16**: 149–162.

16. Myslobodsky M. Metabolic encephalopathies and petit mal epilepsy. In: Myslobodsky M, Mirsky A, eds. Elements of Petit Mal Epilepsy. New York: Lang, 1988.

17. Boccardi M, Laakso MP, Bresciani L, *et al.* The MRI pattern of frontal and temporal brain atrophy in fronto-temporal dementia. *Neurobiol Aging* 2003; **24**: 95–103.

18. Roberge R. The Diogenes syndrome. *Canad Family Physic* 1998; **44**: 812–817.

19. Gispen WH, Biessels G-J. Cognition and synaptic plasticity in diabetes mellitus. *TINs* 2000; **23**: 542–549.

20. Brown R, CD M. Internal versus external cues and the control of attention in Parkinson's disease. *Brain* 1988; **111**: 323–345.

21. Barber J, Tomer R, Sroka H, *et al.* Does unilateral dopamine deficit contribute to depression? *Psychiat Res* 1985; **15**: 17–24.

22. Lloyd A. Comprehension of prosody in Parkinson's disease. *Cortex* 1999; **35**: 389–402.

23. Fuh J, Lee R, Wang S, *et al.* Swallowing difficulty in Parkinson's disease. *Clin Neurol Neurosurg* 1997; **99**: 106–112.

24. Wilson IC, Garbutt JC, Lanier CF, *et al.* Is there a tardive dysmentia. *Schizophr Bull* 1983; **9**: 187–192.

25. Myslobodsky M. Central determinants of attention and mood disorders in tardive dyskinesia (tardive dysmentia). *Brain Cogn* 1993; **23**: 88–101.

26. Dixon R, Bradley K, Budge M, *et al.* Longitudinal quantitative proton magnetic resonance spectroscopy of the hippocampus in Alzheimer's disease. *Brain* 2002; **125**: 2332–2341.

27. Antuono P, Jones J, Wang Y, *et al.* Decreased glutamate plus glutamine in Alzheimer's disease detected in vivo with H-1-MRS at 0.5 T. *Neurology* 2001; **56**: 737–742.

28. Petroff O, Errante L, Rothman D, *et al.* Neuronal and glial metabolite content of the epileptogenic human hippocampus. *Ann Neurol* 2002; **52**: 635–642.

29. Sunderland T, Linker G, Mirza N, *et al.* Decreased beta-amyloid 1–42 and increased tau levels in cerebrospinal fluid of patients with Alzheimer disease. *JAMA* 2003; **289**: 2094–2103.

30. Boccardi M, Laasko MP, Bresciani L, *et al.* Clinical characteristics of frontotemporal patients with symmetric brain atrophy. *Eur Arch Psych Clin Neurosci* 2002; **252**: 235–239.

31. Morello J, Petaja-Repo U, Bichet D, *et al.* Pharmacological chaperones: A new twist on receptor folding. *TIPs* 2000; **21**: 466–469.

32. Mulley J, Scheffer I, Petrou S, *et al.* Channelopathies as a genetic cause of epilepsy. *Curr Opin Neurol* 2003; **16**: 171–176.

33. Hauser W, Morris M, Heston L, *et al.* Seizures and myoclonus in patients with Alzheimer's disease. *Neurology* 1986; **36**: 1226–1230.

34. McVicker R, Shanks O, McClelland R. Prevalence and associated features of epilepsy in adults with Down's syndrome. *Br J Psychiatry* 1994; **164**: 528–532.

35. Puri B, Ho K, Singh I. Age of seizure onset in adults with Down's syndrome. *Int J Clin Pract* 2001; **55**: 442–444.

36. Lalonde FM, Myslobodsky M. Epileptiform syndrome complicates the course of Alzheimer's dementia [In preparation].

37. Mielke R, Schroder R, Fink GR, *et al.* Regional cerebral glucose metabolism and post-mortem pathology in Alzheimer's disease. *Acta Neuropathol* 1996; **91**: 174–179.

38. Johannsen P, Jakobsen J, Gjedde A. Statistical maps of cerebral blood flow deficits in Alzheimer's disease. *Eur J Neurol* 2000; **7**: 385–392.

39. Minoshima S, Giordani B, Berent S, *et al.* Metabolic reduction in the posterior cingulate cortex in very early Alzheimer's disease. *Ann Neurol* 1997; **42**: 85–94.

40. Meguro K, LeMestric C, Landeau B, *et al.* Relations between hypometabolism in the posterior association neocortex and hippocampal atrophy in Alzheimer's disease: A PET/MRI correlative study. *J Neurol Neurosurg Psychiatry* 2001; **71**: 315–321.

41. Theodore W, Gaillard W, De CC, *et al.* Hippocampal volume and glucose metabolism in temporal lobe epileptic foci. *Epilepsia* 2001; **42**: 130–132.

42. Fakhoury T, Abou-Khalil B, Kessler R. Limbic encephalitis and hyperactive foci on PET scan. *Seizure* 1999; **8**: 427–431.

43. Engel JJ, Kuhl DE, Phelps ME, *et al.* Local cerebral metabolism during partial seizures. *Neurology* 1983; **33**: 400–413.

44. Siesjo BK, Wieloch T. Epileptic brain damage: Pathophysiology and neurochemical pathology. In: Delgado-Escueta AV, *et al.*, eds. Advances in neurology. New York: Raven Press, 1986: 813–846.

45. van Gorp W, Mandelkern M, Gee M, Hinkin CH, Stern CE, Paz DK, Dixon W, Evans G, Flynn F, Frederick CJ, *et al.* J. Cerebral metabolic dysfunction in AIDS: Findings in a sample with and without dementia. *Neuropsychiat Clin Neurosci* 1992; **4**: 280–287.

46. Rottenberg D, Moeller J, Strother S, *et al.* The metabolic pathology of the AIDS dementia complex. *Ann Neurol* 1987; **22**: 700–706.

47. Olney J, Wozniak D, Farber N. Glutamate receptor dysfunction and Alzheimer's disease. *Restor Neurol Neurosci* 1998; **13**: 75–83.

48. Olney J. Excitotoxins in foods. *Neurotoxicology* 1994; **15**: 535–544.

49. Stone T. Kynurenines in the CNS: From endogenous obscurity to therapeutic importance. *Prog Neurobiol* 2001; **64**: 185–218.

50. Veliskova J, Velisek L, Galanopoulou A, *et al.* Neuroprotective effects of estrogens on hippocampal cells in adult female rats after status epilepticus. *Epilepsia* 2000; **41**: S30–S35.

51. Sherwin BB. Mild cognitive impairment: Potential pharmacological treatment options. *J Am Geriatr Soc* 2000; **48**: 431–441.

52. Cuajungco MP, Lees GJ. Zinc metabolism in the brain: Relevance to human neurodegenerative disorders. *Neurobiol Dis* 1997; **4**: 137–169.

53. Weiss JH, Sensi SL, Koh JY. Zn^{2+}: A novel ionic mediator of neural injury in brain disease. *TIPs* 2000; **21**: 395–401.

54. Christensen M, Frederickson C. Zinc-containing afferent projections to the rat cortico-medial amygdaloid complex: A retrograde tracing study. *J Compar Neurol* 1998; **40**: 375–390.

55. Zou K, Gong J, Yanagisawa K, *et al.* A novel function of monomeric amyloid beta-protein serving as an antioxidant molecule against metal-induced oxidative damage. *J Neurosci* 2002; **22**: 4833–4841.

56. Jellinger KA. The role of iron in neurodegeneration. Prospects for pharmacotherapy of Parkinson's disease. *Drugs & Aging* 1999; **14**: 115–134.

57. Jaworowski Z. Radiation risk and ethics. *Physics Today* 1999; **September**: 24–29.

58. Dobson C, Itzhaki R. Herpes simplex virus type 1 and Alzheimer's disease. *Neurobiol Aging* 1999; **20**: 457–465.

59. Solerte S, Cravello L, Ferrari E, *et al.* Overproduction of IFN-gamma and TNF-alpha from natural killer (NK) cells is associated with abnormal NK reactivity and cognitive derangement in Alzheimer's disease. *Ann NY Acad Sci* 2000; **917**: 331–340.

60. Cornell-Bell A, Finkbeiner SM. Ca^{2+} waves in astrocytes. *Cell Calcium* 1991; **12**: 185–204.

61. Nourhashemi F, Gillette-Guyonnet S, Andrieu S, *et al.* Alzheimer disease: Protective factors. *Am J Clin Nutr* 2000; **71**: 643S–649S.

62. Gruol DL, Nelson TE. Physiological and pathological roles of interleukin-6 in the central nervous system. *Mol Neurobiol* 1997; **15**: 307–339.

63. Friedman G, Froom P, Sazbon L, *et al.* Apolipoprotein E-epsilon 4 genotype predicts a poor outcome in survivors of traumatic brain injury. *Neurology* 1999; **52**: 244–248.

64. St'astny F, Skultetyova I, Pliss L, *et al.* Quinolinic acid enhances permeability of rat brain microvessels to plasma albumin. *Brain Res Bull* 2000; **53**: 415–420.

65. Michikawa M. The role of cholesterol in pathogenesis of Alzheimer's disease. *Mol Neurobiol* 2003; **27**: 1–12.

66. Friendland R. Lipid metabolism, epidemiology, and the mechanism of Alzheimer's disease. *Ann NY Acad Sci* 2002; **977**: 387–390.

67. Devuyst G, Karapanayiotides T, Hottinger I, *et al.* Prodromal and early epileptic seizures in acute stroke: Does higher serum cholesterol protect? *Neurology* 2003; **61**: 249–252.

68. Jorm A. Subtypes of Alzheimer's dementia: A conceptual analysis and critical review. *Psychol Med* 1985; **15**: 543–553.

69. Tune L, Sunderland T. New cholinergic therapies: Treatment tools for the psychiatrist. *J Clin Psychiatry* 1998; **59**: 31–35.

70. Myslobodsky M. Petit mal epilepsy. A search for precursors of petit mal activity. New York: Academic Press, 1976.

71. Eschle D, Siegel A, Wieser H. Epilepsy with severe abdominal pain. *Mayo Clin Proc:* 2002; **77**: 1358–1360.

72. Schauble B, Britton J, Mullan B, *et al.* Ictal vomiting in association with left temporal lobe seizures in a left hemisphere language-dominant patient. *Epilepsia* 2002; **43**: 1432–1435.

73. Jain K. Evaluation of memantine for neuroprotection in dementia. *Expert Opin Investig Drugs* 2000; **9**: 1397–1406.

74. Loscher W, Honack D. Over-additive anticonvulsant effect of memantine and NBQX in kindled rats. *Eur J Pharmacol* 1994; **259**: R3–R5.

75. Myslobodsky MS, Golovchinsky V, Mintz M. Ketamine — Convulsant or anti-convulsant. *Pharmacol Biochem Behav* 1981; **14**: 27–33.

76. Shi W-X, Zhang X-X. Dendritic glutamate-induced bursting in the prefrontal cortex: Further characterization and effects of phencyclidine. *J Pharmacol Experiment Therapeut* 2003; **305**: 680–687.

77. Farber N, Jiang X, Heinkel C, *et al.* Antiepileptic drugs and agents that inhibit voltage-gated sodium channels prevent NMDA antagonist neurotoxicity. *Mol Psychiatry* 2002; **7**: 726–733.

78. Hogh P, Smith S, Scahill R, *et al.* Epilepsy presenting as AD: Neuroimaging, electro-clinical features, and response to treatment. *Neurology* 2002; **58**: 298–301.

79. Timmons S, Sweeney B, Hyland M, *et al.* New onset seizures in the elderly: Aetiology and prognosis. *Ir Med J* 2002; **95**: 47–49.

80. Flor P, Battaglia G, Nicoletti F, *et al.* Neuroprotective activity of metabotropic glutamate receptor ligands. *Adv Exp Med Biol* 2002; **513**: 197–223.

81. Brandimonte M, Einstein GO, McDaniel MA, (eds). Prospective memory: Theory and applications. Mahwah, NJ: Lawrence Erlbaum Associates Inc., 1996.

82. Moscovitch M. A neuropsychological approach to memory and perception in normal and pathological aging. In: Craik FIM, Trehub S, eds. Aging and cognitive processes. New York: Plenum, 1982: 55–78.

83. Patton GWR, Meit M. Effects of aging on prospective memory. *Exper Aging Res* 1993; **19**: 165–176.

84. McKitrick LA, Camp CJ, Black FW. Prospective memory intervention in Alzheimer's disease. *J Gerontol* 1992; **47**: P337–P343.

85. Huppert FA, Beardsall L. Prospective memory impairment as an early indicator of dementia. *J Clin Exptl Neuropsychol* 1993; **15**: 805–821.

86. Fuster J. The prefrontal cortex. New York: Raven Press, 1989.

87. McCormick P. Orienting attention without awareness. *J Expl Psychol-Human Percept Perform* 1997; **23**: 168–180.

88. McDaniel MA, Einstein GO. The importance of cue familiarity and cue distinctiveness in prospective memory. *Memory* 1993; **1**: 23–41.

89. Park D, Hertzog C, Kidder D, *et al.* Effect of age on event-based and time-based prospective memory. *Psychol Aging* 1997; **12**: 314–327.

90. Craik FIM. A functional account of age differences in memory. In: Klix F, Hagendorf H, eds. Human memory and cognitive capabilities: Mechanisms and performances. Amsterdam: Elsevier, 1986: 409–422.

91. Cherry KE, LeCompte DC. Age individual differences influence prospective memory. *Psychol Aging* 1999; **14**: 60–76.

92. Einstein GO, Smith RE, McDaniel MA, *et al.* Aging and prospective memory: The influence of increased task demands at encoding and retrieval. *Psychol Aging* 1997; **12**: 479–488.

93. Mantyla T. Activating actions and interrupting intentions: Mechanisms of retrieval sensitization in prospective memory. In: Brandimonte M, *et al.*, eds. Prospective memory: Theory and applications. Hillsdale, NJ: Erlbaum, 1995: 93–113.

94. Kliegel M, Martin M, McDaniel M, *et al.* Varying the importance of a prospective memory task: Differential effects across time- and event-based prospective memory. *Memory* 2001; **9**: 1–11.

95. Gibbon J, Malapani C, Dale CL, *et al.* Toward a neurobiology of temporal cognition: Advances and challenges. *Curr Opin Neurobiol* 1997; **7**: 170–184.

96. Malapani C, Fairhurst S. Scalar timing in animals and humans. *Learn Motiv* 2002; **33**: 156–176.

97. Francis-Smythe J, Robertson I. On the relationship between time management and time estimate. *Br J of Psychol* 1999; **90**: 333–347.

98. Harris JE, Wilkins AJ. Remembering to do things: A theoretical framework and an illustrative experiment. *Human Learning* 1982; **1**: 123–136.

99. Kvavilashvili L, Ellis J. Varieties of intention: Some distinctions and classifications. In: Brandimonte M, *et al.*, eds. Prospective memory: Theory and applications. Hillsdale, NJ: Erlbaum, 1997: 23–51.

100. Schultz W. Reward signaling by dopamine neurons. *Neuroscientist* 2001; **7**: 293–302.

101. Graf P, Uttl B. Prospective memory: A new focus for research. *Consciousness and Cognition* 2001; **10**: 437–450.

102. Evans D, Hebert L, Beckett L, *et al.* Education and other measures of socioeconomic status and risk of incident Alzheimer disease in a defined population of older persons. *Arch Neurol* 1997; **54**: 1399–1405.

103. Mortimer J. Brain reserve and the clinical expression of Alzheimer's disease. *Geriatrics* 1997; **52**: S50–S53.

104. Snowdon D, Greiner L, Markesbery W. Linguistic ability in early life and the neuropathology of Alzheimer's disease and cerebrovascular disease. Findings from the Nun study. *Ann N Y Acad Sci* 2000; **903**: 34–38.

105. Snowdon D, Kemper S, Mortimer J, *et al.* Linguistic ability in early life and cognitive function and Alzheimer's disease in late life. Findings from the Nun study. *JAMA* 1996; **275**: 528–532.

106. Graves A, Mortimer J, Larson E, *et al.* Head circumference as a measure of cognitive reserve. Association with severity of impairment in Alzheimer's disease. *Br J Psychiatry* 1996; **169**: 86–92.

107. Das UN. Long-chain polyunsaturated fatty acids in the growth and development of the brain and memory. *Nutrition* 2003; **19**: 62–65.

108. Lessmann V, Gottmann K, Malcangio M. Neurotrophin secretion: Current facts and future prospects. *Prog Neurobiol* 2003; **69**: 341–374.

109. Shaw S, Commins K, O'Mara S. Deficits in spatial learning and synaptic plasticity induced by the rapid and competitive broad-spectrum cyclooxygenase inhibitor ibuprofen are reversed by increasing endogenous brain-derived neurotrophic factor. *Eur J Neurosci* 2003; **17**: 2438–2446.

110. Speeches. Speeches given at the BAFS Friend's dinner: Mercy killing in the new millennium. *Med Soc Sci* 2000; **40**: 193.

c) Self-destructive Behavior: The Cultural Perspective

1. The Surgeon General's call to action to prevent suicide. Washington, DC: Public Health Service, 1999.

2. Bouvard M, Doyen C. Suicide in adolescents *Encephale-Rev. Psychiat. Clin Biol Ther* 1996; **22**: 35–39.

3. Klerman G. Clinical epidemiology of suicide. *J Clin Psychiatry* 1988; **48**: 33–38.

4. Minois G. History of suicide: Voluntary death in Western culture. Baltimore: John Hopkins University Press, 1999.

5. Murphy G, Wetzel R. Suicide risk by birth cohort in the US, 1949–1974. *Arch Gen Psychiatry* 1980; **37**: 519–523.

6. Tolmas HC. Violence among youth: A major epidemic in America: One pediatrician's perspective. *Am Acad Pediatr: Adolescent Health Section Newsletter* 1998; **20**: 18–30.

7. Kline M. Mathematics. The loss of certainty. Oxford: Oxford University Press, 1980.

8. Goldstein K. Human nature in the light of psychopathology. Cambridge, Mass: Harvard University Press, 1940.

9. Harte J. Consider a spherical cow: A course in environmental problem solving. Sausalito, CA: University Science Books, 1988.

10. Bondy B, Kuznik J, Baghai T, *et al.* Lack of association of serotonin-2A receptor gene polymorphism (T102C) with suicidal ideation and suicide. *Am J Med Genet* 2000; **96**: 831–835.

11. Du L, Faludi G, Palkovits M, *et al.* Serotonergic genes and suicidality. *Crisis* 2001; **22**: 54–60.

12. Mann J J, Brent D A, Arango V. The neurobiology and genetics of suicide and attempted suicide: A focus on the serotonergic system. *Neuropsychopharmacology* 2001; **24**: 467–477.

13. Lesch KP, Merschdorf U. Impulsivity, aggression, and serotonin: A molecular psychobiological perspective. *Behav Sci Law* 2000; **18**: 581–604.

14. Heinz A, Mann K, Weinberger D R, *et al.* Serotonergic dysfunction, negative mood states, and response to alcohol. *Alcoholism (NY)* 2001; **25**: 487–495.

15. Caspi A, Sugden K, Moffitt TE, *et al.* Influence of life stress on depression: Moderation by a polymorphism in the 5-HTT gene. *Science* 2003; **18**: 386–389.

16. Brown GW. Genetic and population perspectives on life events and depression. *Soc Psychiatry Psychiatr Epidemiol* 1998; **33**: 363–372.

17. Brown GW. Social roles, context and evolution in the origins of depression. *J Health Social Behavior* 2002; **43**: 255–276.

18. Kety S. Genetic factors in suicide. In: Roy A, ed. Suicide. Baltimore: Williams & Wilkins, 1986.

19. Raine A, Meloy JR, Bihrle S, *et al.* Reduced prefrontal and increased subcortical brain functioning assessed using positron emission tomography in predatory and affective murderers. *Behav Sci Law* 1998; **16**: 319–332.

20. Jenkins IH, Fernandez W, Playford ED, *et al.* Impaired activation of the supplementary motor area in Parkinson's disease is reversed when akinesia is treated with apomorphine. *Ann Neurol* 1992; **32**: 749–757.

21. Brooks D. Motor disturbance and brain functional imaging in Parkinson's disease. *Eur Neurol* 1997; **38**: 26–32.

22. Myslobodsky M, Lalonde F, Hicks L. Are patients with Parkinson's disease suicidal? *J Geriatr Psychiat Neurol* 2001; **14**: 120–124.

23. Merari A. Suicide terrorism. Invited lecture delivered at the APA Convention. Chicago, 2002.

24. Becker E. The denial of death. New York: The Free Press, 1973.

25. Elliott F. The episodic dyscontrol syndrome and aggression. *Neurol Clin* 1984; **2**: 113–125.

26. Runeson B, Beskow J, Waern M. The suicidal process in suicides among young people. *Acta Psychiatr Scand* 1996; **93**: 35–42.

27. Welch S. A review of the literature on the epidemiology of parasuicide in the general population. *Psychiatr Serv* 2001; **52**: 368–375.

28. Jenkins G, Hale R, Papanastassiou M, *et al.* Suicide rate 22 years after parasuicide: Cohort study. *Br Med J* 2002; **325**: 1155.

29. Rudge D. In the mind of a would be suicide bomber. *Jerusalem Post* 2002 May 30.

30. van Praag HM. Anxiety and increased aggression as pacemakers of depression. *Acta Psychiat Scand* 1998; **98**: 81–88.

31. Haj-Yahi M, Tamish S. The rates of child sexual abuse and its psychological consequences as revealed by a study among Palestinian university students. *Child Abuse Negl* 2001; **25**: 1303–1327.

32. Durkheim E. Suicide. Glencoe, Ill: Free Press, 1951.

33. Hamdi E, Amin Y, Abou-Saleh M. Performance of the Hamilton depression rating scale in depressed patients in the United Arab Emirates. *Acta Psychiatr Scand* 1997; **96**: 416–423.

34. Racy J. Psychiatry in the Arab East. *Acta Psychoatrica Scandinavica* 1970; **Suppl 21**: 1–171.

35. Katz P. Conflict of cultures in a state mental hospital system. In: Gaines A D, ed. Ethnopsychiatry: The cultural construction of professional and folk psychiatries. Albany, New York: State University of New York Press, 1992: 355–377.

36. Miller R. On the primacy of embarrassment in social life. *Psychol Inquiry* 2001; **12**: 30–40.

37. Nisbett RE, Cohen D. Culture of honor: The psychology of violence in the South. Boulder: Westview Press, 1996.

38. Gans E. Herostratus forever. Chronicles of love and resentment. *Anthropoetics* 1997: April 5.

39. Kennedy BP, Kawachi I, Brainerd E. The role of social capital in the Russian mortality crisis. *World Dev* 1998; **26**: 2029–2043.

40. Rubio M. Perverse social capital — Some evidence from Colombia. *J Econ Issues* 1997; **31**: 805–816.

41. Beck A. Depression: Clinical, experimental and theoretical aspects. London: Staples, 1967.

42. Sifneos P. Alexithymia: Past and present. *Am J Psychiatry* 1996; **153**: 137–142.

43. Appleby L, Cooper J, Amos T, *et al.* Psychological autopsy study of suicides by people aged under 35. *Br J Psychiat* 1999; **175**: 168–174.

44. Beautrais A, Sassatpoo PM. Suicides and serious suicide attempts: Two populations or one? *Psychol Med* 2001; **31**: 837–845.

45. Vijaykumar L, Rajkumar S. Are risk factors for suicide universal? A case control study in India. *Acta Psychiatr Scand* 1999; **99**: 407–411.

46. Hawton K, Haw C, Houston K, *et al.* Family history of suicidal behaviour: Prevalence and significance in deliberate self-harm patients. *Acta Psychiat Scandinav* 2002; **106**: 387–393.

47. Bourgeois M. Serotonin impulsivity and suicide. *Hum Psychopharmacol-Clin Exp* 1991; **6**: S31–S36.

48. Wolfersdorf M, Kiefer A. Depression and the aggression hypothesis — A comparison of depressed inpatients and non-depressive controls using the Buss-Durkee hostility inventory. *Psychiatr Prax* 1998; **25**: 240–245.

49. Fekete S, Schmidtke A. The impact of mass media reports on suicide and attitudes toward self-destruction: Previous studies and some new data from Hungary and Germany. In: Mishara B, ed. The impact of suicide. New York: Springer Publishing Company, Inc, 1995: 142–155.

Chapter 5
Collective Exaggerated Emotions

1. Bartholomew RE. Ethnocentricity and the social construction of 'mass hysteria'. *Cult Med Psychiatry,* 1990; **14**: 455–494.

2. Kaye JA, Melero-Montes M D, Jick H. Mumps, measles, and rubella vaccine and the incidence of autism recorded by general practitioners: A time trend analysis. *Br Med J* 2001; **322**: 460–463.

3. Lord C, Cook E, Leventhal B, *et al.* Autism spectrum disorders. *Neuron* 2000; **28**: 355–363.

4. Moulder J, LS E, RS M, *et al.* Cell phones and cancer: What is the evidence for a connection? *Radiation Res* 1999; **151**: 513–531.

5. Valberg PA, Kavlet R, Rafferty CN. Can low-level 50/60 Hz electric and magnetic fields cause biological effects? *Radiation Res* 1997; **148**: 2–21.

6. Jones T, Craig A, Hoy D, *et al.* Mass psychogenic illness attributed to toxic exposure at a high school. *NE J Med* 2000; **342**: 96–100.

7. Le Magnen J. Physiologie des sensations — Une cas de sensibilite olfactive se present comme un charactere sexuel secondaire feminin. *CR Acad Sci* 1948; **228**: 947–1048.

8. Myslobodsky M. The origin of radiophobias. *Perspect Biol Med* 2001; **44**: 543–555.

9. Taylor S. Psychiatry and natural history. *Br Med J* 1978; **2**: 1754–1758.

10. Critchley M. The divine banquet of the brain. New York: Raven Press, 1980.

11. Stirn A. Body piercing: Medical consequences and psychological motivations. *Lancet* 2003; **361**: 1205–1215.

12. Mobius P. Uber den begriff der hysterie. *Zent Nervenheilkunde* 1888; **11**: 66–71.

13. Tomes N. The making of a germ panic: Then and now. *Am J Public Health* 2000; **90**: 91–198.

14. Gladwell M. The tipping point. New York: Little, Brown, 2000.

15. Trevarthen C. The tasks of consciousness: How could the brain do them? *Ciba Found Series* 1979; **69**: 187–253.

16. Calman KC. Cancer: Science and society and the communication of risk. *Br Med J* 1996; **313**: 799–802.

17. Rizzolatti G, Fadiga L, Fogassi L, *et al.* Resonance behaviors and mirror neurons. *Arch Ital Biol* 1999; **137**: 85–100.

18. Fadiga L, Fogassi L, Gallese V, *et al.* Visuomotor neurons: Ambiguity of the discharge or 'motor' perception? *Int J Psychophysiology* 2000; **35**: 165–177.

19. Gallese V, Goldman V. Mirror neurons and the simulation theory of mind-reading. *Trends in Cognitive Sciences,* 1998; **2**: 493.

20. Martin A. The organization of semantic knowledge and the origin of words in the brain. In: Jablonski NG, Aiello LC, eds. The origins and diversification of language. San Francisco: California Academy of Sciences, 1998: 69–88.

21. Ramachandran VS. Mirror neurons and imitation learning as the driving force behind 'the great leap forward' in human evolution. *Edge* 2000; **69**.

22. Seger C, Desmond J, Glover G, *et al.* Functional magnetic resonance imaging evidence for right-hemisphere involvement in processing unusual semantic relationships. *Neuropsychol* 2000; **14**: 361–369.

23. Nolde S, Johnson M, D'Esposito M. Left prefrontal activation during episodic remembering: An event-related fMRI study. *Neuroreport* 1998; **9**: 3509–3514.

24. Cheney DL, Seyfarth RM. How monkeys see the world. Chicago: University of Chicago Press, 1990.

25. Berlyne DE. Motivational problems raised by exploratory and epistemic behavior. In: Koch S, ed. Psychology: A study of science. New York: McGraw Hill, 1963: 284–364.

26. Umilta M, Kohler E, Gallese V, *et al.* I know what you are doing: A neurophysiological study. *Neuron 31* 2001; **31**: 155–165.

27. Byrne RW, Whiten A. Machiavellian intelligence. Oxford: Oxford University Press, 1988.

28. Meehl PE. Why I do not attend case conferences. Psychodiagnosis. Selected papers. New York: Norton & Co., 1977.

29. Colden L. Observations on psychotherapy of schizophrenia. In: Fromm-Reichmann F, Moreno JL, eds. Progress in psychotherapy. New York: Grune & Stratton, 1956: 239–247.

30. Slovic P, Fischhoff B, Lichtenstein S. Facts versus fears: Understanding perceived risk. In: Kahneman D, *et al.*, eds. Judgment under uncertainty: Heuristics and biases. Cambridge: Cambridge University Press, 1982: 463–489.
31. Slovic P. The perception of risk. London: Earthscan Publications, 2000.
32. Sidel V, Cohen H, Gould R. Good intentions and the road to bioterrorism preparedness. *Am J Public Health* 2001; **91**: 710–716.
33. Coffey D. The cost of biological terrorism. *Oncologist* 1997; **2**: XI–XII.
34. Weinstein N. Optimistic biases about personal risks. *Am J Public Health* 1989; **246**: 1232–1233.
35. Rechard R. Historical relationship between performance assessment for radioactive waste disposal and other types of risk assessment. *Risk Anal* 1999; **19**: 763–807.
36. Wildavsky A. But is it true? A citizen's guide to environmental health and safety issues: Harvard University Press, 1995.
37. Lewin K. Principles of topological psychology. New York: McGraw-Hill, 1936.
38. Slovic P. Trust, emotion, sex, politics, and science: Surveying the risk-assessment battle-field. *Risk Anal* 1999; **19**: 689–701.
39. Siegrist M, Cvetkovich G, Roth C. Salient value similarity, social trust, and risk/benefit perception. *Risk Anal* 2000; **20**: 353–362.
40. Ziman JM. Public knowledge. Cambridge: Cambridge University Press, 1968.
41. Hettema J, Neale M, Kendler K. A review and meta-analysis of the genetic epidemiology of anxiety disorders. *Am J Psychiatry* 2001; **158**: 1568–1578.

Chapter 6
A Complementary Point of View

1. Cook HJ. The new philosophy and medicine in seventeenth-century England. In: Lindberg D, Westman RS, eds. Reappraisals of the scientific revolution. Cambridge: Cambridge University Press, 1990.
2. Dieppe P. To cure or not to cure, that is not the question. *J RS Medicine* 2000; **93**: 611+.
3. Fox JG. Some practical and legal objections to prescription privileges for psychologists. *Private Practice* 1989; **6**: 23–39.
4. Breiter J, McNamar J. The right to prescribe medicine: Considerations for professional psychology. *Profes Psychol Res Pract* 1991; **22**: 179–187.
5. Burns SM, Chemtob C, DeLeon P, *et al.* Psychotropic medication: A new technique for psychology? *Psychotherapy* 1988; **25**: 508–515.
6. Heiby EM. Concluding remarks on the debate about prescription privileges for psychologists. *J Clin Psychol* 2002; **58**: 709–722.
7. DeNelsky GY. The case against prescription privileges for psychologists. *American Psychologists* 1996; **51**: 207–212.
8. Pies RW. The 'deep structure' of clinical medicine and prescribing privileges for psychologists. *J Clin Psychol* 1991; **52**: 4–8.
9. Weene KA. The psychologist's role in the collaborative process of psychopharmacology. *J Clin Psychol* 2002; **58**: 617–621.

10. Lin KM, Poland RE, Wan YJY, *et al.* The evolving science of pharmacogenetics: Clinical and ethnic perspectives. *Psychopharmacol Bull* 1996; **32**: 205–217.

11. Bertilsson L, Alm C, Carreras CD, *et al.* Debrisoquine hydroxylation polymorphism and personality. *Lancet* 1989; **1**: 555.

12. Karunanithy R, Sumita KP. Undeclared drugs in Chinese antirheumatoid medicine. *Int J Pharmacol Pract* 1991; **1**: 117–119.

13. De Smet PAGM. Drugs used in non-orthodox medicine. In: Dukes NMG, ed. Meyler's side effects of drugs. Amsterdam: Elsevier, 1992: 1209–1232.

14. Lewin RA. More on merde. *Perspect Biology Med* 2001; **44**: 594–607.

15. Jastenberg T, Evans S. Global herbal medicine: A critique. *J Alternat Compl Med* 2003; **9**: 321–329.

16. Eisenberg D, Kaptchuk T. Varieties of healing. 1: Medical pluralism in the United States. *Ann Intern Med* 2001; **135**: 189–195.

17. Fisher AA, Le Couteur DG. Lead poisoning from complementary and alternative medicine in multiple sclerosis. *J Neurol Neurosurg Psychiatry* 2000; **69**: 687–689.

18. Fleming GA. The FDA, regulation, and the risk of stroke. *The NE J Medicine* 2000; **343**: 1886–1887.

19. Milner J. Functional foods: The US perspective. *Am J Clin Nutr* 2000; **71**: 1654S–1659S.

20. Myslobodsky M, Weiner M. Pharmacologic implications of hemispheric asymmetries. *Life Sciences* 1976; **19**: 1467–1478.

21. Myslobodsky M, Weiner M. Pharmacopsychotherapy and aberrant brain laterality. In: Myslobodsky M, ed. Hemisyndromes: Psychobiology, neurology, psychiatry. New York: Academic Press, 1983: 447.

22. Tsai CJ, Kumar S, Ma BY, *et al.* Folding funnels, binding funnels, and protein function. *Protein Sci* 1999; **8**: 1181–1190.

23. Bosshard H. Molecular recognition by induced fit: How fit is the concept? *News Physiol Sci* 2001; **16**: 171–173.

24. Yue G, Cole K. Strength increases from the motor program: Comparison of training with maximal voluntary and imagined muscle contractions. *J Neurophysiol* 1992; **67**: 1114–1123.

25. Feeney D, Gonzalez A, Law W. Amphetamine, haloperidol, and experience interact to affect rate of recovery after motor cortex injury. *Science* 1982; **217**: 855–857.

26. Feeney D, Hovda D. Amphetamine and apomorphine restore tactile placing after motor cortex injury in the cat. *Psychopharmacology (Berl)* 1983; **79**: 67–71.

27. Fox PT, Raichle ME. Stimulus rate dependence of regional cerebral blood flow in human striate cortex demonstrated by positron emission tomography. *J Neurophysiology* 1984; **51**: 1109–1120.

28. Walker-Batson D, Curtis S, Natarajan R, *et al.* A double-Blind, placebo-controlled study of the use of amphetamine in the treatment of aphasia. *Stroke* 2001; **32**: 2093–2098.

29. Berger FM. Introduction: The aim and achievements of psychopharmacology. In: Clark WG, Del Giudice J, eds. Principles of psychopharmacology. 2 edn. New York: Academic Press, 1978: 9–40.

30. Levy SM. Behavioral risk factors and host vulnerability. In: Bridge PT, *et al.*, eds. Psychological, neuropsychiatric, and substance abuse aspects of AIDS. New York: Raven Press, 1988: 225–239.

31. Shapiro A. The placebo effect. In: Clark W, del Giudice J, eds. Principles of psychopharmacology. New York: Academic Press, 1978.

32. Ratai R. The Jewish alchemists. Princeton: Princeton University Press, 1994.

33. Mathabane M. Lobola, AIDS and Africa. Washington Post 2000 March 27.

34. Curtis V, Biran A. Dirt, disgust, and disease — Is hygiene in our genes? *Perspect Biol Med* 2001; **44**: 17–31.

35. Jackson J. Telling the truth. *J Med Ethics* 1991; **17**: 5–9.

36. Rawlinson MC. Truth-telling and paternalism in the clinic: Philosophical reflections on the use of placebos in medicinal practice. In: White L, *et al.*, eds. Placebo. Theory, research and mechanisms. New York: The Guilford Press, 1985.

37. Hróbjartsson A, Gøtzsche P. Is the placebo powerless? An analysis of clinical trials comparing placebo treatment with no treatment. *N Engl J Med* 2001; **344**: 1594–1602.

38. de la Fuente-Fernandez R, Ruth T, Sossi V, *et al.* Expectation and dopamine release: Mechanism of the placebo effect in Parkinson's disease. *Science* 2001; **293**: 1164–1166.

39. Azari N, Nickel J, Wunderlich G, *et al.* Neural correlates of religious experience. *Eur J Neurosci* 2001; **13**: 1649–1652.

40. Myslobodsky M. Awareness salvaged by cunning: Rehabilitation by deception in audio-visual neglect. In: Myslobodsky M, ed. The Mythomanias: The nature of deception and self-deception. Hillsdale: Erlbaum, 1997.

41. Elliott R, Rees G, Dolan R. Ventromedial prefrontal cortex mediates guessing. *Neuropsychol* 1999; **37**: 403–411.

42. Bettoni M, Bettoni MC. Constructivist foundations of modeling — A Kantian perspective. *Internat J Intelligent Syst* 1997; **12**: 577–595.

43. Berlyne DE. Motivational problems raised by exploratory and epistemic behavior. In: Koch S, ed. Psychology: A study of science. New York: McGraw Hill, 1963: 284–364.

44. Uttal WR. The new phrenology. Cambridge, MA: MIT Press, 2001.

45. Szasz T. The myth of psychotherapy. Garden City, NY: Ancor Press/Doubleday, 1979.

46. Gevitz N. Alternative medicine and the orthodox canon. *Mt Sinai J Med* 1995; **62**: 127–131.

47. Burroughs H. Alternative healing: The complete A-Z guide to over 160 different alternative therapies. La Mesa, California: Halcyon, 1993.

48. Jacobs C. Healing and prophecy in the black Spiritual churches: A need for re-examination. *Med Anthropol* 1990; **12**: 349–370.

49. Gardner M. Fads and fallacies in the name of science. New York: Dover Publications, Inc., 1957.

50. Conklin BA. Consuming grief: Compassionate cannibalism in an Amazonian society. University of Texas Press, 2001.

51. Atkins P. Science and religion: Rack of featherbed — The uncomfortable supremacy of science. *Sci Progress,* 2000; **83**: 25–31.

52. Pan PP. Before Olympics, officials confront public expectorations. *The Washington Post* 2001 August 20; A12.

53. Yasuo Y. The Body, Self-cultivation and Ki-energy. Albany, NY: State University of New York Press, 1993.

54. Krieger D, Peper E, Ancoli S. Therapeutic touch: Searching for evidence of physiological change. *Am J Nurs* 1979; **79**: 660–662.

55. Zefron L. The history of the laying-on of hands in nursing. *Nurs Forum* 1975; **14**: 350–363.

56. Harkness EF, Abbot NC, Ernst E. A randomized trial of distant healing for skin warts. *Am J Med* 2000; **108**: 448–452.

57. Walker S, Tonigan J, Miller W, *et al.* Intercessory prayer in the treatment of alcohol abuse and dependence: A pilot investigation. *Altern Ther Health Med* 1997; **3**: 79–86.

58. Sicher F, Targ E, Moore DI, *et al.* A randomized double-blind study of the effects of distant healing in a population with advanced AIDS. Report on a small scale study. *West J Med* 1998; **169**: 356–363.

59. Eberhard J, Geissbuhler V. Influence of alternative birth methods on traditional birth management. *Fetal Diagn Ther* 2000; **15**: 283–290.

60. Fadiman A. The spirit catches you and you fall down. New York: Farrar Straus & Giroux, 1998.

61. Carvalho I, Chacham AS, Viana P. Traditional birth attendants and their practices in the State of Pernambuco rural area, Brazil, 1996. *Intern J Gynecol Obstetr* 1998; **63**: S53–S60.

62. Thapa N, Chongsuvivatwong V, Gafu M, *et al.* Infant death rates and animal-shed delivery in remote rural areas of Nepal. *Soc Sci Med* 2000; **51**: 1447–1456.

63. Lewin RA. Merde. Excursions in scientific cultural, and sociohistorical coprology. New York: Random House, 1999.

64. Graham H. Eternal Eve. The history of gynecology and obstetrics. Garden City, New York: Double Day & Company, Inc., 1951.

65. Shapiro J. Satisfaction with obstetric care. Patient survey in a family practice shared-call group. *Can Fam Physician* 1999; **45**: 651–657.

66. MacDorman M, Singh G. Midwifery care, social and medical risk factors, and birth outcomes in the USA. *J Epidemiol Commun Health* 1998; **52**: 310–317.

67. Biro M, Waldenstrom U, JH. P. Team midwifery care in a tertiary level obstetric service: A randomized controlled trial. *Birth* 2000; **27**: 68–173.

68. Baldwin K. The midwifery solution to contemporary problems in American obstetrics. *J Nurse Midwifery* 1999; **44**: 75–79.

69. Fisher JA. The plague makers. New York: Simon & Shuster, 1994.

70. Ewald PW. Evolution of infectious disease. Oxford: Oxford University Press, 1994.

71. Gupta JK, Nikodem C. Maternal posture in labour. *Eur J Obstet Gynecol Reprod Biol* 2000; **92**: 273–277.

72. Siebzehnrubl E. Natural birth — Modern obstetrics between delivery chair and the operation theater. *Med Welt* 1998; **49**: 275–280.

73. Landau WM. The doctors dilemma — Problems that do not go away. *Perspect Biol Med* 1989; **32**: 505–512.

74. Carmichael A, Ratzan RE. Medicine. A treasure of art and literature. New York: Hugh Lauter Levin Assoc., Inc., 1991.

75. Herink R. The psychotherapy handbook. New York: New American Library, 1980.

76. Astin J. Why patients use alternative medicine: Results of a national study. *JAMA* 1998; **20**: 1548–1553.
77. Foster DF, Phillips RS, Hamel MB, *et al.* Alternative medicine use in older Americans. *J Am Geriatr Soc* 2000; **48**: 1560–1565.
78. Huffman M. Current evidence for self-medication in primates: A multidisciplinary perspective. *Yearbook of Physical Anthropol* 1997; **40**: 171–200.
79. Lozano G. Parasitic stress and self-medication in wild animals. *Stress Behav* 1998; **27**: 291–317.
80. Frasca T, Brett A, Yoo S. Mandrake toxicity. A case of mistaken identity. *Arch Intern Med* 1997; **157**: 2007–2009.
81. Kline M. Mathematics. The loss of certainty. Oxford: Oxford University Press, 1980.
82. Freidson E. Profession of medicine. A study of the sociology of applied knowledge. Chicago: The University of Chicago Press, 1988.

Chapter 7
Holistic Philosophy and a Recipe for Causative Goulash

1. Smuts J. Holism and evolution. London: Macmillan, 1926.
2. Bernard C. Introduction à l'etude de la médicine experiméntale. New York: Dover, 1865/1957.
3. Goldstein K. The organism. New York: American Book, 1939.
4. Harrington A. Reenchanted science: Holism in German culture from Wilhelm H to Hitler. Princeton, NJ: Princeton University Press, 1996.
5. Libbrecht K. Cylindrically symmetric Green's function approach for modeling the crystal growth morphology of ice. *Phys Rev E Stat Phys Plasmas Fluids Relat Interdiscip Topics* 1999; **60**: 1967–1974.
6. Pate-Cornell M. Conditional uncertainty analysis and implications for decision making: The case of WIPP. *Risk Anal* 1999; **19**: 995–1002.
7. Bier VM. Challenges to the acceptance of probabilistic risk analysis. *Risk Anal* 1999; **19**: 703–710.
8. Evans AS. Causation and disease: A chronological journey. New York: Plenum Medical Book Co., 1993.
9. May R. The meaning of anxiety. New York: W.W. Norton & Co., Inc., 1979.
10. Lenzen VF. Causality in natural science. Springfield, Ill: Charles C. Thomas Publisher, 1954.
11. Susser M, Susser E. Choosing a future for epidemiology: I. Eras and paradigms. *Am J Public Health* 1996; **86**: 668–673.
12. Wildavsky A. Doing better and feeling worse. The political pathology of health policy. *Daedalus* 1977; **106**: 105–123.
13. Skolbekken J. The risk epidemic in medical journals. *Soc Sci Med* 1995; **40**: 291–305.
14. Sutter MC. Assigning causation in disease: Beyond Koch's postulates. *Perspect Biol Med* 1996; **39**: 581–592.

15. Susser M, Susser E. Choosing a future for epidemiology: II. From black box to Chinese boxes and ecoepidemiology. *Am J Public Health* 1996; **86**: 674–677.
16. McKinlay JB, Marceau LD. The boldly go. *Am J Public Health* 2000; **90**: 25–33.
17. Thagard P. How scientists explain disease. Princeton: Princeton University Press, 1999.
18. McCormick J. The multifactorial aetiology of coronary heart disease: A dangerous delusion. *Perspect Biol Med* 1988; **32**: 103–108.
19. Meehl PE. Why I do not attend case conferences. Psychodiagnosis. Selected papers. New York: Norton & Co., 1977.
20. Begg CB. The search for cancer risk factors: When can we stop looking? *Am J Public Health* 2001; **91**: 360–364.
21. Delvin K. The math gene. New York: Basic Books, 2000.
22. Satel S. PC, M.D. How political correctness is corrupting medicine. New York: Basic Books, 2000.
23. Reinfrank R. Clinical decision making: Course teaching notes. Hartford, CT: Harford Hospital, 1978.
24. Stettler N, Zemel B, Kumanyika S, *et al.* Infant weight gain and childhood overweight status in a multicenter, cohort study. *Pediatrics* 2002; **109**: 194–199.
25. Adair JS, Cole T. Rapid child growth raises blood pressure in adolescent boys who were thin at birth. *Hypertension* 2003; **41**: 451–456.
26. Collins JJ, David R, Symons R, *et al.* Low-income African-American mothers' perception of exposure to racial discrimination and infant birth weight. *Epidemiology* 2000; **11**: 337–339.
27. Martyn C, Greenwald S. A hypothesis about a mechanism for the programming of blood pressure and vascular disease in early life. *Clin Exp Pharmacol Physiol* 2001; **28**: 948–951.
28. Chapman N, Mohamudally A, Stanton A, *et al.* Abnormal microvascular network geometry — The link between low birth weight and increased cardiovascular risk? *Hypertension* 1996; **28**: 703.
29. Chapman N, Mohamudally A, Cerutti A, *et al.* Retinal vascular network architecture in low-birth-weight men. *J Hypertens* 1997; **15**: 1449–1453.
30. Struijker-Boudier H. Arteriolar and capillary remodeling in hypertension. *Drugs* 1999; **59**: 37–40.
31. Crone C. Oxygen supply to the brain. In: Nicolau C, ed. Oxygen transport in red blood cells. Oxford: Pergamon Press, 1986.
32. Stehbens WE. Coronary heart disease, hypercholesterolemia, and atherosclerosis I. False premises. *Exp Mol Pathol* 2001; **70**: 103–119.
33. Stehbens WE. Coronary heart disease, hypercholesterolemia, and atherosclerosis II. Misrepresented data. *Exp Mol Pathol* 2001; **70**: 120–139.
34. Nieto FJ. Infections and atherosclerosis: New clues from an old hypothesis? *Am J Epidemiol* 1998; **148**: 937–948.
35. Hopkins P, Williams R. Identification and relative weight of cardiovascular risk factors. *Cardiol Clin* 1986; **4**: 3–31.
36. Sargent T, Smith B. Coinage, debasements, and Gresham's laws. *Econom Theory* 1997; **10**: 197–226.

37. Meier C. Antibiotics in the prevention and treatment of coronary heart disease. *J Infect Dis* 2000; **181**: S558–S562.

38. Shoenfeld S. Atherosclerosis as an infectious, inflammatory and autoimmune disease. *Trends in Immunology* 2001; **22**: 293–295.

39. Ornish D, Scherwitz LW, Billings JH, *et al.* Intensive lifestyle changes for reversal of coronary heart disease. *JAMA* 1998; **280**: 2001–2007.

40. Norman R, Malla A. Stressful life events and schizophrenia. *Br J Psychiatry* 1993; **162**: 161–166.

41. Caspi A, Sugden K, Moffitt TE, *et al.* Influence of life stress on depression: Moderation by a polymorphism in the 5-HTT gene. *Science* 2003; **18**: 386–389.

42. Myslobodsky M, Weiner I. Contemporary issues in modeling psychopathology. Boston: Kluwer Academic, 2000.

43. Egan MF, Kojima M, Callicott JH, *et al.* The BDNF val66met polymorphism affects activity-dependent secretion of BDNF and human memory and hippocampal function. *Cell* 2003; **112**: 257–269.

44. Weinberger D, Egan M, Bertolino A, *et al.* Prefrontal neurons and the genetics of schizophrenia. *Biol Psychiatry* 2001; **50**: 825–844.

45. Kuznetsova N, Semenov S. The determination of serum antibrain antibodies in psychiatric patients. *Korsakoff USSR J Neuropathol Psychiatry* 1961; **6**: 869–872.

46. Karlsson H, Bachmann S, Schroder J, *et al.* Retroviral RNA identified in the cerebrospinal fluids and brains of individuals with schizophrenia. *Proc Natl Acad Sci USA* 2001; **98**: 4634–4639.

47. Todd PM, Gigerenzer G. Précis of simple heuristics that make us smart. *Behav Brain Sci* 2000; **23**: 727–780.

48. Wildavsky A. Doing better and feeling worse. The political pathology of health policy. *Daedalus* 1977; **106**: 105–123.

49. Fox JG, Wang TC. Overview of *Helicobacter pylori*. In: Goedert JJ, ed. Infectious causes of cancer: Targets for intervention. Totawa, NJ: Humana Press, 2000.

50. Marshall B, Warren J. Unidentified curved bacilli in the stomach of patients with gastritis and peptic ulceration. *Lancet* 1984; **1**: 1311–1315.

51. Cromer A. Uncommon sense. The heretical nature of science. New York: Oxford University Press, 1993.

52. Ziman JM. Public knowledge. Cambridge: Cambridge University Press, 1968.

53. Fendrick AM, Hirth RA, Chernew ME. Differences between generalist and specialist physicians regarding Helicobacter pylori and peptic ulcer disease. *Am J Gastroenterol* 1996; **91**: 1544–1548.

54. Slovic P, Fischhoff B, Lichtenstein S. Fact versus fears: Understanding perceived risk. In: Kahneman D, *et al.*, eds. Judgment under uncertainty: Heuristics and biases. Cambridge: Cambridge University Press, 1982: 463–489.

55. Cole M, Maltzman I. A handbook of contemporary Soviet psychology. New York: Basic Books, Inc., 1969.

56. Cochran G, Ewald P, Cochran K. Infectious causation of disease: An evolutionary perspective. *Persp Biol Med* 2000; **43**: 406–448.

57. Latour B. The pasteurization of France. Translated by A. Sheridan & J. Law. Cambridge, MA.: Howard University Press, 1988.

58. Roger E, Shoemaker E. Communication of innovation. New York: Free Press, 1971.

59. Schwartz S, Carpenter KM. The right answer for the wrong question: Consequences of type III error for public health research. *Am J Public Health* 1999; **89**: 1175–1180.

60. Levenstein S, Prantera C, Varvo V, *et al.* Long-term symptom patterns in duodenal ulcer: Psychosocial factors. *J Psychosomat Res* 1996; **41**: 465–472.

61. Passaro D, Chosy E, Parsonnet J. Helicobacter pylori: Consensus and controversy. *Clin Infect Dis* 2002; **35**: 298–304.

62. Dormandy T. The white death. New York: New York University Press, 2000.

63. Kline M. Mathematics. The loss of certainty. Oxford: Oxford University Press, 1980.

64. Berger R. Understanding science: Why causes are not enough. *Philosophy Sci* 1998; **65**: 306–332.

65. Stehbens WE. Causality in medical science with particular reference to heart-disease and atherosclerosis. *Perspect Biol Med* 1992; **36**: 97–119.

66. Timmer E, Voorn WJ, Tjiptadi, *et al.* Variability of the duration of life of living creatures. Amsterdam: IOS Press, 2000.

67. Lakey J. Informing the public about radiation — The messenger and the message: 1997 G. William Morgan Lecture. *Health Physics* 1998; **75**: 367–374.

68. Rothman KJ, Greenland S. Modern epidemiology. Philadelphia: Lippinckott-Raven, 1998.

69. Kitcher PS. Explanatory unification and the causal structure of the world. In: al. KPSe, ed. Minnesota studies in the philosophy of science. v. 13. Scientific explanation. Minneapolis: University of Minnesota Press, 1989: 410–505.

70. Popper KR. Conjectures and refutations: The growth of scientific knowledge. New York: Harper & Row, 1968.

71. Medawar PB, Medawar J. Aristotle to Zoos. Cambridge, MA: Harvard University Press, 1983.

72. Motokawa T. Sushi Science and Hamburger Science. *Perspect Biol Med* 1989; **32**: 489–504.

73. Kluckhohn C, Murray H. Personality formation: The determinants. In: Kluckhohn C, Murray H, eds. Personality in nature, society, and culture. New York: Knopf, 1948: 35.

74. Rousseau J-J. Confessions. Harmondsworth: Penguin Books, 1953.

75. Slater E. The neurotic constitution. A statistical study of two thousand neurotic soldiers. *J Neurology and Psychiatry* 1943; **6**: 1–16.

76. Fadiman A. The spirit catches you and you fall down. New York: Farrar Straus & Giroux, 1998.

77. Sumner W. Folkways. A study of the sociological importance of usages, manners, customs, mores, morals. New York: Mentor Book, 1960.

78. Eysenck H. Uses and abuses of psychology. Aylsbury: Hazel Watson & Viney, Ltd., 1974.

79. Glymour C, Stalker D. Sounding board. Engineers, cranks, physicians, magicians. *N Engl J Med* 1983; **308**: 960–964.

80. Cottrell A. Emergent properties of complex systems. In: Duncan R, Weston-Smith M, eds. Encyclopedia of ignorance. New York: Pergamon, 1977: 129–135.

Chapter 8
If Health Psychology is the Answer, What was the Question?

1. King H. The power of paternity: The father of medicine meets the prince of physicians. In: Cantor D, ed. Reinventing Hippocrates. Aldershot: Ashgate, 2001.
2. Allport GW. The historical background of modern social psychology. v. 1. In: Lindzey G, ed. Handbook of social psychology. Reading, Mass.: Addison-Wesley, 1954: 3.
3. Nuland SB. Doctors. The biography of medicine. 2 edn. New York: Vintage Books, 1995.
4. Bates DG. Why not call modern medicine 'alternative'? *Perspect Biol Med* 2000; **43**: 502–508.
5. Lyons J. The American medical doctor in the current milieu — A matter of trust. *Perspect Biol Med* 1994; **37**: 442–459.
6. Simon B. Mind and madness in ancient Greece. The classical roots of modern psychiatry. Ithaca, New York: Cornell University Press, 1978.
7. Meehl PE. Why I do not attend case conferences. Psychodiagnosis. Selected papers. New York: Norton & Co., 1977.
8. Katon W, Kleinman A, Rosen G. Depression and somatization: A review. Part II. *Am J Med* 1982; **72**: 241–247.
9. Murphy E. The normal, and the perils of the sylleptic argument. *Perspect Biol Med* 1972; **15**: 566–582.
10. Normelli H, Sevastik J, Ljung G, *et al.* The symmetry of the breasts in normal and scoliotic girls. *Spine* 1986; **11**: 749–752.
11. Murphy EA. Public and private hypotheses. *J Clin Epidemiol* 1989; **42**: 79–84.
12. Maltzman IM. Alcoholism: A review of its characteristics, etiology, treatments, and controversies. Boston: Kluwer Academic Publishers, 2000.
13. Smith R. In search of "non-disease". *Br Med J* 2002; **324**: 883–885.
14. Kovacs J. The concept of health and disease. *Med Health Care Philos* 1998; **1**: 31–39.
15. Homans G. The human group. New York: Harcourt Brace Jovanovich, 1960.
16. Institute of Medicine. Committee for the study of the future of public health. The future of public health. Washington, DC: National Academy Press, 1988.
17. Grier W, Cobbs P. Black rage. New York: Basic Books, Inc., 1968.
18. Sperber M. Masks of loneliness. Alfred Adler in perspective. New York: Macmillan Publishing Co., Inc, 1974.
19. Dormandy T. The white death. New York: New York University Press, 2000.
20. Myslobodsky MS, Tomer R, Holden T, *et al.* Cognitive impairment in patients with Tardive-Dyskinesia. *J Nerv Ment Dis* 1985; **173**: 156–160.
21. Dieppe P. To cure or not to cure, that is not the question. *J RS Medicine* 2000; **93**: 611+.
22. Pies RW. The 'deep structure' of clinical medicine and prescribing privileges for psychologists. *J Clin Psychol* 1991; **52**: 4–8.

23. Pond C. Adipose tissue, the anatomists' Cinderella, goes to the ball at last, and meets some influential partners. *Postgrad Med J* 2000; **76**: 671–673.

24. Evans R. The evolution of challenges to researchers in health psychology. *Health Psychol* 1989; **8**: 631–639.

25. Belar C. Clinical health psychology: A specialty for the 21st century. *Health Psychol* 1997; **16**: 411–416.

26. Matarazzo J. Behavioral health and behavioral medicine: Frontiers for a new health psychology. *Am Psychol* 1980; **35**: 807–817.

27. Antonovsky A. The implications of salutogenesis: An outsider's view. In: Turnbull A, *et al.*, eds. Cognitive coping: Families and disability. Baltimore: Brooke, 1993.

28. Cohen L, Rothschild H. The bandwagons of medicine. *Perspect Biol Med* 1979; **22**: 531–538.

29. Papas AME. Antioxidant status, diet, nutrition, and health. Boca Raton: CRC Press, 1999.

30. Salganik R, Albright C, Rodgers J, *et al.* Dietary antioxidant depletion: Enhancement of tumor apoptosis and inhibition of brain tumor growth in transgenic mice. *Carcinogenesis* 2000; **21**: 909–914.

31. Fries J. Aging, natural death, and the compression of morbidity. *N Engl J Med* 1980; **17**: 130–135.

32. Landau WM. The doctors dilemma — Problems that do not go away. *Perspect Biol Med* 1989; **32**: 505–512.

33. Vita A, Terry R, Hubert H, *et al.* Aging, health risks, and cumulative disability. *N Engl J Med* 1998; **338**: 1035–1041.

34. Sallis JF, Owen N. Physical activity & behavioral medicine. Thousand Oaks: SAGE Publications, 1999.

35. Meltzer M. Introduction to health economics for physicians. *Lancet* 2001; **358**: 993–998.

36. Strannergård O, Strannergård I-L. The causes of the increasing prevalence of allergy: Is atopy a microbial deprivation disorder? *Allergy* 2001; **56**: 91–102.

37. Curtis V, Biran A. Dirt, disgust, and disease — Is hygiene in our genes? *Perspect Biol Med* 2001; **44**: 17–31.

38. Riedler J, Eder W, Oberfeld G, *et al.* Austrian children living on a farm have less hay fever, asthma and allergic sensitization. *Clin Exp Allergy* 2000; **30**: 194–200.

39. Kilpelainen M, Terho EO, Helenius H, *et al.* Farm environment in childhood prevents the development of allergies. *Clin Exp Allergy* 2000; **30**: 201–208.

40. Bjorksten B. Environment and infant immunity. *Proc Nutr Soc* 1999; **58**: 729–732.

41. Matricardi PM, Bonini S. High microbial turnover rate preventing atopy: A solution to inconsistencies impinging on the Hygiene hypothesis? *Clin Exp Allergy* 2000; **30**: 1506–1510.

42. Busse WW, Lemanske RF. Advances in immunology — Asthma. *NE J Med* 2001; **344**: 350–362.

43. Keys A. Mediterranean diet and public-health — Personal reflections. *Am J Clin Nutr* 1995; **61**: S1321–S1323.

44. Browner WS, Westenhouse J, Tice JA. What if Americans ate less fat? A quantitative estimate of the effect on mortality. *JAMA* 1991; **265**: 3285–3291.

45. Zock PL. Dietary fats and cancer. *Curr Opin Lipidology* 2001; **12**: 5–10.

46. Wildavsky A. Doing better and feeling worse. The political pathology of health policy. *Daedalus* 1977; **106**: 105–123.

47. Frenk H, Dar R. A critique of nicotine addiction. Boston: Kluwer Academic, 2000.

48. Oscarson M. Genetic polymorphisms in the cytochrome P450 2A6 (CYP2A6) gene: Implications for interindividual differences in nicotine metabolism. *Drug Metab Dispos* 2001; **29**: 91–95.

49. Kihara T, Shimohama S, Sawada H, *et al.* Nicotinic receptor stimulation protects neurons against beta-amyloid toxicity. *Ann Neurol* 1997; **42**: 159–163.

50. Linert W, Bridge M, Huber M, *et al.* In vitro and in vivo studies investigating possible antioxidant actions of nicotine: Relevance to Parkinson's and Alzheimer's diseases. *[Biochimica Biophysica Acta] Molec Basis Dis* 1999; **1454**: 143–152.

51. Lambert N, Hartsough C. Prospective study of tobacco smoking and substance dependencies among samples of ADHD and non-ADHD participants. *J Learn Disabil* 1998; **31**: 533–544.

52. Levin E, Conners C, Sparrow E, *et al.* Nicotine effects on adults with attention-deficit/hyperactivity disorder. *Psychopharmacology* 1996; **123**: 55–63.

53. Green J, Evans B, Rhodes J, *et al.* An oral formulation of nicotine for release and absorption in the colon: Its development and pharmacokinetics. *Br J Clin Pharmacol* 1999; **48**: 485–493.

54. Weinstein N. Optimistic biases about personal risks. *Am J Public Health 246* 1989: 1232–1233.

55. Weinstein N. Unrealistic optimism about susceptibility to health problems: Conclusions from a community-wide sample. *J Behav Med* 1987; **10**: 481–500.

56. Slovic P, Fischhoff B, Lichtenstein S. Fact versus fears: Understanding perceived risk. In: Kahneman D, *et al.*, eds. Judgment under uncertainty: Heuristics and biases. Cambridge: Cambridge University Press, 1982: 463–489.

57. Taubes G. The soft science of dietary fat. *Science* 2001; **291**: 2536–2545.

58. Sturm R. The effects of obesity, smoking, and drinking on medical problems and costs. *Health Affairs* 2002; **21**: 245–253.

59. Hegsted D. Dietary standards. *J Am Diet Assoc* 1975; **66**: 13–21.

60. Hegsted D. Optimal nutrition. *Cancer* 1979; **43**: 996–2003.

61. Meadows AB, Abbott C, Lier K. Low cholesterol and noncardiovascular mortality. *Milit Med* 2000; **165**: 466–469.

62. Michikawa M. The role of cholesterol in pathogenesis of Alzheimer's disease. *Mol Neurobiol* 2003; **27**: 1–12.

63. Golier JA, Marzuk PM, Leon AC, *et al.* Low serum-cholesterol level and attempted-suicide. *Am J Psychiat* 1995; **152**: 419–423.

64. Engelberg H. Low serum cholesterol and suicide. *Lancet* 1992; **339**: 727–729.

65. Kaplan JR, Shively CA, Fontenot MB, *et al.* Demonstration of an association among dietary-cholesterol, central serotonergic activity, and social-behavior in monkeys. *Psychosom Med* 1994; **56**: 479–484.

66. Brunner J, Parhofer K, Schwandt P, *et al.* Cholesterol, omega-3 fatty acids, and suicide risk: Empirical evidence and pathophysiological hypotheses. *Fortschr Neurol Psychiatr* 2001; **69**: 460–467.

67. Skolbekken J. The risk epidemic in medical journals. *Soc Sci Med* 1995; **40**: 291–305.

68. Moeller M. History, idea, and present situation of self-help-groups. *Gruppenpsychotherap Gruppendyn* 1997; **33**: 113–129.

69. Love S. Dr. Susan Love's hormone book: Making informed choices about menopause: Crown Publishing Group, Inc., 1998.

70. Knowles J. The responsibility of the individual. *Daedalus:* 1977; **Winter**: 57–80.

71. Miller K. The evolution of professional identity: The case of osteopathic medicine. *Soc Sci Med* 1998; **47**: 1739–1748.

72. Adams T. Dentistry and medical dominance. *Soc Sci Med* 1999; **48**: 407–420.

73. Shortt SED. Physicians, science and status: Issues in the professionalization of Anglo-American medicine in the nineteenth century. *Med Hist* 1983; **27**: 51–68.

74. Richards A, Carley J, Jenkins-Clarke S, *et al.* Skill mix between nurses and doctors working in primary care delegation or allocation: A review of the literature. *Int J Nurs Stud* 2000; **37**: 185–197.

75. Smith G. The future of consultation-liaison psychiatry. *Austral NZ J Psychiat* 2003; **37**: 150–159.

76. Reiser SJ. Technology and the use of the senses in twentieth century medicine. In: Bynum W, Porter R, eds. Medicine and the five senses. Cambridge: Cambridge University Press, 1993.

77. Friedenberg RM. Health care rationing: Every physician's dilemma. *Radiology* 2000; **217**: 626–628.

78. Wartenberg R. Diagnostic tests in neurology. A selection for office use. Chicago: The Year Book Publishers, 1954.

79. Phoon CKL. Must doctors still examine patients? *Perspect Biol Med* 2000; **43**: 548–561.

80. Satel S. PC, M.D. How political correctness is corrupting medicine. New York: Basic Books, 2000.

81. Brooke MH. The Websters' dictionary: The binification of medical and neurologic education. *Neurology* 2000; **54**: 1554–1556.

82. Stanberry B. Legal ethical and risk issues in telemedicine. *Comput Meth Programs Biomed* 2001; **64**: 225–233.

83. Evans R. Health promotion — Science or ideology? *Health Psychol* 1988; **7**: 203–219.

84. Nuland SB. The biography of medicine. New York: Vintage Books, 1988.

85. Whorton J. Crusaders for fitness: The history of American health reformers. Princeton, NJ: Princeton University Press, 1982.

86. Peterson D. Is psychology a profession? *Am Psycholol* 1976; **31**: 572–581.

87. Peterson D. Unintended consequences. Ventures and misadventures in the education of professional psychologists. *Am Psychol* 2003; **58**: 791–800.

Index